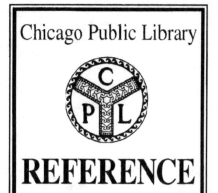

ENVIRONMENTAL

MERCURY CONTAMINATION

ENVIRONMENTAL

MERCURY CONTAMINATION

Rolf Hartung, Ph.D.
Associate Professor of Environmental and
Industrial Health, University of Michigan

Bertram D. Dinman, M.D., Sc.D.
Director, Institute of Environmental and
Industrial Health, University of Michigan

Editors

This volume is based on an
international conference on mercury
held at the University of Michigan,
with additional material, comments
and summaries supplied by the editors

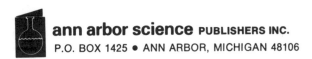
ann arbor science PUBLISHERS INC.
P.O. BOX 1425 ● ANN ARBOR, MICHIGAN 48106

© Copyright 1972 by Ann Arbor Science Publishers, Inc.
P.O. Box 1425, Ann Arbor, Michigan 48106

Library of Congress Catalog Card No. 72-77312
ISBN 0-250-97513-0

Printed in the United States of America

First Impressions 1972
Second Impressions 1972

FOREWORD

Because of the recent discovery of mercury in foods in North America, there has been an almost explosively increasing public awareness of the problem of environmental mercury contamination. We seem repeatedly to have underestimated and are later surprised by the pervasiveness of various environmental toxicants—whether they be DDT, radioactive elements, oil, or mercury.

With respect to mercury contamination, it would appear to the unsophisticated that the scientific community was taken totally by surprise, that no previous investigations had taken place. As with most categorical statements, this is only partially correct, since considerable effort and concern has been directed toward this problem outside North America. Notably, the Japanese have suffered the consequences of disregard by an industrial society of profligate mercury discharge. The Swedish grasped the implications of the Japanese experience and have directed extensive investigations toward understanding environmental mercury contamination.

The Japanese responded to their problem by directing their efforts toward a delineation of the human consequences of organo-mercury absorption and toxicity as well as studying the distribution of mercury in the biota. Since, in Sweden, severe health aberrations in humans had not developed, the Swedish activity was largely directed toward study of the less dramatic but equally important results of mercury's introduction into the environment, *e.g.*, transport, distribution, and subclinical potential effect.

The unanswered question regarding the previous lack of concern for this problem in North America, despite international knowledge of its existence, requires a multifaceted answer. In 1966, Dr. Dinman was explicitly told by Professor Lars Friberg of the Karolinska Institute in Stockholm, Sweden, that if we would but seek out mercury contamination in air, food, and waters, we would most

v

assuredly find the problem lurking there, awaiting discovery. The reason why such suggestions were not pursued stems from the reality that we in North America are a crisis-motivated society. Only after a crisis developed did concern and support for such investigations ensue. Recent history has shown how potent a stimulus crisis proves to be.

Under this stimulus, we now clearly see that, with public support, willing hands and minds are available--and indeed have been applied--toward an understanding of the problem of environmental mercury contamination. Thus, it would be useful if the present state of knowledge concerning this environmental problem could in part be summarized. To help meet this need, the International Conference on Environmental Mercury Contamination was held in Ann Arbor, Michigan, from September 30 to October 2, 1970. This volume is based on that conference, although many of the papers presented have been greatly expanded and discussion materials have been added to papers to improve their content and readability.

The International Conference was organized in the hope of achieving an assessment of our present state of knowledge, and some indication of what is still needed to understand the broad outlines and specific details of the problem. The information developed here is, as yet, fragmentary. However, it should lay to rest the fear that there is total scientific ignorance of many ramifications of the problem.

This compilation of available knowledge should serve partially to reassure but, at the same time, not permit complacency. The broad outlines of approaches to the understanding of this problem regarding mercury can also serve to lay the groundwork for a systematic attack on our still vaguely perceived concerns regarding other metals and trace elements, *e.g.*, arsenic, cadmium, chromium, selenium, and their potential impact upon society and the environment.

Rolf Hartung, Ph.D.
Associate Professor of Environmental and Industrial Health, University of Michigan

Bertram D. Dinman, M.D., Sc.D.
Director, Institute of Environmental and Industrial Health, University of Michigan

A. Geoffrey Norman, Ph.D., Sc.D.
Vice-President for Research, University of Michigan

TABLE OF CONTENTS

PART I
THE OCCURRENCE OF MERCURY IN THE ENVIRONMENT AND MAN

PART II
METHODS OF ANALYSIS

PART III
ENVIRONMENTAL DYNAMICS OF MERCURY

PART IV
BIOLOGICAL EFFECTS OF MERCURY COMPOUNDS

PART I

THE OCCURRENCE OF MERCURY IN

THE ENVIRONMENT AND MAN

CONTRIBUTORS TO PART I

Jack D. Bails, Anadromous Fisheries Management Specialist, Division of Fisheries, Michigan Department of Natural Resources, Lansing, Michigan

Richard A. Copeland, Ph.D., Environmental Research Group, Inc., Ann Arbor, Michigan

O. M. Derryberry, M.D., M.P.H., Manager of Health and Environmental Science, Tennessee Valley Authority, Chattanooga, Tennessee

Frank M. D'Itri, Ph.D., Assistant Professor of Water Chemistry, Institute of Water Research, Michigan State University, East Lansing, Michigan

E. H. Dustman, Ph.D., Patuxent Wildlife Research Center, Division of Wildlife Research, Bureau of Sport Fisheries and Wildlife, Laurel, Maryland

J. B. Elder, Ph.D., Division of Wildlife Services, Bureau of Sport Fisheries and Wildlife, Minneapolis, Minnesota

R. A. Greig, Bureau of Commercial Fisheries, Technological Laboratory, Ann Arbor, Michigan

David H. Klein, Ph.D., Department of Chemistry, Hope College, Holland, Michigan

Stanton J. Kleinert, Biologist and Coordinator of Mercury Studies, Wisconsin Department of Natural Resources, Madison, Wisconsin

John G. Konrad, Ph.D., Supervisor of Special Studies, Wisconsin Department of Natural Resources, Madison, Wisconsin

E. Mastromatteo, M.D., Environmental Health Services Branch, Ontario Department of Health, Toronto, Ontario, Canada

H. L. Seagran, Bureau of Commercial Fisheries, Technological Laboratory, Ann Arbor, Michigan

L. F. Stickel, Ph.D., Patuxent Wildlife Research Center, Division of Wildlife Research, Bureau of Sport Fisheries and Wildlife, Laurel, Maryland

R. B. Sutherland, M.D., Environmental Health Services
    Branch, Ontario Department of Health, Toronto, Ontario,
    Canada
Tadao Takeuchi, M.D., Pathology Department, Kumamoto Uni-
    versity School of Medicine, Kumamoto Prefecture, Japan
William G. Turney, Assistant Chief Engineer, Michigan Water
    Resources Commission, Lansing, Michigan
Kenneth R. Wilcox, Jr., M.D., Department of Public Health,
    State of Michigan, Lansing, Michigan

Sources of Mercury in the Environment

Frank M. D'Itri

As the scope and variety of scientific investigation continues to broaden our understanding of the kind and extent of mercury contamination of the environment, we increasingly recognize this contamination as a widespread and serious threat to man and his ecosystem. Therefore, before we can attack and solve this problem, the various sources of mercury in the environment should be recognized.

In answer to the basic question of where the mercury found in the environment is coming from, two major source divisions can be cited. First, mercury is present in nature, and the sources of this are not a result of man's action. Rather, a general cycle[1,2] is probably involved wherein the mercury is transported to the oceans as a natural result of land erosion. And due to its high vapor pressure, metallic mercury is most likely to be evaporated from the world's soils into the atmosphere. The amount and method of accumulation of mercury by this natural process warrants further exploration, and some meaningful definitions and working techniques should be formulated to extend this research in the future.

In the meantime, the second general division of sources of mercury in the environment involves the direct or indirect result of man's action. And, of course, the subsequent contamination of the ecosystem has aroused much public concern and has generated much interest in the scientific research that has been accomplished so far.

On the basis of this research, it is known that the United States consumed in excess of 5.7 million pounds of mercury in 1968.[3] It has been estimated that more than 163,000,000 pounds of mercury have been consumed by the United States since the turn of the century.[4] Furthermore, the United States has increased its consumption

5

of mercury by approximately 50% during the last ten years,
or from approximately four to six million pounds per year.[3]
While these figures show the amount of mercury consumed in
the United States, it must be emphasized that an unknown
portion of this mercury escapes into the environment by
one route or another, with the most obvious routes listed
below. In addition to listing these routes, it is important to note that these consumption figures include only
the mercury produced in this country or imported; they do
not include mercury contamination sources resulting from
nonmercury-related technology, such as the mercury that is
released to the atmosphere through the burning of fossil
fuels.

Major Mercury-Consuming Industries in the U.S.

The major mercury-consuming industries in the United
States can be tabulated on the basis of their 1968 consumption figures.[3]

1. The electrical apparatus industry was responsible
for the consumption of almost 1.5 million pounds of mercury
or about 26.6% of the total national consumption. In this
category, the largest specific use of mercury is in the
manufacture of mercury batteries and alkaline energy cells.
This use alone consumed an estimated million pounds of mercury.[5] The remainder of the mercury was used in the manufacture of such items as mercury-pool rectifiers and power
tubes, as well as a variety of lamps including fluorescent,
germicidal, photocopying, and high intensity arc discharge
lamps.

2. Industrial control instruments industries consumed
about 606,000 pounds or approximately 10.6% of the mercury
that was used in the manufacture of mercury switches, re-
lays, gauges, pump seals, and valves.

3. General laboratory use consumed about 151,000 pounds,
or approximately 2.6% of the mercury that was expended, for
experimental equipment and general laboratory use in 1968.
The most common laboratory uses of mercury result from its
physical rather than its chemical properties. Therefore,
the most common laboratory uses are found in diffusion
pumps, barometers, manometers, McLeod gauges, thermometers,
and vibration dampers.

4. The chlor-alkali industry uses the continuous flow
mercury cathode cell to produce chlorine and caustic soda.
The 1968 figures indicate that more than 1.3 million pounds
of mercury or 23.1% of the total consumption in the United
States was used to produce over 8.4 million tons of chlorine.[6]

In the United States, the percentage of chlorine and caustic soda that was produced by the continuous mercury cathode cell has steadily increased from 4% in 1946 to 12.5% in 1956, to 21% in 1963, and swelled to 28.5% by 1968. Projected figures suggest that by 1975, 38% of all chlorine will be produced by means of the mercury cell.[5]

Production was switched from diaphragm cells to mercury cells because of the demand for a purer caustic soda--purer in the sense of having fewer chloride ions. Because of mercury's unusual propensity to form an amalgam with the reduced sodium metal derived from salt brine, the mercury cell process results in a very pure grade of caustic soda. While the operating economics have historically favored diaphragm cells, this edge has gradually been narrowed to the point where it will be incidental in the near future. Therefore, still more conversions from diaphragm to mercury cells can be expected.

Mercury losses from the mercury cell process have been estimated in the order of 0.45 pounds of mercury for each ton of chlorine so produced.[4] Therefore, based on the combined figure of 8.4 million tons of chlorine produced in the United States and assuming that 26.2% of the chlorine was produced by the continuous mercury cell method,[7] an estimated amount of mercury in excess of 990,000 pounds was lost throughout the United States in 1968. In addition to this, the Canadian chlor-alkali industry requires an annual mercury acquisition of about 200,000 pounds to replace its mercury loss.[8] Mercury in the chlor-alkali industry can be lost during several phases of the process--through the caustic soda product, through the overall cleaning of the mercury cell room, through the brine solution, through the hydrogen gas byproduct, through the brine saturation, and through the air. The quantity of mercury that ultimately reaches the environment depends, in a large measure, on the overall operating efficiency of the companies that are involved.

Furthermore, it is important to note that caustic soda produced by this method will contain varying amounts of mercury at the trace level, depending on its degree of purification. These traces of mercury can be introduced into the human food cycle if the caustic soda produced by this method is used in the processing of foods for human consumption. And sodium hydroxide or caustic soda has been used as a peeling agent for tubers and fruits, a glazing agent for pretzels, a sour cream-butter neutralizer, a reagent in the refining process for vegetable oils and animal fats, as well as a reagent to adjust alkalinity in the canned vegetable industry.

Paint Manufacture Use of Organo-Mercurials

5. The paint industry was responsible for 14.4% of the nation's mercury consumption or 803,000 pounds of mercury. Organo-mercurial compounds are widely used as bacteriocide-fungicide agents to protect water-based paints from bacterial fermentation prior to application, and to retard fungus attacks upon painted surfaces under damp and humid conditions. The most widely used paint preservatives are phenylmercury derivatives of various organic acids. These mercury compounds are usually added to paint in concentration levels of between 100 and 15,000 parts per million. In addition, organo-mercurial compounds with a very low water solubility are incorporated into marine paints to improve their durability and to increase their resistance to fouling by bacteria and other marine growth.

6. Agriculture accounted for 260,000 pounds, or 4.6% of the mercury consumed, in the manufacture of fungicides in the United States in 1968. Fungicides are needed in agriculture because great crop losses are caused by a wide variety of plant-pathogenic fungi. Since organo-mercurials possess a wider spectrum of fungicidal activity than non-mercurial formulations, they have been used extensively to control fungus diseases through application as seed dressing on the seeds of barley, beans, corn, cotton, flax, millet, milo, oats, peanuts, peas, rice, rye, safflower, sorghum, soybeans, sugarbeets, and wheat. Foliar application of these mercury compounds has been made on strawberries, peaches, apples, cherries, pears, potatoes, and tomatoes. Despite the high toxicity of organic mercury compounds, they have continued to be the chosen fungicides in the seed treatment of cereal grains. Also included in this category are the mercury-containing fungicides which are used by individual homeowners on their lawns, trees, ornamental shrubs, and gardens. Nonetheless, the agricultural demand for mercury fungicides has steadily decreased over the past decade.[9] This demand undoubtedly will continue to decline at an accelerated pace in the United States as a result of recent adverse rulings by the Federal authorities.

7. Dental preparations utilized 4.1% or 234,000 pounds of the mercury consumed in 1968. An amalgam alloy composed of silver, tin, copper, and sometimes zinc is mixed with mercury to form a plastic mass which can be molded to fill tooth cavities.

8. Catalyst needs fulfilled 2.5% or 145,000 pounds of the 1968 mercury consumption. Mercury is used to prepare

various catalytic salts, especially the chloride, oxide, sulfate, acetate, and phosphate salts which, in turn, are used to produce vinyl chloride urethanes, anthraquinone derivatives, and many other chemical manufacturing products which require a mercury-based catalyst.

The catalytic use of mercury initially focused world attention on the environmental mercury problem in the middle and late 1950's. In a chemical plant located near Minamata, Japan, mercuric sulfate and chloride were being used as the catalytic agents for the conversion of acetylene into acetaldhyde and vinyl chloride respectively.[10,11] As a result of these operations, the mercury catalysts were methylated in a side reaction to form the highly poisonous methylmercury chloride which was discharged via the wastewater stream into Minamata Bay and was subsequently accumulated in the fish and shellfish of the bay. The methylmercury chloride in fish and shellfish was found to be the toxic material responsible for severe neurological disorders among inhabitants in the vicinity of Minamata Bay. Today the term "Minamata Disease" describes the chemical and pathological characteristics of this neurological disorder and has become synonymous with methylmercury poisoning specifically and alkyl mercury poisoning in general. From 1953 when the Minamata Disease was first recognized to the present, 121 confirmed cases of the disease resulting in 46 deaths have been recognized in the Minamata area with an additional 47 confirmed cases and 6 deaths in the Nugata, Japan area.[12]

Mercury Compounds as Slimicides

9. The paper and pulp industry required about 0.6% or 32,000 pounds of the 1968 American mercury production. In the process of manufacturing paper, conditions such as favorable temperature, high humidity, and an adequate supply of nutrients in the form of wood fiber, as well as inorganic and organic additives, are ideal for the growth of microbes. Furthermore, if these microbial growths are not controlled during the paper-making process, the results are clogged filters and sieves and, consequently, an inferior product. In addition to clogged filters and sieves, slime deposits that have formed in the water systems of the paper mill can become dislodged and incorporated into the paper pulp. Then, when the pulp is rolled into paper, the slime contaminant leaves discolored and weakened areas in the finished paper. These defects are more susceptible to tearing and result in costly time being lost because the paper-making machines cannot function

smoothly. In addition to controlling microbial growth
during the paper manufacturing process, some of the slimicide is regulated to remain in the finished paper and
serve as a protection from fungal deterioration.

In the 1950's and early 1960's, substantial amounts of
various mercury compounds were used as slimicides in paper
manufacturing systems to control microbial growth. Since
then, however, the amount of mercury compounds used for
this purpose has declined for several reasons. The primary
cause was a Federal Drug Administration ruling that mercury
compounds cannot be used to manufacture the paper or card-
board that comes in direct contact with foodstuffs. Also,
very effective nonmercury biocides such as chloro phenols,
chlorine, bromo ketones, and organic sulfur compounds have
been introduced into this market continually. Finally,
the cost of mercury has risen steadily so that its price
has more than doubled during the 1960's.[9]

It is important to note another source of mercury contamination attributable to the paper and pulp industry.
Because of the increased demand for caustic soda and chlorine gas in the pulping operation, many paper-making operations in the United States and Canada have found it
economical to produce caustic soda and chlorine at the
pulping plant, usually by the continuous mercury cathode
cell method. Since the caustic soda produced by this method
may contain as much as 7 ppm of mercury as an impurity,[13]
mercury is again lost to the environment through the wash
water and entrapment into the final paper product.

   10. The pharmaceutical and cosmetic industries utilized
over 0.5% or 32,000 pounds of the total mercury production.
Mercury and its compounds have been used in medicine from
earliest times. Today, mercury compounds are used in a
variety of well-defined pharmaceutical and cosmetic applications. Phenylmercuric acetate has been used in contraceptive vaginal jellies,[14] and various organo-mercury
compounds have been used as diuretics for many years; but
this use seems to have declined over the past decade, primarily because nonmercury compounds have been found to be
as effective as the mercury compounds. Organo-mercurials,
however, still enjoy wide use as antiseptic products under
such trade names as Merthiolate, Mercurochrome, Metaphen,
and Mercresin. Although mercury and compounds in which it
is included have been used in medicine since antiquity, the
development of efficient antibiotics and the toxicity of
mercury compounds have contributed to a marked reduction
in their use except as diuretics and ointments for topical
application. Finally, because microbial problems often

occur in base emulsions of pharmaceuticals, cosmetics, soaps, and similar products, mercurials in one form or another are often added to act as preservatives.

Applications of Mercury for Amalgamation

11. Amalgamation entails the use of about 0.35% or 20,000 pounds of mercury per year. Except for iron and platinum, most metals can be amalgamated with mercury, and some selected amalgams have great utility in industry. In the chlor-alkali industry electrolytically-formed sodium is amalgamated with the mercury serving as the cathode; and because of the design of the cell, the mercury-sodium amalgam can be mechanically removed from the brine chamber. It is this unique feature of the continuous mercury cathode cell which allows the production of caustic soda containing a very low chloride ion concentration.

Another important use of elemental mercury is the extraction of gold from its ore. As early as the first century B.C., the extraction of gold from its ore or impurities by amalgamation was known and probably represents the first practical nondecorative use of mercury.[15] Furthermore, this same property of mercury was undoubtedly responsible for the initial importation of mercury into the western hemisphere when large quantities of mercury were transported from Almaden, Spain to what is now Mexico, Peru, and Bolivia for many centuries prior to the Industrial Revolution. With the invention of the Patio (amalgamation) process in 1557 for the recovery of gold and silver from its ore, mercury was shipped to the New World under a Spanish crown monopoly that endured nearly 300 years. It was this process and Spanish mercury that permitted the economical extraction of silver and gold from the ores of the New World. Considering the precarious nature of ocean shipping in the period between 1560 and 1860, it would be reasonable to conclude that a great deal of mercury went to the bottom or foundered along the coastlines of the Americas.[16]

One amalgamation method mixes the powdered ore with water and passes the resulting slurry across copper plates coated with a thin layer of mercury. The gold particles adhere to the mercury film to form an amalgam which remains on the plates while the water washes away the rocks and earth. From time to time the gold amalgam is scraped off. The gold is recovered by heating the amalgam to vaporize the mercury leaving the gold behind. In 1965, the largest gold producer in the United States recovered

approximately 64% of its gold from the ore by amalgamation.
The consumption of mercury in this operation was about 5.75
grams per ton of ore milled and 32.2 grams of mercury per
ounce of gold recovered by amalgamation.[17]

12. Another 11%, or slightly more than 628,000 pounds,
of the total mercury consumption is expended in a variety
of diversified uses. Undoubtedly, most of the mercury in
this category has been used in the installation and expansion of caustic soda plants throughout the United States.
Also, all mercury consumption not assigned into one of the
above categories is included here. These miscellaneous uses
of mercury can be quite extensive. For example, engines
have been designed which utilize mercury vapor instead of
steam in the boiler. Mercury's boiling point (357°C),
higher than water, theoretically makes a great increase
in efficiency possible, but problems with cost, weight,
and corrosion have hindered such development.[18]

In addition to the uses already mentioned, mercury in
some form is used in preserving wood, etching metals, tan-
ning leather, preserving hides and skins at meat packing
plants, manufacturing felt, in photography, sintering
plants, iron and steel works, ceramics and glass industries,
in manufacturing artificial jewelry, the bronzing industry,
the explosive industry, photoengraving, and tattooing.
Also, mercury and especially the phenylmercurials are used
as preservatives or fungustats in consumer and industrial
products such as floor waxes, furniture polishes, fabric
softeners, air conditioner filters, toothbrushes, metal
cutting, oil emulsions, mattress inner components, cellu-
lose sponges, rope, canvas, dry wall products, wall plaster,
adhesives, scatter rugs, brooms, furniture polishing rags,
dust rags, dust mops and a variety of dust-control preparations. Mercury is commonly used as an antimicrobial agent
in many consumer products manufactured with plastics,
rubber, leather or textile components.

In addition to the practical application and utilization
of mercury technology, there are many experimental applications of mercury in rather exotic uses. For example,
the use of mercury has been proposed for liquid flywheels
and gyroscopes for spacecraft stabilization, ion engines
for rockets, nuclear-reactor coolants, fuel cells, and
turboelectric power systems.[19] The list of mercury uses
is quite extensive. Bailey and Smith have estimated that
while most of the mercury consumed in the United States
has been confined to a relatively small number of general
purpose categories, there are almost 3000 distinct
applications within these categories.[20]

In addition to recognizing the kinds and extent of industrial mercury consumption, it is important to ascertain how mercury and its various compounds are lost to the environment. Virtually all operations that involve the use of mercury provide the opportunity for its escape. While the route of mercury contamination sometimes can be involved and complex, the introduction of mercury into the environment through man's actions can be grouped into the two main categories of mercury or nonmercury related technology.

Direct Sources of Mercury Contamination

As a result of man's utilization and exploitation of mercury and mercury-related technology, many forms of mercury have been released directly or indirectly into the environment. Direct sources can be defined as those that release mercury into the environment when this release could be prevented at the source through the application of appropriate pollution abatement systems. By and large, virtually all manufacturing operations that utilize mercury fall into this subcategory, primarily because the current market price of mercury is usually much less than its eventual recovery cost. "Direct source" contamination most frequently occurs when trace amounts of mercury in one form or another are released into rivers and streams through wastewater discharges and/or are vented into the atmosphere as a resource which is not economically recoverable in the manufacturing operation.

While mercury-containing fungicidal and slimicidal compounds used in agriculture and industry contribute to the overall mercury problem because of the mercury lost during the manufacture of these chemicals, this is a paradoxical contribution because these compounds are expressly produced to be applied to the environment. Considering the overall mercury burden on the environment, this group of chemicals, although responsible for only 4.6% of the United States consumption in 1968, may have singular significance because of the importance of alkyl mercury compounds to the overall mercury problem. For this reason, they have been included as a direct source. The agricultural uses of mercury include seed dressings, foliage sprays, and lawn and garden applications, whereas some industrial applications of these compounds are found in commercial laundries, cooling towers, and in the paper and pulp industry to suppress mold and microbial growth. All of these uses apply the mercury directly to the environment.

Indirect Sources of Mercury Contamination

The indirect sources associated with mercury-related technology are defined as the inadvertent or accidental releases of mercury into the environment, resulting from the use, misuse and disposal of mercury and mercury-containing industrial and consumer products.

Undoubtedly, the most dangerous indirect route of mercury contamination results when its misuse affects man directly. With the exception of occupational or industrial mercury intoxication, this human threat is most commonly associated with the accidental or uninformed misuse of mercury-containing agricultural formulations. Since the introduction of organic mercury compounds for the prevention of seed-borne diseases in 1914, a relatively large number of people have been fatally poisoned or severely incapacitated. The most common cases of individual human poisoning usually result from eating food products such as bread or porridge made from cereal grains treated with some form of alkyl mercury fungicide.[21-26] An alternate route of human poisoning involves the slaughter and consumption of livestock fed waste grain treated with a fungicide.[21] Known mercury poisoning epidemics occurred in the Guatemalan Highlands in 1965,[22] Pakistan in 1961,[26] Northern Iraq in 1956 and Central Iraq in 1961.[24] These epidemics resulted when farmers and their families ate bread made from alkyl mercury-treated wheat that was given to them for planting. Undoubtedly many of the farmers were not adequately warned of the potent poisonous nature of the seed-dressing agent; however, other farmers had been warned against eating or feeding livestock the treated grain, but must not have felt that the threat was real. This feeling may have come about because some farmers washed the grain to remove the poisonous agent, and then fed the grain to chickens that appeared completely normal, even after days of eating the washed grain. The farmers who were hesitant about using the grain for food were misled by villagers, known to have eaten the dressed wheat in the form of bread, who appeared healthy and well for days or weeks afterward.[21]

The accidental or inadvertent as well as intentional feeding of waste dressed seed grain to farm livestock may be more prevalent than has been previously realized. The literature has reported a disturbing number of cases of organo-mercurial poisoning of livestock severe enough to warrant investigation,[27-35] but one can only speculate on the number of organo-mercurial poisonings which were not severe enough to warrant the farmer's calling the veterinarian.

Another example of indirect environmental mercury contamination was the result of utilization of 55-gallon steel drums which once held a slimicide formulation containing phenylmercuric acetate. During five days in July, 1968, more than 500,000 fish were killed in the Watauga arm of Boone Reservoir, Tennessee.[36] The cause of the fish-kill was difficult to determine, but after most common causes of fish-kills were eliminated, the cause was found to be a slime control preparation containing phenylmercuric acetate and 2,4,6-trichlorophenol. This substance was introduced into the reservoir because supposedly empty 55-gallon steel barrels that had contained phenylmercuric acetate were used for flotation purposes at the boat docks. It was subsequently determined that the phenylmercuric acetate was transformed into diphenylmercury which was responsible for the fish-kill. The actual amount of the phenylmercuric acetate that had remained in the barrels was not determined.

In addition, an undetermined amount of mercury is also lost to the nation's watercourses through the wastewater discharges of tens of thousands of hospitals, dental offices, and the various chemical laboratories in the United States that use mercury. One example of this type of mercury loss is the direct result of the continual use of mercuric chloride as a fixative for tissues in many of our hospitals. After examination of the tissue has been completed, the excess fixative solution is usually flushed down the sink and the treated tissues either incinerated or ground up in a disposal unit. The actual number of hospitals using this technique is not known, but the use of mercury to prepare the fixative solution is still advocated.[37,38]

Since mercury is purposely incorporated into many industrial or consumer products such as paints, pharmaceuticals, paper products, fluorescent lamps, mercury batteries, and many other products too numerous to list, the indiscriminate disposal of these products by an uninformed population represents an important environmental mercury contamination route, especially of our nation's rivers, streams, and lakes. In addition, burning products that contain mercury can volatilize the mercury and introduce its vapors into the atmosphere; considering the large number of mercury-containing consumer products, this could also be a significant source of environmental mercury contamination. Lundholm reported that in the mid-1960's, when phenylmercuric acetate was more widely used as a slimicide in the paper and pulp industry, an estimated 1100 pounds of mercury were added to the Swedish atmosphere annually through the burning of newspaper.

Sewer System Disposal of Unwanted Chemicals

While the introduction of toxic materials into the nation's waterways through the manufacturing operations of our nation's industries has been widely acknowledged, the sanitary sewer systems of this nation also serve as a convenient disposal system for many unwanted chemicals, including many mercury-containing consumer products. Quite understandably, the respective mercury sources that enter the sewer system are individually small enough to be considered insignificant, but the problem assumes larger proportions when the total amounts and variety of sources are considered. The total mercury content of the sewage system is the result of all the incidental uses of mercury-containing compounds by individuals and businesses. These include the mercury found in water-based paints, paper products, cosmetics, broken thermometers, mercury amalgam tooth fillings, discarded pharmaceuticals, household and laundry disinfectants, as well as the runoff of mercury lawn and garden fungicides. On the average, the mercury concentration of the sewage effluent is one order of magnitude greater than the watercourse that receives it.[40] These data are also substantiated by the work of Klein and Goldberg[41] who reported that the mercury concentration in surface sediment samples near municipal sewer ocean outfalls is eight to ten times higher than in similar deposits that are farther from the outfall. This could amount to mercury concentrations in sewage treatment plants of from 0.5 ppb to 1.0 ppb. Based on these approximate figures, it would not be unreasonable to expect from 400 to 800 pounds of mercury per year per million population in an urban environment.

Even though the concentrations of mercury in the sewage treatment plant effluent are higher than in the watercourses that receive them, substantial amounts of mercury appear to be removed by the sewage treatment plant. Andersson[42] found that decayed sludge from Swedish sewage treatment plants contained 6 ppm to 29 ppm of mercury on a dry weight basis. Therefore, it would appear that substantial amounts of mercury are prevented from being released into the aquatic environment. However, this mercury can be indirectly released by the terrestrial environment if the sludge is recycled as fertilizer. Assuming the sludge is applied to fields in the same amounts that are usually recommended for stable manure (2 to 4 tons per acre), between 12 and 110 grams of mercury would be added per acre. This value is substantially higher than the 0.4 to 0.9 grams of mercury added per acre through the application of typical stable manure. If, on the other hand, the sludge is processed through a multiple hearth furnace which reduces it to an easily disposable insoluble sterile ash, the mercury entrapped and removed through the action of the sludge will be volatilized and redistributed into the environment.

So far only the most obvious direct and indirect environmental mercury contamination sources have been mentioned, but less obvious, complex and involved routes also exist. One such direct route involves the experimental use of phenylmercuric acetate applied as an airborne spray for the control of transpiration in forests.[43-45] Mercuric chloride has been used experimentally as a disinfectant chemical for impounded waters that are used to recharge underground aquifers in California's San Joaquin Valley.[46]

Mercury Release from Fossil Fuels

In addition to the mercury lost into the environment as a result of man's utilization and exploitation of mercury and mercury-related technology, an undeterminable but potentially large source of environmental mercury contamination results from the inadvertent release of mercury through the utilization and exploitation of the world's mineral resources other than mercury. In this category, undoubtedly the largest single source contributor to the environmental release of mercury results when fossil fuels such as coal and crude oil are burned or converted into other products.

Coal typically contains many of the known elements, in very small amounts which are not commonly reported as part of the standard ash analysis. Furthermore, it is an established fact that many coal and brown coal ashes contain exceptionally high amounts of certain trace elements relative to their average content in the earth's crust.[47-49] In a survey of the literature involving the occurrence of rare and uncommon elements in coal, Gibson and Selvig[50] reported that more than half the known elements, including mercury, have been found in coal. V. M. Goldschmidt[51] explained the enrichment of mercury and other trace elements in coal and the uptake of nutrient and ballast elements by the living plants from the soil, subsoil, and water. These trace elements are ultimately translocated into the roots, twigs, and leaves. Goldschmidt offers another possible explanation--that the normally soluble trace elements are precipitated as the respective sulfides by the special local chemical environment which develops hydrogen sulfide associated with the anaerobic rotting of plant materials.

The available data concerning the concentration of mercury in coal is very limited. Goldschmidt and Peters[40] have reported the presence of mercury in different kinds of coal, peats, and shales from Germany and England, while Inagaki[52] qualitatively found mercury present in some Japanese coals. In a report on the spectrographic analysis for 38 different elements of 596 spot samples from 16 coal seams in West Virginia, Headlee and Hunter[53] found that the mercury content in coal ash ranged from less than 100 ppm to 280 ppm with an average value of 130 ppm. While these values appear inordinately high for coal ash, the presence of mercury is apparent.

The very limited available information on mercury concentrations in coal indicates that most of the current data is in the Russian literature. The distribution of mercury in coal in various parts of the USSR has been reported to range between 0.02 ppm and 300 ppm.[54-60] In addition, up to 3000 ppm of mercury has been reported in the solid bitumens of the Sevan-Akerin zone of the Lesser Caucasus.[61] While these high values of mercury in coals have been reported, it is important to recognize that, as a rule, coal deposits containing more than 1.0 ppm mercury are usually located in or adjacent to known mercury mineralizations. When mercury-containing coals are used in the coking process, free mercury and mercuric sulfide have been recovered as byproducts in the subsequent distillation of the coal tar.[62 65]

Pakter[66,67] reported that coal charges from 80% of the byproduct coking plants in the USSR were analyzed for their respective mercury contents, and mercury was detected in practically all of them. The overall average mercury concentration for all the plants was 0.28 ppm.

Mercury Content in Crude Oil

The data are even more sparse with respect to information about the mercury content in crude oil than that found for coal. In the Wilbur Springs District, California, which includes the important Abbott mercury mine as well as four or five smaller mercury deposits, White[68] reported that hydrocarbons and methane are frequently associated with mercury deposits. Also, the Mt. Diablo District, California, is known for the association of mercury with petroleum, hydrocarbon gases, and saline oilfield waters. Bailey et al. reported that native mercury and possibly other forms of mercury occur in petroleum, natural gas, and the brine of the Cymric oil field, Kern County,

California.[69] A quantitative spectrographic analysis of
the metal content was made on the ash of three Cymric field
crude oils. The analyses showed that these crude oils contained remarkably large amounts of mercury, with the reported values ranging from 1.9 ppm to 21 ppm. The latter
value is one of the highest reported for any natural fluid
and compares with the value of 21 ppm for Santa Barbara
crude oil reported by Trost.[70] The Cymric oil field natural gas that separates from the petroleum and brine upon
release in pressure is saturated with mercury vapor at the
oil field, but the mercury evidently combines with hydrogen
sulfide from "sour" natural gases released from the other
oil fields, and is precipitated in the pipe lines. Also,
some native mercury separates from the crude oil at the
pumping station.

The mercury content in brines associated with oil producing wells has been reported to be from less than 0.02
ppm to 0.2 ppm. It has been estimated that the total
quantity of mercury discharged from all fluids during the
existence of the Cymric oil field would probably be equivalent to many thousands of flasks of 76 pounds each.[71]

Although the mercury content of fossil fuels may appear
to be insignificantly small, if the total amounts of coal
and oil that are consumed in the world since the industrial
revolution are considered, proportionately, the amount of
mercury released into the environment would conceivably exceed the amounts of mercury lost to the environment through
the exploitation of mercury-related technology. In order
to appreciate the significance of this source relative to
other sources of mercury contamination in the environment,
it is interesting to note that, in the United States alone,
the production of coal and crude oil in 1968 was in excess
of 500 and 488 million tons respectively.[72-74] Assuming
that these fossil fuels contained between 10 ppb and 1 ppm
mercury, this represents from 20,000 to 2,000,000 pounds
of additional mercury which could ultimately be lost into
the environment each year.

Finally, another environmental mercury contamination
source, admittedly small, occurs in the recovery or use
of raw materials which contain small amounts of mercury.
Usually traces of mercury are present in many sulfide ores
in concentrations which are not economically feasible to
recover the mercury. When these ores are roasted, especially those of gold, copper, lead, and zinc, the mercury
is vaporized and is driven off with the evolved sulfur
dioxide; even though the gas is cooled, scrubbed, and
filtered, some of the mercury escapes into the atmosphere.[75]

In special cases, however, significant quantities of mercury have been recovered as a byproduct of copper, gold and zinc production.[76]

References

1. Stock, A. and F. Cucuel. "The Occurrence of Mercury," Naturwissenschaften, *22*, 390 (1934); Chem. Abstr., *28*: 7086, in German.
2. Goldschmidt, V. M. "Geochemical Distribution Laws of the Elements. IX. The Relative Abundances of the Elements and the Atomic Species," Skrifter Norske Videnskaps – Akad. Oslo., I. Mat. – Naturv. Klasse No. 4 (1937); Chem. Abstr., *33*:4918, in German, 148 pp.
3. West, J. M. "Mercury," 1968 Minerals Yearbook. (Washington, D. C.: U. S. Government Printing Office, 1969), Vol. L-II, p. 693.
4. Kolbye, A. C. Statement presented at the "Hearing on the Effects of Mercury on Man and the Environment," Senate Committee on Commerce, Subcommittee on Energy, Natural Resources and the Environment (May 8, 1970).
5. Maykuth, D. M., Chairman. "Trends in Usage of Mercury," Report of the National Materials Advisory Board. (Washington, D. C.: National Research Council, September, 1969).
6. Anon. "Chlorine Gas," Chemicals, 17(2), 35 (1970). Published quarterly by the U.S. Department of Commerce.
7. Sommers, H. A. "The Chlor-alkali Industry," Chem. Engr. Prog., *61*, 94 (1965).
8. Fimreite, N. "Mercury Uses in Canada and Their Possible Hazards as Sources of Mercury Contamination," Environmental Pollution, *1*(1970).
9. Anon. "Mercury," Commodity Year Book, 1969, H. Jiler, Ed. (New York: Commodity Research Bureau, Inc., 1970), p. 217.
10. Irukayama, K. "The Pollution of Minamata Bay and Minamata Disease," Advan. Water Pollution Res., Proc. 3rd Int. Conf., Munich, Germany, September, 1966, *3* 153 (1967).
11. Kurland, L. T., S. N. Faro, and H. Siedler. "Minamata Disease," World Neurology, *1*, 370 (1960).
12. Takeuchi, T. "Biological Reactions and Pathological Changes of Human Beings and Animals under the Condition of Organic Mercury Contamination." Reprint of a paper presented at the International Conference on Environmental Mercury Contamination, Ann Arbor, Michigan, September, 1970.

13. Bouveng, H. O.   "The Chlorine Industry and the Mercury Problem," Modern Kemi, *3*, 45 (1968), *Swedish*.
14. Eastman, N. J. and A. B. Scott.   "Phenylmercuric Acetate as a Contraceptive," Human Fertility, *9*, 33 (1944).
15. Stillman, J. M.   The Story of Early Chemistry.   (New York: D. Appleton and Company, 1924), p. 30.
16. Flawn, P. T.   Personal communication.
17. Wise, E. M.   "Gold and Gold Compounds," Kirk-Othmer Encyclopedia of Chemical Technology, Second Edition. (New York: John Wiley and Sons, Interscience Publishers, 1966), Vol. 10, p. 683.
18. Anon.   "Mercury Vapor and Steam Power Turbines Save Fuel," Science Newsletter, *57*, 56 (January 28, 1950).
19. Engel, G. T.   "Mercury," Kirk-Othmer Encyclopedia of Chemical Technology, Second Edition.   (New York: John Wiley and Sons, Interscience Publishers, 1966), Vol. 13, p. 218.
20. Bailey, E. H. and R. M. Smith.   "Mercury, Its Occurrence and Economical Trends," U. S. Geol. Surv. Circ. *496*, 11 (1964).
21. Roueche, B.   "Annals of Medicine - Insufficient Evidence," New Yorker Magazine (August 22, 1970), p. 64.
22. Ordonez, J. V., J. A. Carrelo, and M. M. Carrelo. "Epidemiological Study of a Disease in the Guatemalan Highlands Believed to be Encephalitis," Boletin de la Oficina Sanctaria Panamericana, *60*(6), 510 (1966), *Spanish with English summary*.
23. Engleson, G. and T. Herner.   "Alkyl Mercury Poisoning," Acta Paedratrica, *41*, 289 (1952).
24. Jalili, M. H. and A. H. Abbasi.   "Poisoning by Ethyl Mercury Toluene Sulphonanclide," Brit. J. Ind. Med., *18*, 303 (1961).
25. Chatskii, G. I.   "Chemical Aspects of Granozan Poisoning," Sb. Nauch. Tr. Kafedry Fak. Kher. Agmi. Vrach Kaz Zhelez Doroga., *3*, 184 (1966); Biological Abstracts, *49*:34850, *Russian*
26. Haq, I. U.   "Agrosan Poisoning in Man," Brit. Med. J., 1579 (1963).
27. Boley, L. E., C. C. Morrill, and R. Graham.   "Evidence of Mercury Poisoning in Feeder Calves," N. Amer. Vet., *22*, 161 (1941).
28. Gorton, B.   "Mercurial Poisoning," Vet. Jour., *80*, 48 (1924).
29. Sonoda, M., R. Nakamura, K. Too, and A. Matsuhashi. "Chemical Studies on Mercury Poisoning in Cattle," Jap. J. Vet. Res., *4*, 5 (1956).

30. Fujimoto, Y., K. Ohshima, H. Satoh, and Y. Ohta. "Pathological Studies on Mercury Poisoning in Cattle," Ibid., *4*, 17 (1956).
31. Merberg, W. W. "Mercury Poisoning in a Dairy Herd," Vet. Med., *49*, 401 (1954).
32. Taylor, E. L. "Mercury Poisoning in Swine," Am. Vet. Med. Assoc. J., *111*, 46 (1947).
33. Jungherr, E. "Mercury Poisoning in Chinchillas," Ibid., *130*, 16 (1957).
34. McEntee, K. "Mercurial Poisoning in Swine," Cornell Vet., *40*, 143 (1950).
35. Loosmore, R. M., J. D. J. Darding, and L. Lewis. "Mercury Poisoning in Pigs," Vet. Record, *81*, 268 (1967).
36. Tennessee Valley Authority, Division of Health and Safety, Water Quality Branch. "Fish-Kill in Boone Reservoir, July 9-13, 1968." Chattanooga, Tennessee (December, 1968).
37. Meadows, R. and H. Schoemaker. "Improved Processing Technique for Renal Biopsies for Light Microscopy," J. Clinical Pathology, *23*, 548 (1970).
38. Marshall, C. E. Personal communication.
39. Lundholm, B. "Background Information: A Survey of the Situation in Sweden," Mercury Problem, Oikos Supp., *9*, 48 (1967).
40. Klein, D. H. Personal communication.
41. Klein, D. H. and E. D. Goldberg. "Mercury in the Marine Environment," Enviro. Sci. Tech., *4*, 765 (1970).
42. Andersson, A. "Mercury in Decayed Sludge," Grudfor-battring, *20*, 149 (1967); Chem. Abstr., *69*:45867d, *Swedish*.
43. Granger, R. L. and L. J. Edgerton. "The Effects of Two New Petroleum Spray Oils and Phenylmercuric Acetate on the Stomata of Apple Leaves," Proc. Amer. Soc. Hort. Sci., *88*, 48 (1966).
44. Hart, G. E., J. D. Schultz, and G. B. Coltharp. "Controlling Transportation in Aspen with Phenylmercuric Acetate," Water Resources Research, *5*, 407 (1969).
45. Waggoner, P. E. and B. A. Brando. "Stomata and the Hydrological Cycle," Proc. Nat. Acad. Sci., *57*, 1096 (1967).
46. Anon. "Mercuric Chloride for Better Watered Farms," Science News Letter, *58*, 59 (July 22, 1950).
47. Goldschmidt, V. M. and C. Peters. "The Concentration of Rare Elements in Coal," Nachr. Ges. Wiss. Gottengen,

Math.-Physik, Klasse (1933), pp. 371-86, *German*; Chem. Abstr., *27*:5690.
48. Goldschmidt, V. M. "Rare Elements in Coal Ashes," Ind. Eng. Chem., *27*, 1100 (1935).
49. Fuchs, W. "Rare Elements in German Brown-Coal Ashes," Ibid., *27*, 1099 (1935).
50. Gibson, F. H. and W. A. Selvig. "Rare and Uncommon Chemical Elements in Coal," Technical Paper 669 (Washington, D.C.: U.S. Government Printing Office, 1944), 23 pp., Chem. Abstr., *39*:1272.
51. Goldschmidt, V. M. "The Principles of Distribution of Chemical Elements in Minerals and Rocks," J. Chem. Soc. (1937), p. 655.
52. Inagaki, M. "Spectroscopic Analysis of Inorganic Matters in Coal. I," J. Coal Research Institute, *2*, 229 (1951), *Japanese*; Chem. Abstr., *49*:7221a.
53. Headlee, A. J. W. and R. G. Hunter. "Elements in Coal Ash and Their Industrial Significance," Ind. Eng. Chem., *45*, 548 (1953); also "The Inorganic Elements in Coal," West Virginia Geol. Survey 13 A, 36 (1955), Chem. Abstr., *50*:551h.
54. Karasik, M. A., O. G. Dvornikov, and V. Y. Petrov. "Distribution of Mercury in Coals in the Southeastern Parts of the Donets Basin," Mineralog. i Geokhim. Pivdenno-Skhidnoi. Chastini Ukr. RSR, Akad. Nauk Ukr. RSR (1963), 53-67, *Russian*; Chem. Abstr., *61*:5399d.
55. Karasik, M. A., A. E. Vasilevs'ka, V. Y. Petrov, and E. A. Ratekhin. "Distribution of Mercury in Coals of the Central and Donets-Makeevka Regions of the Donets Basin," Geol. Zh., Akad. Nauk Ukr. RSR,*22*(2), 53 (1962), *Russian*; Chem. Abstr., *57*:2513f.
56. Dvornikov, A. G. "Some Mercuriferous Characteristics of Coals of the East Donets Basin (Rostov Region)," Dokl. Akad. Nauk SSSR, *172*(1), 199 (1967), *Russian;* Chem. Abstr., *66*:57653g.
57. Dvornikov, A. G. "Mercury Geochemical Anomaly in Coals of the Endogenic Dispersion Halo Near the Nikotovka Mercury Deposit," Dopov. Akad. Nauk Ukr. RSR, Ser. B, *30*(8), 732 (1968), *Ukranian*; Chem. Abstr., *70*:13512p.
58. Vasilevs'ka, A. E., and V. P. Sheherbakov. "Forms of Mercury Compounds in Donets Basin Coals," Dopovodi Akad. Nauk Ukr. RSR (11), 1494-6 (1963), *Russian*; Chem. Abstr., *60*:10433b.
59. Karasik, M. A., A. G. Dvornikov, G. K. Talalaev, and K. K. Zemblevskii. "Mercury Content in Donbass Coals and Their Coking Products," Koks Khim (9), 14-16 (1967), *Russian*; Chem. Abstr., *67*:110361j.

60. Bol'shakov, A. P. "On the Role of Coal in Ore Deposition of the Nikitovskoyl Quicksilver Deposits," Geochemistry International, No. 3, 459-462 (1964). Transl. from Geokhimiya, No. 5, 477-480 (1964).
61. Kashkai, M. A. and T. N. Nasibov. "Mercury-Containing Solid Bitumens of the Lesser Caucasus," Geokhimiya, No. 9, 1132-4 (1968), *Russian*; Chem. Abstr., *69*: 108745k.
62. Holdsworth, E. C. "Mercury Pollution from Coal Combustion," Chemical Age (London, March 27, 1970).
63. Aston, F. W. "The Constitution of Mercury Derived from Coal Tar," Nature, *119*, 489 (1927).
64. Kirby, W. "Mercury from Coal Tar," J. Soc. Chem. Ind. *46*, 422R (1927).
65. Dvornikov, A. G. "Mercury Distribution in Gas Coal of the Northern Small Folding Area (Donbass)," Dopov. Akad. Nauk Ukr. RSR, Ser. B, *29*(9), 828 (1967), *Ukranian*; Chem. Abstr., *67*:110396z.
66. Pakter, M. K., D. P. Dubrovskaya, A. V. Pershin, and G. K. Talalaev. "Mercury in Chemical Products of Coking," Koks Khim. (11), 43-46 (1968), *Russian*; Chem. Abstr., *70*:70038n.
67. Pakter, M. K., D. P. Dubrovskaya, A. V. Pershin, and G. K. Talalaev. "Mercury in Coal Charges in Byproduct Coking Plants," Khim. Tverd. Topl. (6), 145-50 (1967), *Russian*; Chem. Abstr., *68*:71081s.
68. White, D. E. "Magmatic, Connate, and Metaphorphic Waters," Bull. Geol. Soc. Am., *68*, 1659 (1957).
69. Bailey, E. H., P. D. Snavely, and D. E. White. "Chemical Analyses of Brine and Crude Oil, Cymric Field, Kern County, California," U. S. Geol. Surv. Prog. Paper 424-D, D306-D309 (1961).
70. Trost, P. B. Statement made at the International Conference on Environmental Mercury Contamination, Ann Arbor, Michigan, September 30, 1970.
71. White, D. E. "Mercury and Base-Metal Deposits with Associated Thermal and Mineral Waters," Geochemistry of Hydrothermal Ore Deposits. Ed. by H. L. Barnes (New York: Holt, Rinehart, and Winston, Inc., 1967).
72. Institute of Geological Sciences. "Statistical Summary of the Mineral Industry 1963-1968," Natural Environmental Research Council. (London: Her Majesty's Stationery Office, 1970), p. 240.
73. Young, W. H. and J. J. Gallagher. "Coal - Bituminous and Lignite," 1968 Minerals Yearbook. (Washington: D. C.: U. S. Government Printing Office, 1969), Volume II, p. 301.

74. Lorenz, W. C. "Coal - Pennsylvania Anthracite," Ibid., p. 379.
75. Komlev, G. A., T. N. Kleandrov, V. S. Chakhotin, L. K. Udalov, and V. F. Makarov. "Decrease in Metal Loss During the Treatment of Mercury Ores in Rotary Kilns," Izv. Akad. Nauk. Uz. SSR, Ser. Takhn, Nauk. 8(4), 66-69 (1964), Russian; Chem. Abstr., 62:8727h.
76. Bureau of Mines. "Mercury Potential of the United States," Bureau of Mines Information Circular 8252. (Washington, D. C.: U. S. Government Printing Office, 1965).

Some Estimates of Natural Levels of Mercury
in the Environment

David H. Klein

The sparse geochemical data which are available indicate that the natural weathering process transfers mercury through the environment--from the continents, via rivers, to the oceans--at a rate of about 5000 tons per year.[4] Of the total mercury mined annually, half is apparently released into the environment. This man-controlled transport mechanism--from mines, via industry, to various waterways--also involves about 5000 tons per year. In addition, natural mercury evaporates from soils and rocks, moves through the atmosphere, and subsequently rains out; industrially-derived but unmined mercury, as from the burning of fossil fuels, follows a similar pattern. It is not at present possible to make even rough guesses about the quantities of mercury transported through the atmosphere, although it is probably reasonable to suppose that man and nature contribute about equally to the total.

In considering mercury as a pollutant it is important to distinguish the mercury present due to natural processes from that which is present due to industrial contamination. Mercury is widely distributed by nature, almost always in quite low concentrations; mercury as a contaminant enters the environment in only a few locations, but in relatively large amounts. To diagnose mercury contamination it is necessary to have estimates of the natural concentrations of mercury in various segments of the environment.

Mercury Concentrations in the U. S. Atmosphere

Mercury concentrations in the U. S. atmosphere are now being studied by the National Air Pollution Control Administration. Eriksson[3] estimates a world average of 20 ng/m³. This is appreciably higher than the values reported by Williston,[7] who measured the concentration of the elemental vapor in the atmosphere of the San Francisco Bay region. At 10,000 feet altitude, 20 miles offshore, concentrations averaged slightly below 1 ng/m³. On land, the observed values ranged from 1 to 50 ng/m³, with an average of perhaps 3 ng/m³. The measurements were made in the geologic province within which are found most of California's mercury mines, which may explain the observed strong dependence of the mercury concentration on wind direction.

Mercury concentrations in rainfall and in surface soils, together with atmospheric concentrations, would be of value in quantifying the atmospheric transport mechanisms of mercury, but again, few numbers are available. Stock and Cucuel[6] report seventeen rainwater analyses. Five of these showed mercury concentrations indistinguishable from the blank, while the other twelve ranged from 0.05 to 0.48 mg/l. The average of the 17 values is 0.14 mg/l.

The concentration of mercury in air, and thus in rainwater, is expected to be appreciably higher in industrialized areas, due to increased consumption of fossil fuels and to evaporative and mechanical losses from mercury-consuming industries. Results of the analyses of a few surface soil samples taken around the St. Clair River-Lake St. Clair-Detroit River industrial complex suggest that this is true. The sampling locations and results are shown in Figure 1. The mercury concentrations in soils distant or windward from the industrialized areas average around 0.03 ppm, while in the northern and southern industrialized regions the concentrations are elevated as much as ten-fold. The value 0.03 ppm may represent the natural concentration in these soils. Andersson[1] reports a range from 0.020 to 0.920 ppm, with an average of 0.07 ppm, for 200 soil samples, and Martin[5] gives the natural mercury content of English soils as between 0.01 and 0.06 ppm. Appreciably higher values are often found near mineral deposits, and so do not necessarily reflect environmental contamination.

Concentration of Mercury in Fresh Waters

The concentration of mercury in fresh waters is quite variable. Stock and Cucuel[6] report a range of 0.02 to 0.07

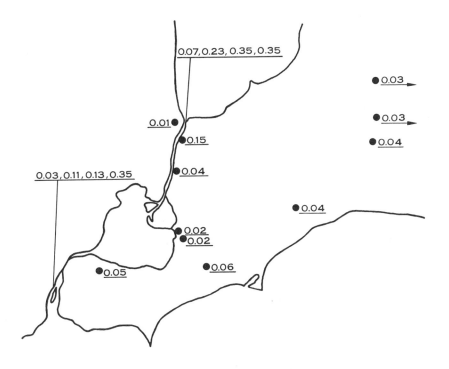

Figure 1: Mercury Sampling Locations and Results, St. Clair River/Lake St. Clair/Detroit River Industrial Complex

ppb for samples from Germany, and Dall'Aglio[2] reports normal groundwater values in Tuscany ranging from 0.01 to 0.05 ppb. Again, much higher values may be observed in mineralized regions. The results of the analyses of 67 samples from lakes, ponds, and rivers of the northeastern United States are shown in Figure 2, as a concentration-frequency diagram. The diagram suggests a rather narrow Gaussian distribution of concentrations around a mean of about 0.05 ppb, with a superimposed, apparently orderless, array of higher values ranging up to 2.8 ppb. The Gaussian distribution probably represents the natural levels in the region, with the higher values indicating contamination. This interpretation is supported by using some discrimination in the selection of samples to be represented. Samples

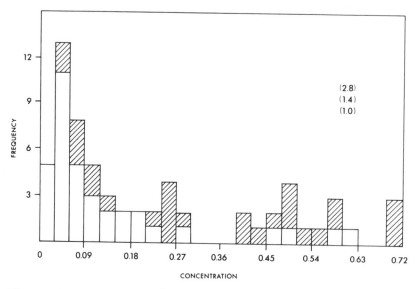

Figure 2:   Concentration-Frequency Diagram of 67 Samples
from Northeastern United States

expected to be polluted by mercury may be rejected, using
the following criteria: (a) samples taken within a mile
downstream from a municipal sewage outfall,   (b) samples
taken within a mile downstream from a chemical plant or
paper mill,   (c) samples taken from waters known to contain fish with high mercury content,   (d) samples with
anomalously high electrical conductivity. The 31 samples
rejected by these criteria are shown on Figure 2 by shaded
bars. Of the 36 samples with mercury contents above 0.12
ppb, 24 are thus rejected, while of the 31 samples below
0.12 ppb, only 7 are rejected. Assuming a cutoff of the
Gaussian distribution of the retained samples at 0.02 ppb,
the mercury concentration of the natural waters in the
northeastern U.S. is 0.055 ppb, with a standard deviation
of 0.035.

Most of the values presented above are subject to further refinement, especially since natural levels may vary
appreciably with the geology of the region. The figures
do, however, serve at least as rough baselines, to aid in
identifying the magnitude and sources of mercury as an
environmental contaminant.

References

1. Andersson, A. "Mercury in Swedish Soils," Oikos Supplementum, *9*, 13 (1967).
2. Dall'Aglio, M. "The Abundance of Mercury in 300 Natural Water Samples from Tuscany and Latuim," Origin and Distribution of the Elements, L. H. Ahrens, Ed. (Pergamon Press, 1968), p. 1065.
3. Eriksson, E. "Mercury in Nature," Oikos Supplementum, *9*, 13 (1967).
4. Goldberg, E. D. "Chemical Invasion of the Ocean by Man," McGraw-Hill Yearbook of Science and Technology (1970), p. 66.
5. Martin, J. T. "Mercury Residues in Plants," Analyst, *88*, 413 (1963).
6. Stock, A. and F. Cucuel. "Die Verbreitung des Quecksilbers," Naturwissenschaften, *22*, 390 (1934).
7. Williston, S. H. "Mercury in the Atmosphere," Journal of Geophysical Research, *73*, 7051 (1968).

The Mercury Pollution Problem in Michigan

William G. Turney

After Michigan learned about the mercury problem in February, 1970, the Michigan Water Resources Commission began a rather extensive review of all industries and communities around the state, trying to find whether or not there were any point discharges going into the waters of the state. It originally found two; one was Wyandotte Chemical, which has a chlor-alkali plant located on the Detroit River. Before a control program was instituted, Wyandotte Chemical was discharging approximately 10 to 20 pounds of mercury per day. The other point discharge source of mercury was General Electric Company, a small manufacturing plant located in the middle of the state near Edmore, Michigan. This company manufactures magnets for electronic components, and they are the sole manufacturer of this particular type of magnet, used by the U.S. Department of Defense. Their discharge was approximately 1,500 pounds of mercury per year, most of which was released as elemental mercury. The effect on the environment was very isolated in and around the plant location and there was no real damage to the fishery in the area.

In August, 1970, the Michigan Water Resources Commission investigated a fish-kill near Caspian in the Upper Peninsula of Michigan. It found no apparent cause for the fish-kill, but analyzed the fish for mercury and found that they contained about 2.5 ppm. It was found that a small laundry nearby was using a mildew inhibitor containing phenylmercuric acetate. The laundry had been discharging this compound for the past five years at approximately a quarter of a pound of mercury per day. It never was determined that the mercury was the cause of the fish-kill, but there was no other apparent cause. All three of these points source discharges have been stopped.

Phenylmercuric acetate (PMA) is used throughout the country for many purposes. In Michigan, there was one formulator of an algaecide or slimicide that was used extensively by communities and industries in air conditioning cooling towers. The U. S. Department of Agriculture withdrew their registration for such compounds, which are no longer being manufactured in Michigan.

The Commission also made an extensive survey of paper mills, because the paper industry had used PMA for slime control in their production processes. There are 35 mills in Michigan; however, no mills in Michigan use PMA, and none have used it since about 1959. The use of PMA was stopped at that time due to inquiries from the U. S. Food and Drug Administration and restrictions imposed upon paper that was used in the food industry as food wrappers. Thus, the paper mills in Michigan voluntarily ceased the use of that material at that time.

It has been mentioned that there are many incidental uses of mercury. One of these incidental uses is in water treatment plants. Mercury seals containing more than ten pounds of mercury in each seal are used extensively in many of these plants. Underwater grinders may also contain mercury seals. In the past, seals have broken and have released mercury. Switches and other instruments may account for 50 to 60 pounds of mercury in some moderately-sized water treatment plants.

Mercury is also found in the soil, especially in residues from sand and gravel processing. These residual gravels are being mined experimentally for gold in Michigan, and the operators of the process report that they are also recovering mercury.

In relation to the interest expressed in fossil fuels, a limited number of coal samples from southeastern Ohio have been tested recently on behalf of the two major power companies in Michigan, the Detroit Edison and Consumer's

Power. The analyses indicate that this particular coal
contains about 0.5 ppm mercury. I hope that other investigators will contribute more information on this aspect
of the mercury problem.

To put this into perspective, the Dow Chemical Company
plant on the St. Clair River at Sarnia, Ontario, had an
average discharge of about 50 to 60 pounds a day during the
past few years before the control system was instituted,
which could amount to 22,000 to 23,000 pounds a year. The
Detroit Edison Company and Consumer's Power in Michigan
consumed about 20,000,000 tons of coal in 1969. At 0.5
ppm mercury, this amount of coal would contain about 20,000
pounds of mercury per year, which would be approximately
equivalent to the discharge from the Dow plant. Analyses
of the ashes from these fossil fuel plants and analyses of
the pond overflows from the wet-ash handling systems contained no detectable mercury, which supports our suspicions
that the mercury is probably going out of the stacks.

Mercury in Fish in the Great Lakes

Jack D. Bails

On March 24, 1970, Canada announced that 12,000 pounds
of commercially caught walleye from Lake St. Clair were to
be destroyed because of mercury contamination. This set
off a chain reaction of fishing closures and restrictions
which eventually encompassed 26 states and four provinces.
It soon became clear that Lake St. Clair was the center of
the crisis, and that we needed to analyze the degree of
mercury contamination of the environment in this location
(Figure 3).

The Canadian Wildlife Service initiated a study of environmental mercury contamination in 1968. After several
attempts to utilize laboratories within Canada during
early 1969, the mercury analysis was finally accomplished
in California. The first results, including a few fish
from Lake St. Clair, were reported by the Ontario Water
Resources Commission in February, 1970, at a meeting of
the Great Lakes International Joint Commission. Since the
major consumers of mercury have been identified within
Michigan, it is unlikely that any major new problem areas
will be discovered around Lake St. Clair.

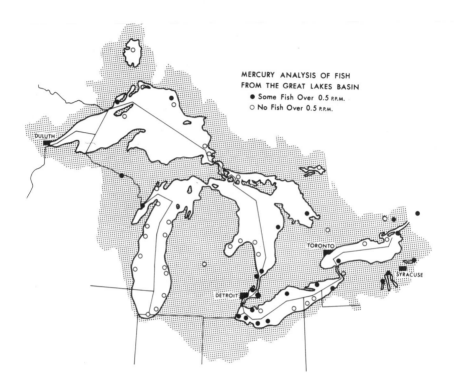

Figure 3:   Mercury Analysis of Fish from the Great Lakes
    Basin

Fish Sampling on Lake St. Clair

Since March of 1970, extensive fish sampling has occurred on Lake St. Clair. Until July, 1970, much of the
sampling was done on "shotgun" approach to determine the
species affected and the number that exceeded 0.5 ppm mercury. While this screening approach to sampling provided
immediate information needed to institute fishing closures
to protect public health, it did not provide the detailed
data on any given species necessary to understand the
problem. Walleye analyzed for mercury from Lake St. Clair
exemplify the highly variable results that have been observed when no effort was made to reduce possible sources
of variability (Figure 4).

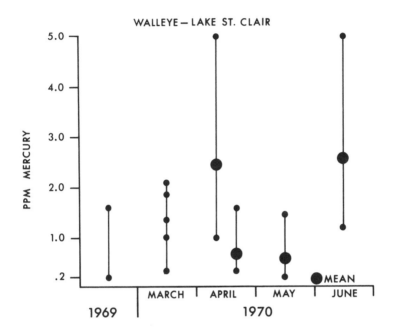

Figure 4: Mercury Concentrations in Walleye from Lake St. Clair

In July, 1970, sampling stations in Michigan waters were established, along with standards for sample size, species, and the portions of specimens to be analyzed. Fish of uniform size were taken. The range and mean for the July, 1970, sampling of walleye in Lake St. Clair indicated that sampling error was largely responsible for the wide range of values reported previously. This July, 1970, sampling provides the first solid baseline from which we can determine whether or not, and at what rate, mercury levels decline in fish. No clear trends are yet apparent.

Locations of Sampling Stations

Five sampling stations were established in the area of concern shown on Figure 5. Station #1 is located in the

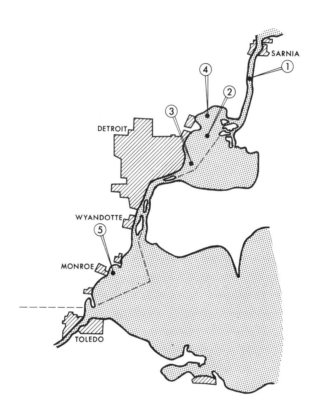

Figure 5: Sampling Stations Established in Michigan and Ontario

St. Clair River below Sarnia, Ontario. Station #2 is located near the middle of Lake St. Clair, at a point where the major channels of the St. Clair River enter. Station #3 is located near the outlet of the lake at the head of the Detroit River. Station #4 is in Anchor Bay, and station #5 is off Monroe, Michigan, in Lake Erie. Walleye, yellow perch, catfish, and rock bass were chosen as index species.

Figure 6 indicates that, comparing mercury concentration in walleye from the five sites, the levels appear to be lower in Lake Erie. This would seem reasonable since

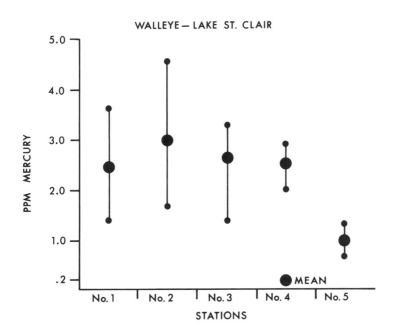

Figure 6: Mercury Concentration in Walleye from Five Sampling Stations Near Lake St. Clair

the largest source of mercury input was located at Sarnia, Ontario. The highest levels of mercury were found in walleye taken at station #2 in the middle of the lake, where most of the flow of the St. Clair River enters. The mean values of mercury content in walleye range from a high of 3 ppm to a low of 1 ppm, which is still twice the acceptable level for human consumption now recognized in the United States and Canada.

Mercury levels in yellow perch generally follow the same trends as the ones seen in walleyes (Figure 7). The levels of mercury were highest in fish taken from station #2 in the middle of the lake and lowest in station #5 in Lake Erie. The mean mercury values in perch were as high as 2.2 ppm but dropped to 0.2 ppm in Lake Erie.

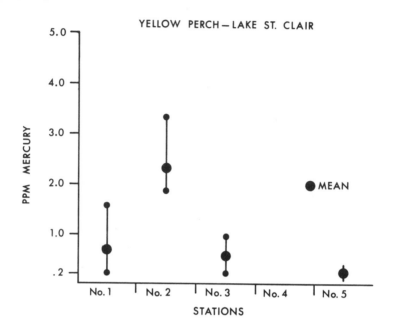

Figure 7: Mercury Concentrations in Yellow Perch from
   Five Sampling Stations Near Lake St. Clair

There are many factors which complicate understanding
of the problem of mercury contamination in fish. Some of
the more important species of fish in Lake St. Clair are
migratory. Walleye sampled in Lake Erie may have just re-
turned from Lake St. Clair. Walleye analyzed from southern
Lake Huron may have resided for some time in the St. Clair
River. Previous tagging studies confirmed these migration
patterns for walleye, and mercury levels of walleye reflect
these movements. Feeding habits of each species change
with size and season, which may have an effect on the observed levels if mercury is being concentrated through the
food chain. Predators like smallmouth bass, walleye, northern pike, and muskellunge generally show high levels of
mercury in Lake St. Clair, but so do sturgeon and freshwater drum. Carp, suckers, and the small forage species
generally show low mercury levels in Lake St. Clair and
Lake Erie. It has been generally observed that larger and
older fish of a species show higher levels of mercury.

Studies in Decline of Mercury Levels

Monitoring of mercury levels in fish from Lake St. Clair is continuing at regular intervals; and, with the baseline established in July, 1970, we should be able to detect significant decreases if they occur. In addition, catfish and rock bass from Lake St. Clair are being held in uncontaminated ponds to determine whether or not mercury levels decline more rapidly when the fish are removed from the lake.

Recent radioactive tracer studies in Finland indicate it may take up to 400 days for perch and pike to purge half the mercury from their muscle tissue once contamination has stopped.[1,2] This brings up one of the most crucial questions concerning the contamination in Lake St. Clair. Are fish still concentrating mercury which is being methylated from the bottom deposits? Or, did the fish concentrate mercury only when soluble inorganic mercury was being released by industries into the lake? Until this question is answered, there is no way of predicting how long it will take for mercury in fish to drop to safe levels. At this point in time, it is probably safe to assume that, instead of a matter of months, we are talking about the number of years necessary before fish from Lake St. Clair are safe to eat.

We have just completed a preliminary study of freshwater mussels in Lake St. Clair. We originally thought that mussels would concentrate mercury at much higher levels than fish, and would serve as an excellent biological indicator for detecting mercury uptake and purging rates; however, results have been negative. Freshwater mussels from three sampling locations in Lake St. Clair averaged less than 0.2 ppm mercury. Mussels from uncontaminated lakes were found to have the same level of mercury. Mussels from "clean" sources were placed in cages in Lake St. Clair but showed no increase in mercury concentrations with time. Fish seem to be a much better indicator of mercury contamination than mussels.

References

1. Miettinen, J. K., M. Tillander, K. Rissanen, V. Miettinen, and E. Minkkinen. <u>Nordiskt. kvicksilver</u> symposium, Lindigo 10-11 (October 1968).
2. Miettinen, J. K., M. Tillander, K. Rissanen, V. Miettinen, and Y. Ohmomo. "Distribution and excretion rate of phenyl- and methylmercury nitrate in fish, mussels, mollusks, and crayfish," <u>9th Japan Conf.</u> <u>Radiosotop</u>. B/II-17 (May 1969).

Survey of Mercury Concentrations in Fishes of Lakes St. Clair, Erie, and Huron

R. A. Greig and H. L. Seagran

Introduction

Following the disclosure in late March, 1970, of mercury contamination in fish taken from Canadian waters of Lake St. Clair, the Bureau of Commercial Fisheries Technological Laboratory, on a cooperative basis with other agencies in the Great Lakes area, carried out a preliminary survey of mercury concentrations in fish taken from suspected areas. This report summarizes the findings on fish collected over the period from March 27 to May 8, 1970, from U. S. waters of Lakes Huron, St. Clair, and Erie.

The data collected are discussed from two aspects: (1) the levels of mercury in fish in relation to geographical area--both within a lake and between lakes examined, and (2) the variation of mercury concentrations related to species differences.

Mercury concentrations were greatly different for the various species of fish examined. Data are presented that show the order of highest to lowest accumulation of mercury in these various species of fish.

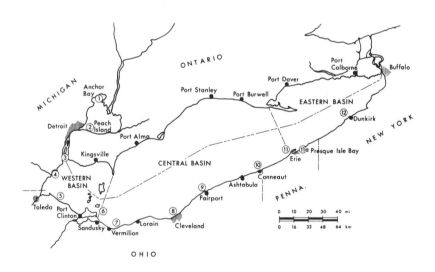

Figure 8: Sampling Areas for Lake Erie and Lake St. Clair

Experimental Methods

Fish samples were collected from the areas indicated by field biologists of our Bureau and the Michigan Department of Natural Resources, either from research vessels or, on-site, from commercial fishermen (Figures 8 and 9).

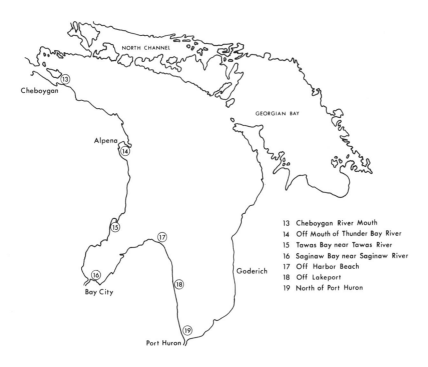

13 Cheboygan River Mouth
14 Off Mouth of Thunder Bay River
15 Tawas Bay near Tawas River
16 Saginaw Bay near Saginaw River
17 Off Harbor Beach
18 Off Lakeport
19 North of Port Huron

Figure 9: Sampling Areas for Lake Huron

Composite samples for analysis were prepared by thorough mixing of the ground, edible portions (that is, headed, eviscerated, scaled and tail removed) from a number of fish (generally 3 to 15, depending on size) taken randomly from one lot, each lot representing a given location and catch date for a species.

At the time this survey study was initiated, our laboratory did not have the analytic capability to perform mercury determinations. Samples were therefore sent to three different cooperating laboratories for analysis for total mercury content. These laboratories and the methods they employed were as follows: (1) Wisconsin Alumni Research Foundation (WARF), Madison, Wisconsin--atomic absorption spectrophotometry following hot acid digestion and dithizone extraction; (2) Environmental Health Laboratories (EHL), Farmington, Michigan--mercury vapor meter detection of mercury vapor released from the sample matrix by pyrolysis; and (3) Phoenix Memorial Laboratory (PML), Ann Arbor, Michigan--neutron activation analysis; i.e. low-temperature acid digestion of the irradiated sample (including a non-radioactive mercury carrier), followed by removal of interfering metals by ion exchange and measurement of radioactivity by gamma ray spectrometry.

As an indication of the relative agreement among these three laboratories, Table 1 summarizes their data on two replicated check samples which were also analyzed by four other laboratories. On an individual laboratory basis, the relative standard deviation of replicates averaged about 10%.

Table 1

Interlaboratory Comparison of Check Samples

Laboratory	Method	Check Sample 1	Check Sample 2
WARF	AA	–	1.8 (2)
EHL	AA	0.74 (5)	1.5 (5)
PML	NAA	0.62 (1)	1.3 (2)
A	AA	0.64 (2)	1.4 (2)
B	AA	0.64 (2)	1.6 (1)
C	AA	0.60 (1)	1.5 (1)
D	NAA	–	1.2 (2)

All values: ppm on wet, ground fish sample

Results and Discussion

Lake St. Clair

The data obtained for Lake St. Clair show that essentially all fish examined contained concentrations of mercury considerably in excess (2 to 4 times) of the U. S. Food and Drug Administration's 0.5 ppm "action level." Samples came largely from the Anchor Bay area. Walleye taken near the head of the Detroit River at Peche Island were also relatively high (1.9 ppm), as were goldfish (0.3 ppm) and carp (0.6 ppm) taken in the Detroit River proper connecting Lakes St. Clair and Erie (Table 2).

Table 2

Mercury Levels in Lake St. Clair Fish

Species		
Muskellunge (16 pounds)		6.7
Muskellunge (1.5 pounds)		1.2
Northern pike		0.7
Rainbow trout		0.4
Walleye	1.9	2.5
White sucker		1.5
Yellow perch		1.5

All values: ppm on wet, ground fish sample

Lake Erie

A large number of fish were collected from Lake Erie from a range of sampling stations; only the most extensive data available for drum, walleye, white bass, and yellow perch, are summarized here (Table 3).

Table 3

Mercury Levels in Lake Erie Fish

Species		Western Basin	Central Basin	Eastern Basin
Freshwater drum	Ave.	0.54	0.20	0.23
	Range	0.4-0.6	0.1-0.4	0.2-0.3
Walleye		1.48	--	0.59
		0.9-2.0		0.4-0.7
White bass		0.90	0.35	0.49
		0.7-1.0	0.3-0.4	0.3-0.7
Yellow perch		0.57	0.22	0.37
		0.3-1.0	0.1-0.5	0.2-0.5

All values: ppm on wet, ground fish sample

For drum, the mercury concentration is greatest in the western basin. Comparing similar size fish, the mercury concentration in drum of approximately one pound was about 0.6 ppm for the western basin, 0.2 ppm to 0.4 ppm for the central basin, and 0.3 ppm for the eastern basin. The Fairport Harbor drum ("downstream" from Cleveland) appeared to contain the highest levels (0.42 ppm) outside the western basin.

Walleye were obtained only from the western and eastern basins. The mercury concentration for walleye in the 2-3 pound size averaged 1.5 ppm for the western basin, whereas fish of a similar size from the eastern basin averaged only 0.6 ppm.

White bass samples of a similar size (about 1/2 pound) had an average mercury concentration of 0.7 ppm for the western basin, 0.35 ppm for the central basin, and 0.3 ppm for the eastern basin. White bass of about one pound in size, however, contained about 1 ppm for the western basin and 0.7 ppm for the eastern basin.

Yellow perch samples obtained from the western basin showed a large variation, apparently decreasing progressively from west to east (0.75 ppm to 0.25 ppm). Comparing

similar size fish (approximately 10 in.), perch from the
eastern basin had mercury concentrations similar to the
eastern portion of the western basin; that is, 0.2 ppm to
0.4 ppm. Again, except for the Fairport Harbor fish (0.46
ppm), perch of the central basin had lower values (0.1 ppm
to 0.2 ppm) than for the other two basins. Slight differences in size of fish may account for some of this difference, however.

Comparison of Species

Beyond these four species just described in some detail,
an effort was also made to rank all species, using fish
collected from the western basin of Lake Erie where more
varieties were collected. Figure 10 shows the relative

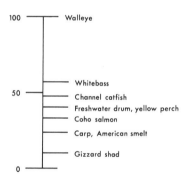

Figure 10: Relative Mercury
Concentration of Species
of Fish from the Western
Basin of Lake Erie (Based
of an Arbitrary Scale of
100)

placement of the various species of fish examined from the
western basin of Lake Erie on an arbitrary scale of 100;
that is, walleye was assumed to have the highest value.
The scale was constructed according to the average mercury
concentration for all samples for a given species. The
scale shows, for example, that white bass and channel catfish had an average mercury concentration approximately
one-half that of walleye, the coho about one-third that of
walleye. Although this method of comparison gives an indication of the relative ability of these fish to accumulate
mercury, a more accurate comparison probably could be made
for fish of the same age or by using a narrow size range
based on the predominant size that appears in the commercial fishery for each species.

Lake Huron

   Although data on Lake Huron fish are relatively limited,
the mercury concentrations again appear to vary among species and between sizes. Of 21 samples analyzed from Lake
Huron, only nine had a concentration of 0.3 ppm or greater.
The highest value (6.8 ppm) was for a northern pike sample
collected near the head of the St. Clair River. Other
samples in the range 0.3 ppm to 0.5 ppm generally came
from his same area or from bays near river drainages
(Table 4).

Table 4

Mercury Levels in Lake Huron Fish

Species	Northern Section	Central Section	Southern Section
American smelt	0.11	--	--
Coho salmon	--	--	0.07
Northern pike	--	0.27 / 0.1 - 0.4	0.2 & 6.8
Rainbow trout	0.06	--	--
Walleye	0.35	--	--
White sucker	0.06	0.05	0.38
Yellow perch	0.26	0.32 / 0.1 - 0.5	--

All values: ppm on wet, ground fish sample

Comparison of Lakes

   Table 5 attempts to compare levels in fish from the
three lakes; yellow perch was selected for this purpose
because it was most broadly sampled. The highest levels
for this species were found in Lake St. Clair (1.5 ppm)
and off Monroe in the extreme western part of Lake Erie
(0.75 ppm). Lake Huron samples showed relatively low concentrations, similar to those found in most Lake Erie
samples. In addition to the relatively high levels found
in perch of St. Clair and western Erie, concentrations of

Table 5

Comparison of Mercury Levels in Yellow Perch

Catch Location		*Average*
Lake St. Clair		
Anchor Bay	8-12	1.5 (3)
Lake Erie		
Monroe	7-9	0.75 (2)
Bono	8-10	0.40 (3)
Sandusky	8-11	0.25 (3)
Vermilion	7-9	0.16 (1)
Cleveland	8-10	0.12 (1)
Fairport	9-12	0.46 (1)
Conneaut	8-9	0.20 (1)
Erie	8-12	0.3 (1)
Dunkirk	11-13	0.47 (3)
Lake Huron		
Thunder Bay	11-13	0.26 (1)
Tawas Bay	9-13	0.12 (1)
Saginaw Bay	–	0.45 (1)

All values: ppm on wet, ground fish sample

mercury close to 0.5 ppm occurred in the extreme eastern
end and in the Fairport areas of Lake Erie, and in Saginaw
Bay of Lake Huron.

Conclusions

The general conclusions of the work were: Fish from
Lake St. Clair and the western basin of Lake Erie have
fairly similar mercury concentrations (from 0.4 ppm to 3
ppm, depending on species), and fish from these areas had
mercury concentrations considerably greater than fish from
Lake Huron and the rest of Lake Erie. Lake Huron fish
were most similar to fish of the central basin of Lake
Erie with regard to their mercury concentrations; fish of
the eastern basin of Lake Erie had slightly higher mercury
concentrations than fish from Lake Huron and the central
basin of Lake Erie.

Mercury in Wild Animals, Lake St. Clair, 1970

E. H. Dustman, L. F. Stickel
and J. B. Elder

Introduction

Following the Canadian discovery of high mercury levels
in the fish of Lake St. Clair, the Bureau of Sport Fisheries and Wildlife undertook a preliminary assessment of
mercury residues in a variety of birds and their eggs, and
in a few other species of animals. The objective was to
sample animals that depend on the Lake and its marshlands
for food and shelter.

The animals were collected on the St. Clair Flats Public
Hunting Grounds. Most of them came from Harsen's Island,
with smaller numbers from Dickinson Island, Little Muscamoot Bay, Big Muscamoot Bay, Goose Bay, and nearby areas.

Mercury was measured in 147 samples from 17 waterfowl
of 4 species, 26 birds of 11 other species, 3 gartersnakes,
and 7 frogs of 2 species. The samples were composed of
body tissues, eggs, and food items removed from stomachs
of some of the collected specimens. Analyses were made of
breast muscle, liver, and kidney of waterfowl, and of liver
and carcass (skinned body minus gastrointestinal tract,
feet, legs, wings, and head) of other birds. Snakes were
skinned but their intestinal tracts were removed. Analyses
for total mercury were made by WARF (Wisconsin Alumni Research Foundation) Institute, employing atomic absorption
spectrophotometry with a "boat modification." All results
are expressed on a wet weight basis.

Acknowledgments

A genuine team effort made these collections and analyses possible. We greatly appreciate the help of W. Fuchs,
W. Shake, J. Frye, and G. Bober of our Bureau in the collection of specimens and the cooperation of the several
persons of the Michigan Department of Natural Resources
who helped with arrangements and permits.   M. A. Ross,
L. N. Locke, and L. Hall of the Patuxent Center performed
the very considerable tasks of autopsy and sample
preparation.

Results and Discussion

Results are shown in Tables 6 through 8, from which the following summary observations were made.

Table 6

Mercury in Waterfowl, Lake St. Clair, 1970

Specimen number	Sex	*Mercury Residues (ppm wet weight)* Breast muscle	Liver	Kidney
Mallard *(Anas platyrhynchos)*				
3-115	F[1]	1.15	4.8	3.5
3-116	F[1]	0.80	3.2	1.6
3-110	F[2]	0.65	1.5	1.4
3-111	M[2]	0.62	1.4	1.2
3-108	M	0.22	0.84	0.53
3-119	F	0.20	0.45	0.30
3-121	M	0.16	0.58	0.49
3-102	F	<0.10	0.23	<0.10
Blue-winged teal *(Anas discors)*				
3-128	F	2.3	5.0	4.4
3-104	F	0.18	0.50	0.63
3-107	F	0.14	0.26	0.31
3-118	F	0.10	0.35	0.27
Lesser scaup *(Aythya affinis)*				
3-127-3	F	1.2	3.4	2.3
3-127-4	M	0.91	5.6	2.6
3-127-2	M	0.58	1.8	0.96
3-127-1	M	0.54	1.9	2.2
Canada goose *(Branta canadensis)*				
3-131	F	<0.10	0.18	<0.10

[1]Egg E-13 was from nest of mallard 3-115 and egg E-14 from 3-116 (see Table 8).
[2]Mallards 3-110 and 3-111 were a mated pair.

Table 7

Mercury in Wild Animals, Lake St. Clair, 1970

Specimen Number	Sex	Mercury Residues (ppm wet weight)		
		Carcass	Liver	Stomach Contents

Great blue heron *(Ardea herodias)*

3-126-2	M	23.0	136	Golden shiner *(Notemigonus crysoleucas)*, 1.8 Minnow *(Cyprinidae)*, 3.6
3-126-1	M	21.2	175	Yellow perch *(Perca flavescens)*, 3.6
3-126-3	F	8.3	66	
3-126-4	M	5.3	14.6	

Black-crowned night heron *(Nycticorax nycticorax)*

3-134	M	2.8	14.0	

Common egret *(Casmerodius albus)*

3-135	F	0.74	6.3	

American bittern *(Botaurus lentiginosus)*

3-105	F	0.55	1.75	Hellgrammite *(Corydalus sp.)* 0.34 Dace *(Semotilus sp.)*, 0.42

Common tern *(Sterna hirundo)*

3-117	M	7.5	39.0	Lake emerald shiner *(Notropis atherinoides)*, 3.8
3-112	M	2.3	13.2	
3-114	F	0.41	2.1	

Black tern *(Chlidonias niger)*

3-133	M	1.3	2.6	
3-120	M	0.61	3.5	
3-122	F	0.41	1.3	

Ring-billed gull *(Larus delawarensis)*

3-113-1	F	0.70	1.8	Herring *(Clupeidae)*, 0.33
3-113-2	F	0.39	1.2	Beetles *(Scarabaeidae)*, <0.10
3-113-3	F	0.14	0.65	

Table 7, cont.

Specimen Number	Sex	Mercury Residues (ppm wet weight)		
		Carcass	Liver	Stomach Contents
Common gallinule *(Gallinula chloropus)*				
3-132	M	0.41	1.4	
Killdeer *(Charadrius vociferous)*				
3-129-1	M	0.68	2.3	
3-129-2	F	0.52	3.7	
3-103	M	0.14	0.5	
Spotted sandpiper *(Actitis macularia)*				
3-130	F	0.55	2.8	
Dunlin *(Erolia alpina)*				
3-106-5	M	0.20	1.3	
3-106-4	F	0.16	0.97	
3-106-1	F	0.16	0.79	
3-106-3	M	0.16	0.70	
3-106-2	F	<0.10	0.99	
Gartersnake *(Thamnophis sirtalis)*				
3-136	F	0.20	0.60	Earthworms *(Lumbricidae)*, 0.27
3-109	F	0.20	0.45	
3-123	F	<0.10	0.60	
Leopard frog *(Rana pipiens)*				
3-125	F	0.18	0.61	
3-101-1	M	<0.10	1.1	
3-101-2	M	<0.10	0.51	
Bullfrog *(Rana catesbeiana)*				
3-124	F	<0.10	0.28	Crayfish *(Cambarus sp.)*, <0.10

Table 8

Mercury in Eggs of Wild Birds, Lake St. Clair, 1970

Specimen number[1]	*Mercury residues (ppm wet weight)*
Mallard *(Anas platyrhynchos)*[2]	
E-1	2.7
S-2	1.2
E-7	1.1
E-13	0.74
E-12	0.57
E-14	0.41
S-1	0.23
S-3	0.22
S-4	0.22
Pied-billed grebe *(Podilymbus podiceps)*	
E-15	4.0
Common tern *(Sterna hirundo)*	
E-4	6.25
E-11	4.0
E-3	1.5
E-2	1.25
E-10	0.63
Black-crowned night heron *(Nycticorax nycticorax)*	
S-7	1.1
S-9	1.05
S-8	0.74
S-5	0.48
S-6	0.46

[1]Each egg was from a different nest.
[2]Egg E-13 was from nest of mallard 3-115 and E-14 was from 3-116 (see Table 6).

Results and Discussion

Results are shown in Tables 6 through 8, from which the following summary observations were made.

(1) Mercury levels in two fish eaters, great blue herons and common terns, far exceeded those in any other species. Lowest residues were in frogs, snakes, and dunlins. Concentrations in one of the herons reached 175 ppm in liver and 23 ppm in carcass; maximum residues in a term were 39 ppm in liver and 7.5 ppm in carcass. These residues are comparable to those in Sweden in birds that died under experimental dosage with methylmercury and in birds that died under field conditions in several Scandinavian countries with signs of mercury poisoning.[1-3] Our analyses were for total mercury; therefore the portion in the methyl form is unknown. Swedish studies, however, have shown that all or almost all of the mercury in fish tissue is methylmercury.[4] Birds are also known to be capable of converting inorganic mercury compounds to methylmercury.[5]

(2) Fish from the stomachs of two great blue herons contained 3.6 ppm, 1.8 ppm, and 3.6 ppm mercury; a fish from a common tern had 3.8 ppm mercury. These high residues in food items are consistent with the high residues in the bodies and livers of these birds.

(3) Mercury in the eggs of three of five terns, the grebe, and one mallard was in the range of residues (1.3-2.0 ppm) in eggs of pheasants whose reproductivity was reduced by mercury in experimental studies.[1] Harmful levels in chicken eggs may be somewhat higher.[6]

(4) Mercury in breast muscle of waterfowl exceeded 0.5 ppm in four of eight mallards, in one of four blue-winged teal, and in all four lesser scaup. It exceeded 1.0 ppm in one bird of each species. Residues in liver were higher; the maximum for each species was 5-6 ppm.

(5) Mercury residues in many of the birds at Lake St. Clair appear to be undesirably high when compared with known harmful amounts. Data are unavailable for a comparison of levels of mercury that could be considered normal for these species, or for a full appraisal of hazard to the birds from the mercury levels in Lake St. Clair.

Our research plans include further surveys of mercury residues in a variety of birds in different localities, including areas not suspected of being polluted by mercury. We have initiated experimental studies of mercury kinetics in birds and of effects of mercury on bird reproduction to provide a basis for understanding the significance of the mercury levels carried by wild birds.

Conclusions

Many birds dependent upon water areas in the Lake St. Clair region have high residues of mercury in their tissues and eggs, demonstrating the extension of the water pollution problem into the marshland environment. Since many of the birds are migratory, mercury from Lake St. Clair will find its way to areas far distant from the source.

References

1. Borg, K., H. Wanntorp, K. Erne, and E. Hanko. "Alkyl Mercury Poisoning in Terrestrial Swedish Wildlife," Viltrevy, *6* (4), 301-379 (1969).
2. Henriksson, Kurt, Elva Karppanen, and Matti Helminen. "High Residue of Mercury in Finnish White-Tailed Eagles," Ornis Fennica, *43* (2), 38-45 (1966).
3. Holt, Gunnar. "Mercury Residues in Wild Birds in Norway 1965-1967," Nord. Vet.-Med., *21*, 105-114 (1969).
4. Westöö, G. "Determination of Methyl Mercury Compounds in Food Stuffs," Acta Chem. Scand., *20*, 2131-2137 (1966).
5. Kiwimäe, Arnold, Åke Swensson, Ulf Ulfvarson, and Gunnell Westöö. "Methyl Mercury Compounds in Eggs From Hens After Oral Administration of Mercury Compounds," Journal of Agricultural and Food Chemistry, *17* (5), 1014-1016 (1969).
6. Tejning, Stig. "Biological Effects of Methyl Mercury Dicyandiamide-Treated Grain in the Domestic Fowl *Gallus gallus* L.," Oikos. Supplementum, *8,* 116 (1967).

Mercury Contents of Bottom Sediments From Wisconsin Rivers and Lakes

John G. Konrad

In May, 1970, the Wisconsin Department of Natural Resources initiated a program to survey bottom sediments from major drainage basins in the State, public surface water supplies, and municipal sewage treatment plants for mercury content. These investigations were conducted to determine the location of mercury deposits and to elucidate the natural background levels in bottom sediments.

Mercury deposits in bottom sediments reflect past and present discharges of mercury and have been found to be
responsible for the long-term mercury contamination of the
aquatic environment in Sweden.[1] This paper discusses the
results of the initial survey.

Experimental Methods

Sediment samples were obtained with either an Eckman
or Petersen Dredge and transported to the laboratory in
200 ml bottles. Public water supply and sewage treatment
plant samples were collected with the aid of the various
plants involved.

Analyses for total mercury content of bottom sediments
and sewage treatment plant sludges were conducted on the
wet (not previously dried) sample as follows: The sample
(10 g) was digested in a mixture of $H_2SO_4 \cdot HNO_3$ by the
standard Association of Official Analytical Chemists procedure.[2] The digest was oxidized with 5% $KMnO_4$ (drop-wise
to a persistent color), prior to reduction with $SnCl_2$ and
analysis by the flameless atomic absorption procedure of
Rathje.[3] Moisture content of the sample was determined
separately, and mercury content expressed on a dry weight
basis. Water samples (25 ml) were analyzed in the same
way except for the omission of the digestion step. A
Perkin-Elmer Model 303 atomic absorption spectrometer,
equipped with a 10 cm x 2 cm flow cell and rapid response
recorder, was used for all analyses.

Alkalinity and pH were determined by the methods described in Standard Methods for the Examination of Water
and Waste Water.[4]

Results of Survey

Bottom sediments were collected from 168 locations on
27 rivers and streams in Wisconsin. These locations were
chosen to reflect the discharges of various industrial and
municipal wastes and to determine the natural background
levels of the waterways. Mercury concentrations were found
in all samples, with the level being somewhat dependent on
the texture of the sediment; that is, higher levels were
found in samples with larger organic matter and clay contents. In areas which receive no identifiable additions
of mercury, a level of mercury ascribable to natural sources can be defined as a background level. This background
level ranged from <0.01 ppm to 0.05 ppm in sandy sediments
and from 0.05 ppm to 0.15 ppm in organic and clayey sediments. Background levels were slightly higher in the

northern part of the state, probably due to the leaching
of unknown geologic deposits in the acid soils of the area.
    The location of mercury deposits in the bottom sediments
of Wisconsin rivers is shown in Figure 11.   Locations 2, 3,

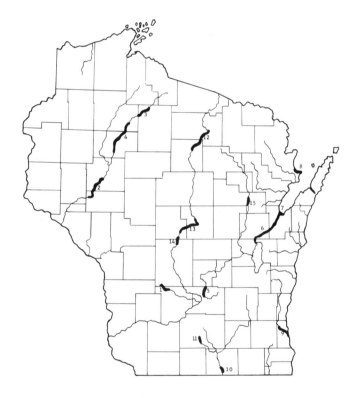

Figure 11:   Location of Mercury Deposits in Bottom
    Sediments of Wisconsin Rivers

4, 6, 7, 8, 12, 13 and 15 on the Chippewa, Flambeau, Fox, Wisconsin, and Wolf Rivers reflect the influence of paper and pulp operations. Use of mercury slimicides in the paper industry has decreased since 1958 when the FDA banned mercury from paper used for food wraps. However, some paper mills were still using phenylmercuric acetate for slime control and in the production of coated papers as late as May, 1970. Deposits from these sources are associated with fibrous organic-type sediments and tend to be steadily moved downstream.

Sewage treatment plant effluents have produced deposits at locations 1, 5 and 11 on the Baraboo, Fox and Rock Rivers. These effluents have resulted from the acceptance and subsequent discharge of industrial wastes containing mercury by several municipal sanitary sewage systems.

Deposits at locations 9, 10 and 14 are the result of industrial effluents; however, the specific sources of those at 9 and 10 have not been identified. The largest mercury deposit found in any Wisconsin river bottom sediment is below a mercury cell chlorine-caustic soda plant at Port Edwards on the Wisconsin River (location 14). This deposit is largely metallic mercury, and ranges from a high of 684 ppm just below the outfall to 12 ppm approximately one mile downstream. This plant began operation in June, 1967; thus, these deposits represent an accumulation of approximately three years of mercury discharges.

The rate of release of mercury from these deposits and the subsequent absorption by fish are of primary concern to safeguarding the public health. High concentrations of mercury in fish have been detected only in the Flambeau-Chippewa River system from above Ladysmith to below Eau Claire, and on the Wisconsin River from Rhinelander to the Mississippi River.[5] It appears that various characteristics of the water and bottom sediments control the release of mercury from the bottom sediments. Table 9 shows a comparison of mercury content in sediments and fish with the alkalinity and pH of the waters. Mercury accumulation in fish was found in waters which had an alkalinity less than 50 ppm and a pH less than 7.5. This is consistent with the Swedish findings of Jernelov[6] that the formation of monomethylmercury is enhanced by slightly acid conditions. Much additional research is required along these lines before any conclusions regarding the parameters controlling release of mercury from sediment deposits can be made.

To determine the effect of municipal sewage treatment effluents on the accumulation of mercury in sediments and on the quality of surface water supplies, samples were

Table 9

Location of Mercury Deposits in Bottom Sediments of Wisconsin Rivers

River	Location of Deposit (No. Corresponds to Sample Location on Figure 11)	Source of Deposit	Average Mercury Content ppm	Average Alkalinity	Average pH	ppm Fish Accumulation
Baraboo	1. Below Wonewoc	Sewage treatment plant effluent	0.5	–	7.6	N.A.
Chippewa	2. Chippewa Falls-Eau Claire	Paper mill	1.2	33	7.1	0.60
Flambeau	3. Below Park Falls	Paper mill	0.6	20	6.9	0.41
	4. Ladysmith area	Paper mill	1.4	25	7.2	1.07
Fox	5. Below Portage	Sewage treatment plant effluent	0.8	–	7.6	N.A.
	6. Neenah-Menasha to mouth	Paper mills and Sew. trt. plt. eff.	2.0	139	7.8	0.36
Menominee	7. Lower Green Bay	Paper mills	1.5	–	7.2	0.21
	8. Marinette area	Paper mills	1.2	81	7.6	0.45
Milwaukee	9. Above mouth and Milwaukee Harbor	Industrial (?)	1.5	168	7.8	0.13
Rock	10. Below Janesville	Industrial (?)	0.4	225	8.3	0.11
	11. Below Madison Sewage Outfall-Badfish Creek	Sewage treatment plant effluent	11.5	–	7.5	N.A.
Wisconsin	12. Rhinelander-Tomahawk	Paper mills	1.5	20	6.7	0.95
	13. Stevens Point-Wis. Rapids	Paper mills	2.7	30	6.8	0.51
	14. Port Edwards-Nekoosa	Chlorine plant	684	36	6.8	1.24
Wolf	15. Below Shawano	Paper mills	0.8	92	7.8	N.A.

obtained from 25 sewage treatment plants and 17 public surface water supplies. Sewage treatment plants which accept sewage containing mercury were found to have elevated mercury levels in the sludge and, in several cases, in the final effluents. Sludges from Kaukauna, Portage, Green Bay, Kimberly, Madison, and Appleton contained 3.7, 5, 6, 16, 20 and 29 ppm mercury, respectively. Of these, however, only Madison, Appleton, and Portage were found to discharge mercury-contaminated effluent. Madison and Portage accept mercury-containing discharges from the manufacture of electrical batteries, while Appleton has received the waste from a coated-paper operation. As a consequence of these discharges, deposits of mercury have been found in the sediments of the Madison outfall ditch and the Fox River below Portage and Appleton. The discharge of mercury from a large municipal sewage treatment plant may be as high as 0.5 pounds per day and, therefore, cannot be overlooked in any survey of mercury sources.

All public surface-water supplies sampled contained no detectable mercury in raw and finished waters (lower limit of detection of about 0.5 ppb). These represent all water supplies from Lake Michigan and Lake Winnebago. Surface waters associated with mercury deposits in the bottom sediments were also generally below the sensitivity of the analytical method used.

In general, it can be concluded that all bottom sediments contain at least trace amounts of mercury. The highest mercury deposits were found below industrial discharges (chlorine-caustic soda and pulp and paper production). However, significant amounts of mercury were found below several sewage treatment plants which accept mercury-containing wastes. Alkalinity and pH may have an important role in the release of mercury from bottom sediments and the subsequent accumulation in fish. Extensive research is needed to elucidate these mechanisms and pathways.

Acknowledgment

Appreciation is expressed to T. A. Gibson for his laboratory analyses and to the field personnel of the Department of Natural Resources for sample collection.

References

1. Jensen, S. and A. Jernelov. "Biological Methylation of Mercury," *Nature Land*, *223*, 753-754 (1969).
2. Association of Official Analytical Chemists. *Official Methods of Analysis*, *10*, 375-377 (1965).

3. Rathje, A. O. "A Rapid Ultraviolet Absorption Method for the Determination of Mercury in Urine," Am. Ind. Hy. Assoc. J., *30*, 126-132 (1969).
4. American Public Health Assoc., American Water Works Assoc. Standard Methods for the Examination of Water and Wastewater. (New York: Water Pollution Control Fed., 1965), 767 pp.
5. Kleinert, S. J. "Mercury Levels in Wisconsin Fish," Conf. on Environmental Mercury Contamination, Ann Arbor, Michigan (September 30-October 2, 1970).
6. Jernelov, A. Personal communication.

Mercury Levels in Wisconsin Fish

Stanton J. Kleinert

The Wisconsin Department of Natural Resources began a survey of mercury residues in fish in April, 1970. These investigations were initated to determine mercury levels in fish from a variety of Wisconsin waters, including waters receiving industrial and municipal wastes, waters draining agricultural areas, lakes and streams removed from the urban population centers, and waters situated in the various soil and bedrock provinces of the state. The investigation followed Swedish[1] and Canadian[2] reports of mercury contamination of fish. The Wisconsin survey was undertaken to see if problems of mercury contamination were also evident in the Wisconsin fishery.

Experimental Methods

Fish collections were made by field personnel of the Wisconsin Department of Natural Resources during the period April through September, 1970. Samples most commonly consisted of one fish, but ranged up to 20 fish of the same species. Almost all samples consisted of medium and larger fish of sufficient size for use as human food or for commercial processing. Field personnel were instructed to wrap each fish species in separate plastic bags and freeze until delivery could be made to the laboratory.

Fish filets or, more specifically, fish muscle tissue excluding bone was processed for mercury analysis. Analysis was made on the wet (not previously dried) sample as

follows: The sample (10 g) was digested in a mixture of
$H_2SO_4 \cdot HNO_3$ by the standard Association of Official Analytical Chemists procedure.[3] The digest was oxidized with
5 percent $KMnO_4$ (drop-wise to a persistent color), prior
to reduction with $SnCl_2$ and analysis by the flameless
atomic absorption procedure of Rathje.[4] A Beckman Model
DU atomic absorption spectrometer, equipped with a 10 x 2
cm flow cell and rapid response recorder, was used for
analysis. Mercury values were expressed as ppm of total
mercury on a wet weight animal tissue basis. Extraction
procedures were checked by adding mercuric chloride to
the samples; subsequent digestions yielded mercury recoveries ranging from 92 to 102 percent.

Alkalinity and pH in river waters were determined by
the methods described in Standard Methods for the Examination of Water and Waste Water.[5]

Findings

Mercury determinations were made on 1,115 samples of
fish filet representing 2,144 fish taken from 103 locations
covering 44 of Wisconsin's 70 counties and Wisconsin's
boundary waters of Lake Michigan, Green Bay, Lake Superior
and the Mississippi River (Figure 12). The species composition of the collections generally reflects the fish
populations of the waters sampled. Thirty-six percent of
the fish sampled were rough fishes and 64% were game and
panfishes (Table 10).

All Wisconsin fish analyzed contained mercury (Table
11). Mercury levels in fish from waters removed from any
known source of mercury use averaged 0.19 ppm and ranged
between 0.01 and 0.60 ppm (Sites 1, 2, 3, 4, 11, 17, 25,
65, 66, 52 in Table 11). These values are believed to
indicate normal background levels of mercury present in
Wisconsin fish. Different species vary in mercury content,
and the larger fish contain higher concentrations of mercury than do smaller fish of the same species taken from
the same water. Northern pike, walleye, sucker, large-
mouth bass, smallmouth bass, and channel catfish frequently
showed high mercury concentrations, while the panfishes,
including bluegill, pumpkinseed, and yellow perch, often
showed low concentrations.

Fish samples taken over the 350-mile stretch of the
Wisconsin River extending below Rhinelander, the 40-mile
stretch of the Flambeau River extending below Cedar Rapids,
and the 50-mile stretch of the Chippewa River extending
from the junction with the Flambeau to Eau Claire contain

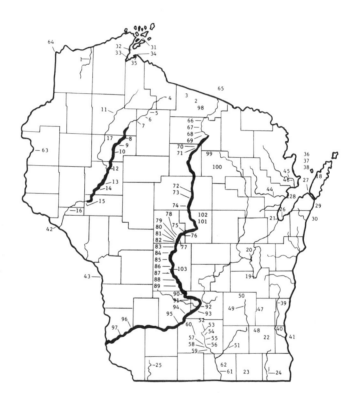

Figure 12: Location of Fish Samples and Fish Consumption
Warning Areas

Table 10

Fish Species Collected and Analyzed for Mercury

Fish Species		Letter Code	Percent of all Samples
Common Name	Scientific Name		
Rough Fish and Minnows			
Sucker	*Catostomus* spp.	S	15
Redhorse	*Moxostoma* spp.	R	3
Buffalo	*Ictiobus* spp.	BF	M
Quillback	*Carpiodes cyprinus*	Q	1
Freshwater Drum	*Aplodinotus grunniens*	D	4
Carp	*Cyprinus carpio*	C	12
Goldfish	*Carassius auratus*	GF	M
Shiner	*Notropis* spp.	SH	M
Mooneye	*Hiodon tergisus*	MO	M
Burbot	*Lota lota*	BB	M
Bowfin	*Amia calva*	BW	M
Alewife	*Alosa pseudoharengus*	A	M
Game Fish and Pan Fish			
Largemouth Bass	*Micropterus salmoides*	LMB	6
Smallmouth Bass	*Micropterus dolomieui*	SMB	3
Bluegill	*Lepomis macrochirus*	B	4
Crappie	*Pomoxis* spp.	CR	5
Pumpkinseed	*Lepomis gibbosus*	P	2
Rockbass	*Ambloplites rupestris*	RB	2
Muskellunge	*Esox masquinongy*	M	M
Northern Pike	*Esox lucius*	NP	9
Bullhead	*Ictalurus* spp.	BU	3
Channel Catfish	*Ictalurus punctatus*	CC	3
Yellow Perch	*Perca flavescens*	YP	6
Sauger	*Stizostedion canadense*	SA	M
Walleye	*Stizostedion vitreum vitreum*	W	13
Cisco	*Coregus artedii*	CI	M
Brook Trout	*Salvelinus fontinalis*	BT	1
Lake Whitefish	*Coregonus elupeaformis*	LW	M
Brown Trout	*Salmo Trutta*	BR	1
Rainbow Trout	*Salmo gairdneri*	RT	1
Lake Trout	*Salvelinus namaycush*	LT	1
Coho Salmon	*Oncorhynchus kisutch*	CS	1
White Bass	*Roccus chrysops*	WB	2
Yellow Bass	*Roccus mississippiensis*	YB	1

*M denotes minor use in the survey, constituting less than 0.5% of all fish samples.

Table 11

Magnitude of Mercury Levels in Fish Muscle Tissue from Various Wisconsin Waters

	Sample Location			Species Sampled	Average ppm Mercury
Basin	County	Water	Site		
Brule River	Douglas	Brule River	1. T49N, R10W, S10	4S, R, 6W, 4BR, 2RT	0.16
Chippewa–Flambeau River Drainage	Vilas	Escanaba Lake	2. Escanaba Lake	YP, W	0.08
	Vilas	Trout Lake	3. Trout Lake	S, R, BB, 2SMB, 4B, 4P, 4RB, 2NP, M, 3YP, 5W, LW, LT	0.11
	Iron	Flambeau River	4. Flambeau Flowage	2R, BB, P, 4RB, 5NP, 5YP, 6W	0.38
	Price	Flambeau River	5. In Park Falls	10S, R, 2M, 5NP, YP, W	0.26
	Price	Flambeau River	6. Below Park Falls	5S, 2CR, P, BU, YP, W	0.39
	Price	Flambeau River	7. Crowley Flowage	CR, 3P, 2BU, 2YP	0.44
	Rusk	Flambeau River	8. Big Falls Flowage	4S, 6R, 2CR, RB, 2NP, 2BU, 2W	0.63
	Rusk	Flambeau River	9. Above Ladysmith	3S, 7BU, 10W	0.97
	Rusk	Flambeau River	10. Below Ladysmith	3S, 3R, 3BU, W	1.28
	Sawyer	Chippewa River	11. Chippewa Flowage	5S, 8W	0.14
	Chippewa	Chippewa River	12. Holcombe Flowage	10S, 3C, B, 9CR, 4NP, 5W	0.55
	Chippewa	Chippewa River	13. Lake Wissota	9S, 4CR, 2RB, 5NP, 3W	0.66
	Chippewa	Chippewa River	14. Below Lake Wissota	5NP	1.09

Drainage/Region	County	Water body	Location	Species	Value
	Eau Claire	Chippewa River	15. Below Eau Claire	8S, R, 4C, 3CC	0.43
	Pepin	Chippewa River	16. Below Durand	5S, 8C, 4MO, SMB, CR, 5W, CC	0.32
Door Drainage	Rusk	Murphy Flowage	17. Murphy Flowage	B, NP	0.36
	Door	Kangaroo Lake	18. Kangaroo Lake	B, YP, W	0.15
Fox River Drainage	Fond du Lac	Fond du Lac R.	19. River Mouth	S	0.20
	Winnebago	Lake Winnebago	20. Asylum Bay	5D, 6CR, 2NP	0.17
	Brown	Fox River	21. River Mouth	S, D, 3C, 2W, 2WB	0.36
Fox (Illinois) River Drainage	Waukesha	Pewaukee Lake	22. Pewaukee Lake	S, B, NP, YP	0.13
	Walworth	Lake Geneva	23. Lake Geneva	4S, 2C, SH, SMB, 5LMB, B, RB, 2NP, YP, 3W, 2BR	0.37
	Racine	Fox River	24. Below Burlington	4S, R, 2C, 3SMB, 3CR, RB, NP, 4CC, YP, WB	0.29
Galena River	Lafayette	Galena River	25. T2N, R1E, S27	2S, 3SMB	0.06
Green Bay	Brown	Green Bay	26. East of Fox River Mouth	8C, NP, BU, YP, W	0.21
	Door	Green Bay	27. N. of Sturgeon Bay Canal	S, BF, A, 4CI, 3LT	0.30
	Oconto	Green Bay	28. East of Oconto	5S, SMB, B, CR, 2NP, 2BU, YP, 2W, 2BR	0.36
Lake Michigan	Door	Lake Michigan	29. East of Algoma	2BR, 2RT, CS	0.08
	Kewaunee	Lake Michigan	30. East of Kewaunee	A, BT, 3BR, RT, CS	0.21
Lake Superior	Bayfield	Lake Superior	31. Apostle Islands	3S, 2LW, 2BR, 2LT	0.30
	Bayfield	Lake Superior	32. Off Boyd Creek	5S, 5W	0.44

Table 11, cont.

Sample Location					Species Sampled	Average ppm Mercury
Basin	County	Water		Site		
Lake Superior	Ashland	Lake Superior	33.	Lower Chequamegon Bay	5S, 2YP	0.09
	Ashland	Lake Superior	34.	Oak Point	5SMB, 5W	0.44
	Ashland	Lake Superior	35.	Kakagon Slough	2C, SMB, RB, BU, YP	0.30
Menominee River	Marinette	Menominee River	36.	Above Marinette	R, NP, 2YP	0.53
			37.	In Marinette	R, 2SMB, 3RB, 2NP, YP	0.44
			38.	River Mouth	2S, 2C, 2BW, A, 3LMB, 5P, 2NP, 4BU, 3YP, 8W	0.44
Milwaukee River	Ozaukee	Milwaukee River	39.	At Thiensville	2S, R, 3C, P, 3NP, 2BU	0.35
	Milwaukee	Milwaukee River	40.	Above North Avenue	3C, GF	0.15
	Milwaukee	Milwaukee River	41.	Milwaukee Harbor	S, 2C, CC, CS	0.11
Mississippi	Pepin	Mississippi R.	42.	Lake Pepin	S, C, 4LMB, 2B, 6CR 3NP, BU, 9CC, YP, 5W	0.33
	La Crosse	Mississippi R.	43.	Below Stoddard	S, C, LMB, B, CR, NP, BU, CC, W	0.30
Oconto River	Oconto	Oconto River	44.	Above Oconto Falls	S, B, CR, 2NP, BU, 2YP	0.12
Peshtigo River	Marinette	Peshtigo River	45.	Above Peshtigo	S, R, SMB, 2RB, 4NP, BU, 3YP	0.29

County	Drainage	River	No.	Location	Species	
Marinette		Peshtigo River	46.	Below Peshtigo	S, C, A, NP, BU, YP	0.22
Washington	Rock River Drainage	Rubincon River	47.	Below Hartford	3C	0.14
Waukesha		Lake LaBelle	48.	Lake LaBelle	BF, C, B, CR, W	0.13
Dodge		Rock River	49.	Lake Sinnissippi	5C, W	0.04
Dodge		Rock River	50.	Horicon	C, 6NP	0.12
Jefferson		Rock River	51.	Lake Koshkonong	4C, 3CC	0.08
Dane		Nevin Hatchery	52.	Hatchery Ponds	10RT	0.10
Dane		Lake Mendota	53.	Lake Mendota	4D, 4C, 3LMB, SMB, 5B, RB, 2NP, 3YP, 3W, 4WB	0.25
Dane		Yahara River	54.	Below Lake Mendota	5D, 2C, 2LMB, B, 2RB, 2NP, 3W, WB	0.22
Dane		Lake Monona	55.	Lake Monona	3D, 5C, 4LMB, B, P, RB, NP, 2W, 2YP, WB	0.22
Dane		Yahara River	56.	Below Lake Monona	6D, 7C, 13LMB, 5B, 3P, 2NP, 3YP, 3W, 3WB	0.25
Dane		Lake Kegonsa	57.	Lake Kegonsa	3D, 4C, 2LMB, B, CR, P, NP, YP, 2W, 3WB, 4YB	0.16
Dane		Starkweather Creek	58.	Creek Mouth	3D, 3C, B, CR, P, YP, 4W, WB, YB	0.17
Dane		Lake Waubesa	59.	Lake Waubesa	D, 2C, 6LMB, B, CR, P, 2NP, W, 2YP, WB, 4YB	0.38
Dane		Lake Wingra	60.	Lake Wingra	5C, BF, 5LMB, B, 2CR, P, NP, YP, YB	0.20
Rock		Rock River	61.	Below Janesville	R, 2C, 2CR, NP, CC, 2YB	0.11
Rock		Spaulding Pond	62.	Spaulding Pond	LMB, NP	0.07
Polk	St. Croix River	St. Croix River	63.	Below St. Croix Falls	BF, 6S, 5D, 4C, 6SMB, 2CR, NP, 2CC, 2SA, W, WB	0.43

Table 11, cont.

	Sample Location			Species Sampled	Average ppm Mercury
Basin	County	Water	Site		
St. Louis River	Douglas	St. Louis River	64. River Mouth	6S, BU, 2YP, 3W	0.62
Wisconsin River Drainage	Vilas	Wisconsin River	65. Lac Vieux Desert	S, NP, 3YP, 5W	0.12
	Oneida	Wisconsin River	66. Rainbow Flowage	R, CR, RB, NP, BU, YP, 3W	0.29
	Oneida	Wisconsin River	67. Above McNaughton	RB, NP, BU, 4YP	0.24
	Oneida	Wisconsin River	68. Below McNaughton	2S, M	0.35
	Oneida	Wisconsin River	69. Boom Lake	S, B, CR, NP, BU, YP, W	0.28
	Lincoln	Wisconsin River	70. Lake Alice	S, LMB, B, CR, BU, W	0.92
	Lincoln	Wisconsin River	71. Lake Mohawksin	S, B, CR, NP, BU, YP, W	0.97
	Marathon	Wisconsin River	72. Lake Wausau	S, C, LMB, B, NP, YP, W	0.62
	Marathon	Wisconsin River	73. Below Mosinee Dam	S, C, W	0.36
	Marathon	Wisconsin River	74. Lake DuBay	S, NP, BU, YP	0.28
	Wood	Wisconsin River	75. Above Biron Dam	S, C, B, NP, W	0.42
	Wood	Wisconsin River	76. Below Biron Dam	S, 2C, NP	0.50
	Wood	Wisconsin River	77. Above Centralia Dam	C	0.56
	Wood	Wisconsin River	78. Above Wyandotte Chemical	S, C, NP, W	0.54

County	Water	Location	Species	Value
Wood	Wisconsin River 79.	Below Wyandotte Chemical	S, C, W	0.58
Wood	Wisconsin River 80.	Moccasin Cr. Mouth	2S, C	0.50
Wood	Wisconsin River 81.	Highway 73 Bridge	S, C	0.61
Wood	Wisconsin River 82.	Below Nekoosa Dam	S, Q, W	1.62
Adams-Juneau	Wisconsin River 83.	Upper Petenwell Flowage	3C, B, 2CR, 2NP, 4W	2.36
Adams-Juneau	Wisconsin River 84.	Petenwell Flowage	C, B, NP, YP	0.94
Adams-Juneau	Wisconsin River 85.	Below Petenwell Dam	C, CR, NP, YP, SH	1.14
Adams-Juneau	Wisconsin River 86.	Buckhorn Bridge	2S, C, LMB, B, CR, WB	0.38
Adams-Juneau	Wisconsin River 87.	Above Castle Rock Dam	C, W	2.22
Adams-Juneau	Wisconsin River 88.	Below Castle Rock Dam	2C, NP, 2W	0.38
Adams-Juneau	Wisconsin River 89.	Above Dells Dam	S, C, CR, W	1.23
Sauk	Wisconsin River 90.	Below Dells Dam	3S, R, Q, B, 3W	1.09
Sauk	Wisconsin River 91.	Below Dells Creek	S, R, Q, 2C, W	1.83
Columbia	Wisconsin River 92.	Below I-94 Bridge	S, 3C, LMB, NP	0.53
Columbia-Sauk	Wisconsin River 93.	At Merrimac	D, YP, W	0.83
Dane-Sauk	Wisconsin River 94.	Below Prairie du Sac Dam	BF, D, 2C, SMB, LMB, W, WB	0.48
Iowa-Sauk	Wisconsin River 95.	Spring Green	S, 3Q, C, NP, SA, 2W	1.01
Grant-Crawford	Wisconsin River 96.	Boscobel	2R, 5Q, 4D, LMB, YP	1.07
Grant-Crawford	Wisconsin River 97.	Bridgeport	4R, 3C, 2W, WB	0.84
Vilas	Stormy Lake 98.	Stormy Lake	5CS	0.16

Table 11, cont.

| Basin | Sample Location | | Site | Species Sampled | Average ppm Mercury |
	County	Water			
Wisconsin River Drainage	Langlade	E. Eau Claire	99. Ackley Township	S, BT	0.13
	Langlade	Spring Brook	100. Antigo	S, 3BT	0.32
	Portage	Little Plover River	101. Plover Township	5BT	0.14
	Portage	Lower Tomorrow River	102. Amherst Township	S, 3C	0.22
	Juneau	Yellow River	103. Above Bullhorn Bridge	W	0.25

The number preceding the letter code indicates the number of separate fish samples taken. Site 1 in Douglas County, for instance (4S, R6W, 4BR, 2RT), amounts to 17 separate fish samples. Each sample consisted of muscle tissue from 1 to 20 fish composited into a single sample. Mercury determinations were made on each of the 17 samples.

mercury residues averaging above the 0.5 ppm guideline
established by the U. S. Food and Drug Administration as
an "action level" for banning fish from interstate markets.
The Wisconsin Department of Health and Social Services
warned against the frequent consumption of these fish, but
advised that one meal of fish per week would not constitute
a health hazard. These warnings have been communicated to
the public; no other Wisconsin waters are included in the
fish consumption warnings. The Chippewa, Flambeau and
Wisconsin Rivers receive waste waters from pulp and paper
mills. A mercury cell process chlor-alkali plant is located on the Wisconsin River. Mercury levels in fish taken
from sections of the three rivers located below these industries (Sites 5-10, 12-14, 70, 71, 84-89) averaged 0.80
ppm and ranged from 0.06 ppm to 4.62 ppm.

Mercury levels in fish samples taken from sections
(Sites 21, 36-38, 26-28) of the Fox and Menominee Rivers
and Green Bay averaged 0.38 ppm. These waters also receive
waste waters from pulp and paper mills, but contain waters
of higher alkalinity and pH than occur in the Chippewa,
Flambeau and Wisconsin Rivers. The Chippewa, Flambeau and
Wisconsin Rivers have an alkalinity of less than 50 ppm
and a pH usually of 7.0 or less.

Mercury levels in fish samples (Sites 47-62, 22-24)
taken from the Rock and Fox (Illinois) River systems in
southern Wisconsin averaged 0.22 ppm mercury. These waters
commonly exceed 200 ppm alkalinity and pH values of 8.0.
They drain areas of extensive agricultural development in-
terspersed with areas of urban development. No pulp or
paper mills are located on either the Rock or Fox (Illinois)
River systems.

Samples from the other waters sampled averaged below 0.5
ppm mercury; however, individual fish samples occasionally
exceeded this level. Samples from Lake Superior and the
Lake Superior Basin (Sites 1, 31-35, 64) averaged 0.34 ppm.
Samples from Lake Michigan (Sites 29 and 30) averaged 0.15
ppm. Samples from the Mississippi River (Sites 42 and 43)
averaged 0.32 ppm.

In general, higher levels of mercury in fish can be related to exposure to waste waters from pulp and paper mills
and chlor-alkali plants. Water chemistry also appears to
play a role. The more alkaline waters of southern and
eastern Wisconsin contain fish of lower mercury content,
even where mercury compounds have been used in the past
and can be found above background levels in the sediments.[6]

Since April, 1970, Wisconsin pulp and paper mills have
reported replacing mercury compounds with other chemicals.

Losses of mercury from the Wyandotte Chemicals Corporation
plant (Wisconsin's only mercury cell chlor-alkali plant)
to the Wisconsin River have been reduced to trace amounts.
However, mercury deposits occur below these industries.[6]
Swedish reports[7] suggest that the continuous release of
mercury from such deposits in the Chippewa, Flambeau, and
Wisconsin Rivers may produce elevated levels in fish for
many years.

Acknowledgment

Appreciation is expressed to P. E. Degurse for his
laboratory analyses, J. G. Konrad for his early involvement with the laboratory analysis and the field personnel
of the Department of Natural Resources for sample
collection.

References

1. Hannerz, L. Experimental Investigation on the Accumulation of Mercury in Water Organisms. Report No. 48
   (Drottningholm, Sweden: Institute of Freshwater Research, 1968), pp. 120–176.
2. Bligh, E. G. Mercury and the Contamination of Freshwater Fish. Fisheries Research Board of Canada. Manuscript Report Series No. 1088 (1970), 27 pp.
3. Association of Official Analytical Chemists. Official
   Methods of Analysis, 10, 375–377 (1965).
4. Rathje, A. O. "A Rapid Ultraviolet Absorption Method
   for the Determination of Mercury in Urine," Am. Ind.
   Hy. Assoc. J., 30, 126–132 (1969).
5. American Public Health Assoc., American Water Works
   Assoc. Standard Methods for the Examination of Water
   and Wastewater. (New York: Water Pollution Control
   Fed., 1965), 767 pp.
6. Konrad, J. G. "Mercury Contents of Bottom Sediments
   from Wisconsin Rivers and Lakes," Conf. on Environmental
   Mercury Contamination, Ann Arbor, Michigan (September
   30–October 2, 1970).
7. Hasselrot, T. B. Report on Current Field Investigations
   Concerning the Mercury Content in Fish, Bottom Sediment
   and Water. Report No. 48 (Drottningholm, Sweden:
   Institute of Freshwater Research, 1968), pp. 102–111.

Mercury in the Lake Michigan Environment

Richard A. Copeland

Introduction

In 1969, the Great Lakes Research Division of the University of Michigan began research for various electric utility companies who were interested in conducting an environmental study on Lake Michigan in connection with their nuclear power plants. The Great Lakes Research Division established a grid system containing 21 stations on Lake Michigan, and sampled these stations for phytoplankton, zooplankton, benthos, water, and sediment three times during 1969 and 1970. These samples have been analyzed for some 30 elements including mercury.

Experimental Methods

The plankton samples were obtained by towing a number 5 and number 20 plankton net, usually for about 1 hour, but for up to 10 hours where plankton were sparse. The number 5 net is fine enough to collect zooplankton but coarse enough that almost all the phytoplankton is washed on through. The number 20 net is fine enough to collect all plankton.

Benthos were collected by means of a bottom-riding sled for *Mysis* and by use of a "Ponar" grab sampler for *Pontoporeia*. In both cases, the benthos were separated from the sediment by sieving through a number 5 plankton net.

After a single rinse with distilled water, the biological samples were placed in washed polyethylene bags and frozen. They were kept frozen until prepared for analysis (usually two to ten months later).

The sediments were also collected by means of the "Ponar" sediment sampler. Since the "Ponar" is made of metal, extreme care was taken to sample only that part of the sediment which in no way had touched the sides of the sampler. In all cases, the sample taken represented the top 1 cm or less of the sediment. These samples were also placed in polyethylene bags and frozen.

All of the biological samples were removed from the polyethylene bags in a frozen state and placed on watch glasses for 24 hours in an oven set at 75°C. The dried samples were thoroughly mixed and a representative 0.5 gram sample was removed for analysis.

The sediment samples were thawed at room temperature and sieved through a 200 μ nylon sieve. An aliquot of the fraction which passed through the sieve was analyzed after drying and mixing. Only the sub 200 μ fraction was analyzed for several reasons. First, a much more representative and homogeneous sample could be obtained. Second, we felt that almost all the mercury entering Lake Michigan was going to be in solution, organically complexed, or associated with very fine particulate matter. Thus the sub 200 μ fraction was the logical place to look for mercury. Finally, we were interested in examining that part of the sediment which was small enough to pass through the gut of a sediment-dwelling animal and possibly be incorporated in the food chain. All of the samples were analyzed nondestructively for mercury by neutron activation analysis, following the procedure outlined by Copeland.[1]

Results and Conclusions

During 1970 there was extensive mercury analysis conducted in the United States on fish, water, and sediment. Very few analyses have been done on other members of the food chain, such as plankton. This is probably due to the difficulty in obtaining samples of aquatic creatures other than fish, and the fact that fish are the last member of the food chain before man and thus the most important.

Figures 13 through 15 show the dry weight mercury values we obtained for phytoplankton, zooplankton, and benthos respectively. The average value of mercury for phytoplankton was 2.2 ppm, for zooplankton 0.9 ppm, and for benthos 1.4 ppm. Our work indicates about 80% weight loss during the drying process, so these values would approximate 0.44, 0.2, and 0.3 ppm if the samples were run wet. Mercury analyses of fish in Lake Michigan were performed by Lucas, Edgington, and Colby[2] who report that wet weight values of less than 10 ppb were found. Since these values are all below the 0.5 ppm level of mercury which has been proposed as a maximum permissible concentration, it appears that Lake Michigan is still relatively free of mercury pollution. The distribution of mercury levels throughout Lake Michigan in plankton and benthos does not tend to indicate any isolated sources of pollution entering the lake. This is not unreasonable, since most of the mercury is probably entering the lake via surface runoff, and there are over 20 major streams emptying into the lake at various points.

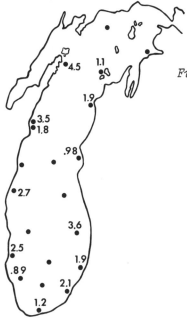

Figure 13: Dry Weight Mercury Concentrations (ppm) in Phytoplankton

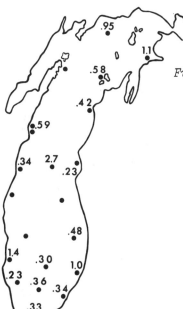

Figure 14: Dry Weight Mercury Concentrations (ppm) in Zooplankton

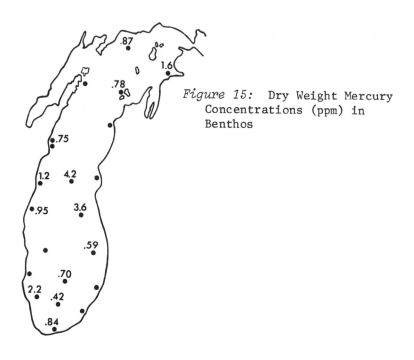

Figure 15:   Dry Weight Mercury
Concentrations (ppm) in
Benthos

The possibility of mercury being an airborne pollutant
can also be considered. If the burning of fossil fuels
released considerable mercury into the air, then mercury
levels in the southern end of Lake Michigan should be high
since the prevailing winds over Chicago blow from the
southwest. Figure 14 shows several mercury values for the
southern part of the lake; these levels are among the lowest encountered anywhere, suggesting that there is little
airborne mercury input into Lake Michigan.

Figure 16 shows mercury levels which have been measured
in the sub 200 µ fraction of the sediment. The average
value obtained is about 1 ppm. Analyses made on bulk
sediment indicate that mercury levels for the bulk material
will run from 1 to 4 times lower than the reported values,
the difference depending on the amount of sub 200 µ material
in the bulk sediment.

Mercury levels in sediment of 0.3 to 1 ppm are not
unusual.   Landstrom et al.[3] found 0.36 ppm in sediment
from a Swedish lake while Bowen[4] reports 0.4 ppm as a
shale average. Values as high as several hundred ppm have

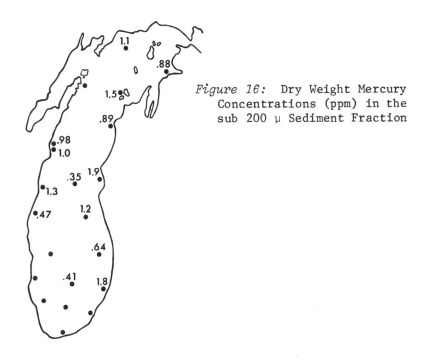

Figure 16: Dry Weight Mercury Concentrations (ppm) in the sub 200 μ Sediment Fraction

been reported in sediment below the Dow Chemical outfall at Sarnia, Ontario.*

It is interesting to note that the lowest mercury values in sediment are in the center of the lake while the highest values are near to shore. This supports the concept of general runoff as the source of mercury, and also tends to indicate that mercury is quite quickly bound up in the sediment when it enters the lake.

Acknowledgments

The author would like to thank Consumers Power Company, American Electric Power Service Corp., Commonwealth Edison Company, Wisconsin Public Service Corp., Northern Indiana Public Service Company, and Wisconsin Electric Power Company for their financial assistance in making this work possible.

---

*Testimony presented at Senator Phillip Hart's (D.-Michigan) hearing on mercury contamination at Clinton Gables, Mt. Clemens, Michigan, May 8, 1970.

References

1. Copeland, R. A. "Determination of Mercury by Non-Destructive Neutron Activation Analysis," published in Part II of this volume.
2. Lucas, H. F., D. N. Edgington, and P. J. Colby. "Concentrations of Trace Elements in Great Lakes Fishes," Journal of Fisheries Research Board of Canada, 27(4), 677-684 (1970).
3. Landstrom, I., K. Samsahl, and C. Wenner. "An Investigation of Trace Elements in Marine and Lacustrine Deposits by Means of a Neutron Activation Method," Modern Trends in Activation Analysis. NBS Spec. Pub. 312, Vol. 1, 353-367 (1969).
4. Bowen, H. J. M. Trace Elements in Biochemistry. (London and New York: Academic Press, 1966), p. 16.

Investigation of Mercury Contamination
in the Tennessee Valley Region

O. M. Derryberry

The first recognized incidence of environmental mercury contamination in the Tennessee Valley region was a fish-kill in Boone Reservoir in upper east Tennessee in July, 1968. After much painstaking investigation, this fish-kill was traced to a mercury compound, diphenylmercury, a degradation product of phenylmercuric acetate, formerly contained in certain derelict steel drums. Phenylmercuric acetate was used by some industries in the area as a desliming agent, and the drums had been sold or given away for use in floating docks and houseboats on the lake. As the drums rusted through or were punctured, the residue escaped to the lake water. Though so diluted as to be scarcely detectable in water, the diphenylmercury was sufficiently toxic to kill fish within a few hours. Specimens of fish sent to laboratories of the Federal Water Quality Administration in Athens, Georgia, and of the U. S. Fish and Wildlife Service in Auburn, Alabama, and Columbia, Missouri, did not reveal the presence of mercury. The diphenylmercury present in the lake water apparently was so acutely toxic to fish as to preclude its accumulation in fish flesh to detectable concentrations by analytical methods then in use.

Mercury Detected in Fish Flesh

In the spring of 1969, a Tennessee Valley Authority (TVA) investigation of a fish-kill on the lower Hiwassee River in eastern Tennessee revealed the presence of a mercury compound--although it was not found to be the cause of the kill. A few months later, using improved analytical techniques, our laboratory examined the flesh of fish taken from the Hiwassee River following the April, 1969, kill and found small amounts of mercury. A check with the U. S. Food and Drug Administration revealed that no concentration limits in fish flesh had been established at that time. FDA did establish guidelines in the spring of 1970, and the recommended limits were lower than the concentrations found earlier in the Hiwassee fish. TVA took new fish samples from this same reach of the river; these samples showed concentrations well below the FDA guidelines.

TVA scientists now have collected and analyzed samples of fish, water, and sediment from 26 reservoirs and 4 stream reaches. No significant levels of mercury have been found in the flesh of fish from these areas, except Pickwick Reservoir in northern Alabama and the North Fork Holston River in southwest Virginia. Fish flesh from Pickwick was found to have mercury content ranging from essentially zero up to 2.4 ppm, the latter well above the working guideline of 0.5 ppm established by FDA. Because of this, the health departments and fish and game agencies of Alabama, Mississippi, and Tennessee acting in concert closed the lake to commercial fishing and advised that mercury presented no hazards to water supplies or to those using the lake for water-contact sports. TVA tested the mercury content of the water--as distinct from the fish-- of Pickwick and found it well below the tentative safety guide of 5.0 ppb recently proposed by the U. S. Public Health Service.

The North Fork Holston River does not support a commercial fishery. Hence, it was necessary only that the Virginia agencies close the river to sport fishing and warn against consumption of fish from this stream.

Mercury Sources in the Tennessee Valley

The major known sources of mercury in the Tennessee Valley are three large caustic-chlorine plants. In most instances these manufacturing processes are such that the industries, within a short period of time, can divert their mercury wastes to artificial ponds to take other action

substantially reducing their discharge into the streams.
We have been advised by the state regulatory agencies that
the plants in the Tennessee Valley region have taken such
action. Although lacking regulatory authority as such,
TVA maintains a regular exchange of information with the
state agencies on these matters, and in addition will continue its monitoring to determine conditions in the TVA
lakes affected.

Figure 17 and 18 indicate the distribution throughout
the Tennessee Valley of sampling points for fish, water,
and mud, and show the location of Pickwick Reservoir and
the North Fork Holston River where concentrations of mercury in fish flesh were found to be higher than the guidelines established by the Food and Drug Administration.

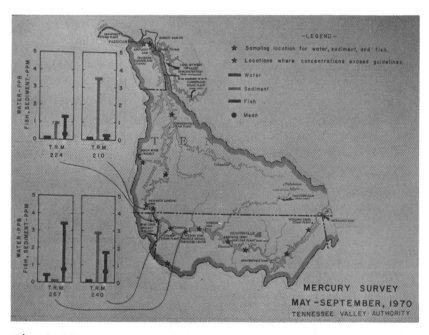

Figure 17: Results of Tennessee Valley Region Mercury
Survey, Tennessee River (T.R.M. = Tennessee River Mile
Number)

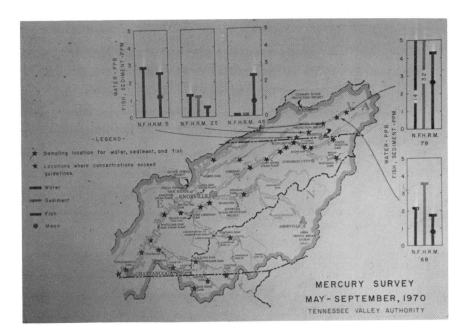

Figure 18: Results of Tennessee Valley Region Mercury Survey, North Fork Holston River (N.F.H.R.M. = North Fork Holston River Mile Number)

Distribution of Mercury in the Environment of Minamata Bay and the Inland Ariake Sea

Tadao Takeuchi

In 1959, the clinical signs, pathological changes, and environmental investigations strongly suggested that an organomercurial compound[1] was the causative agent of Minamata disease. At that time, extremely large concentrations of mercury were contained in the sediment of Minamata Bay (1 x 2 km). Near the drainage channel that leads into the bay from several chemical plants, a maximum concentration of 2010 ppm (wet weight) mercury was found

in sediment using the dithizone method.   Detailed investigation[2] revealed that the concentrations of mercury in
the sediment dropped sharply as a function of the distance
from the effluence point of the factory drainage channel
into Minamata Bay.   The central portion of the bay contained mercury concentrations from 40 ppm to 59 ppm.   But
at the mouth of Minamata Bay that leads to the sea, samples taken approximately 1.0 and 1.5 km from the discharge
point contained 22 ppm and 12 ppm (wet weight) of mercury
respectively (Figure 19).

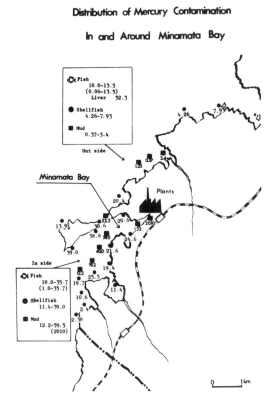

Figure 19: Distribution of Mercury Contamination In and
    Around Minamata Bay

As the distance from the channel entrance increased, the mercury concentrations in the sediments continued to decrease rapidly until, finally, the sediment directly outside Minamata Bay contained only 0.4 ppm to 3.4 ppm mercury. At greater distances into the Shiranui Sea from the mercury source in Minamata Bay, the mercury concentrations in the bottom sediments decreased into the range of 0.06 ppm to 0.55 ppm (wet weight).

The concentration of mercury in shellfish was also found to be a function of distance from the point of effluence. Shellfish from the Bay contained 11.4 ppm to 39.0 ppm of mercury (wet weight), whereas shellfish taken directly outside of the Bay ranged from 2.4 ppm to 20.4 ppm of mercury (wet weight). Furthermore, shellfish caught near the coast of the Shiranui Sea, approximately 6 km north of Minamata Bay contained from 4 ppm to 8 ppm of mercury.

Fish and other seafoods, such as crab and lobster, that were caught in Minamata Bay contained from 1.0 ppm to 36 ppm of mercury, whereas the same seafoods caught outside Minamata Bay in the Shiranui Sea contained from 1.0 ppm to 13.5 ppm. The same seafoods caught in other Japanese waters that were uncontaminated by mercury were always found to contain less than 1.0 ppm of mercury.

These data are significant not only because no parallel relationship exists between the mercury content in the sediments and the shellfish which contain biological concentrations of mercury, but because the same biological concentration mechanism probably occurs in other aquatic organisms as well.

References

1. Takeuchi, T. *Acta Neuropathologica*, *2*, 40-57 (1962).
2. Kitamura, S. "Determination of Mercury Content in Bodies of Inhabitants, Cats, Fishes and Shells in Minamata District and in the Mud of Minamata Bay," *Minamata Disease*. (Shuhan Co., 1968), pp. 257-266.

Mercury Levels in a Sample of Michigan Residents

Kenneth R. Wilcox, Jr.

The following is a brief description of information
collected concerning the distribution of mercury levels in
some residents of Michigan. Although the number of subjects in this study was very limited, the data are useful
in that they tend to confirm our prior expectations rather
than create new problems for us.

When the information concerning the findings of mercury
in fish in the St. Clair area became known to the Michigan
Department of Public Health, we responded on the basis of
our past knowledge and capabilities. We obtained urine
samples from individuals who were known to eat fish frequently that had been taken from the affected waters. We
collected urines from 24 individuals, and in 2/3 of them,
no mercury was detected. Three additional individuals had
a trace of mercury, and 5 had from 0.01 ppm to 0.06 ppm.
After we had obtained these rather negative results, we
learned that the compounds in question were not to be expected in the urine to any extent, and that this form of
screening was not very useful.

We next turned our attention to the determination of
blood levels in similar individuals. Since our department
had no experience with these determinations, a private
laboratory was used to run the blood specimens. We obtained blood and urine from 20 individuals who were known
to be frequent fish-eaters, and obtained hair from 5 of
them. None of the individuals had any symptoms compatible
with methylmercury intoxication. The blood levels in these
individuals, expressed in nanograms per milliliter (ng/ml),

Table 12

Blood Mercury Levels in Michigan Residents

	No. Persons	Extremes (ng/ml)	Mean (ng/ml)
Total	20	7 - 51.5	17.8
Eating fish	6	13 - 51.5	26.6
Stopped	14	7 - 32	14.1

which is approximately parts per billion (ppb), ranged from
7 to 51.5, with a mean of 17.8 (Table 12). In this group
the men tended to have higher levels than the women, with
the men having a mean of 22 ppb and the women, 12.8 ppb.

In reviewing the stated history of fish consumption, 6
of the 20 individuals still (at the time of the blood determination) ate fish taken from Lake St. Clair, and 14
had stopped eating fish approximately two months previously,
when Ontario first announced its ban on fishing. The mean
mercury value for the 6 individuals still eating fish was
26.6 ppb, while that for the 14 who had stopped was 14.1
ppb. Thus there was an apparent effect of continued eating
on the blood mercury level, as one would expect. In addition, since the interval between the blood sampling and the
time the individual stopped consuming fish was approximately
two months, the difference in mean levels would correspond
roughly to the two-fold decrease one would expect if one
considers the excretion rate of methylmercury. Again, the
urine samples proved difficult to correlate with the blood
results. Of the 20 individuals, 9 had no detectable mercury in the urine (Table 13). Five had a trace, 3 had 0.01

Table 13

Urine Mercury Levels in Michigan Residents

| | | *No. of persons having:* | | |
	Total	*<0.01 mg/l*	*0.01 mg/l*	*>0.01 mg/l*
Total	20	14	3	3
Eating fish	6	3	0	3
Stopped	14	11	3	0

ppm, and 3 had from 0.01 ppm to 0.025 ppm mercury. If a
division is made by dietary history, of the 6 still eating
fish, 3 had levels greater than 0.01 ppm; and of the 14
who stopped eating at the time of the ban, 3 had levels of
0.01 ppm and none had levels greater than this.

An attempt was made to measure the mercury content of
the hair of 5 of these individuals, and of 3 individuals
who did not eat fish from the lake (Table 14). However,

Table 14

Hair Mercury Levels in Michigan Residents
(Relative Values)

Stopped eating fish	- 1.0
No fish	- 1.9, 2.0, 2.1
Eating fish	- 3.0, 7.1, 7.2, 8.5

the laboratory doing the analysis by neutron activation used unsuitable standards. We were therefore able to obtain only the relative values of mercury in the hair samples. These samples have been submitted to other laboratories so that eventually we should have definite values for them. One individual in the group of 14 who stopped eating fish at the time of the ban had the lowest value, and was given the relative value of 1. The 3 control individuals had relative values of 1.9, 2.0, and 2.0, so that we can assume a control value twice that of the first subject. The relative values of the 4 individuals who continued to eat fish up to the time of the sampling were higher.

Based on a small number of individuals, the expected higher mercury levels occurred in those having greater exposure. There is no direct correlation between the blood level and hair level, but the 3 individuals having blood levels of approximately 13 ppb had an average relative value of 3.7, while 2 individuals having blood levels of 22 ppb and 25 ppb had an average relative value of 7.8. The data presented here are consistent with what one would expect from the literature, but are insufficient to add much to our knowledge.

To summarize, our findings indicate that the level of mercury found in those individuals who ate fish from the affected waters were not high enough to cause symptomatic illness, but that continued eating was associated with higher levels. The difference in average levels between those who continued to eat fish and those who stopped with the fishing ban was consistent with the half-life of excretion of methylmercury. Based on a few samples obtained, the relative value of mercury in the hair of those eating fish from affected waters was higher than those who did not. We hope that these data can add to the information collected by others, so that we may better define and understand our position in relation to mercury in fish (Table 15).

Table 15

Summary Table of Blood and Urine Mercury Values
for Fish-Eaters in the Lake St. Clair Area

Subjects	Stated Frequency of Fish Meals	Blood Mercury (ng/ml) Lab. Values+	Values Used*	Urine Mercury (mg/l)
Still eating fish				
1	1x/wk	13	13	0.025
4	2x/wk	25	25	trace
6	2x/wk	48, 55	51.5	0.018
2	every other week	8, 18	13	0
5	1x/wk	35	35	0.02
3	every other week	22	22	0
Stopped eating fish 2 months before sampling				
18	2-3x/wk	15, 18	16.5	0
12	2-3x/wk	8, 15	11.5	trace
11	2-3x/wk	10, 12	11	0
13	1x/wk	8, 17	12.5	0.01
14	1x/wk	13	13	0
16	1x/wk	15, 15	15	trace
17	1x/wk	15	15	0.01
9	seldom	5, 15	10	0
10	frequent	10	10	0
7	2x/wk	7, 7	7	0
8	1x/wk	5, 12	8.5	trace
20	1x/wk	32, 32	32	trace
19	1x/wk	18, 35	21.5	0.01
15	2x/wk	5, 22	13.5	0

+ = Some specimens submitted as blind duplicates to
laboratory.
* = Single value or average of duplicates.

Mercury in Humans in the Great Lakes Region

E. Mastromatteo and R. B. Sutherland

The first assessment of mercury as an environmental contaminant in Canada was undertaken by Mr. Norvald Fimreite,
a Norwegian student doing graduate study in the Department
of Zoology, University of Western Ontario. This study,
which was supported financially by a grant from the Canadian
Wildlife Service, was published in March, 1969, as Manuscript Report No. 17 of the Service, under the title "Mercury Uses in Canada and Their Possible Hazards as Sources
of Mercury Contamination."

In his assessment, Mr. Fimreite attempted, through review of published reports and commercial statistics, and by
direct enquiry, to estimate the total amount of mercury
contributed annually to the environment in Canada, particularly to water and soil. Though samples of fish and birds
had been taken in 1968, the results were not then available
for inclusion in his report.

While not presenting any definite evidence or data indicating the existence of mercury contamination, the report
did stimulate government to consider the problem. During
1969, the Ontario Water Resources Commission instituted
enquiries to assess the losses of mercury from chlor-alkali
plants in the province, and undertook some sampling of
streams, waste waters, and bottom muds. Fish were also
taken for analysis. At the same time, Mr. Fimreite continued his sampling of fish and birds.

Interest in mercury pollution was further stimulated in
the summer of 1969 by the finding of increased mercury
levels in wildfowl in Alberta which had eaten mercury-
treated grain. This was followed by the finding of high
levels of mercury in fish from the Saskatchewan River.

In Ontario, the first reports on the fish samples (which
were analyzed using neutron activation analysis by Gulf
Atomic Incorporated and by Professor R. E. Jervis at the
University of Toronto) showed high levels in fish taken
from the St. Clair River, Lake St. Clair, and the Detroit
River. More extensive sampling of fish, both by the Province and by the federal government, was undertaken early
in 1970 with the establishment of additional facilities at
the Ontario Water Resources Commission Laboratory, at the
University of Guelph, and in the Federal Fisheries Research
Board in Winnipeg.

Mercury Tolerance Levels

In the meantime, health authorities at the two levels of government were giving consideration to setting an acceptable residue level for mercury in fish. The Canadian Food and Drug Directorate and the U. S. Food and Drug Administration had both adopted a concentration of 0.5 ppm in fish muscle as a tentative maximum for commercial fish; catches exceeding this level are destroyed. Ontario adopted the same level with respect to sports fishing. This level is lower than that adopted by Sweden (1 ppm in a kilogram pike) but was felt to be desirable in view of the uncertainty which exists as to the minimum dose of alkyl mercury which is teratogenic for humans.

Application of the 0.5 ppm tolerance level has resulted in the closing to all commercial fishing of the St. Clair and Detroit Rivers, Lake St. Clair, the Ottawa River below Ottawa, the St. Lawrence River below Cornwall, and in northwestern Ontario in the following regions: the Wabigoon and English Rivers below Dryden and the Winnipeg River below Kenora.

In addition, commercial fishing has been closed for white bass and pickerel in the western basin of Lake Erie, pickerel in the southern part of Lake Huron, and pickerel, pike, perch, and eel in the upper St. Lawrence River and eastern end of Lake Ontario.

Sports fishing is permitted in the waters listed, but anglers are warned against eating the fish, and the lakes are posted with "Fish for Fun" signs.

Mercury concentrations in fish taken from the Lake St. Clair region range from 0.3 ppm to over 5 ppm, the higher values usually occurring in larger fish and in the predacious species. In the Wabigoon-English River area, levels of over 10 ppm have been encountered.

Mercury Accumulation in Humans

In a preliminary attempt to determine whether there was any accumulation of mercury in humans who had eaten fish from the contaminated waters, local medical officers of health were asked to collect urine specimens for analysis. The results from the first 135 samples submitted are shown in Table 16. These results, while accepted as being within the normal range of mercury excretion, were not considered to eliminate the possibility of increased human absorption, since Japanese and Swedish investigators had earlier reported:

Table 16

Urinary Mercury Concentration Among
135 Great Lakes Residents

Concentration Micrograms/Liter	*Number*	*Per Cent*
<20	90	66.7
20	26	19.3
30	9	6.7
40	8	5.9
50	0	–
60	2	1.4
>60	0	–
Total	135	100.0

(a) that the mercury in fish was present largely as a methylmercury compound
(b) that excretion of mercury following methylmercury intake was very slow in most species, with an estimated half-life in man of up to 70 days and less than 10% of that excreted being via the kidneys
(c) that absorption of methylmercury was more accurately reflected by determination of mercury in hair and blood, particularly the red cells.

Hair and Blood Sample Analysis

In early May, 1970, a visit was made to the English River in northwestern Ontario, where mercury residues in fish had been found to be generally higher than in the Lake St. Clair region. Samples of hair, blood and urine, as well as brief histories of fish consumption, were obtained from Indians and white guides who had been taking fish from contaminated waters, and also from a number of residents whose fish were from unaffected lakes. In all, 30 hair samples from the Kenora-Dryden area were analyzed by Professor Jervis, using the neutron activation technique.

For 9 persons who did not eat fish from the contaminated waters, the concentrations of mercury in the hair samples ranged from 2 ppm to 14 ppm. In the remaining 21 persons who did consume fish from contaminated waters at some time or other during the past year, 5 showed levels of less than

10 ppm, 9 had levels between 10 ppm and 25 ppm, 3 had levels between 25 ppm and 50 ppm, and 4 had levels between 50 ppm and 100 ppm. In most of the individuals tested, the consumption of fish occurred mainly between May and October, with much less fish being eaten during the winter months. The levels of mercury in the hair correlated fairly closely with the number of meals of fish which were eaten per week.

According to Professor Jervis, the higher levels found in the hair were "about one-half of the level at which the first clinical symptoms of mercury poisoning can occur (*viz*. 150 ppm to 200 ppm), based on similar hair analyses of persons who were victims of mercury poisoning in Sweden and Japan."

Mercury determinations were carried out on 29 blood samples by Atomic Energy of Canada Ltd., again using neutron activation analysis. In the 9 persons who seldom ate any fish, or who ate fish only from uncontaminated waters, the mercury levels were below 35 ppb. In those who ate fish from contaminated lakes more than four times per week during May to October, but who seldom ate fish during the following five months, the mercury levels ranged from 20 ppb to 85 ppb. Allowing for mercury excretion during the winter (with no further intake), it is probable that had blood samples been taken last fall on persons eating fish from contaminated lakes, the levels would have been several times higher than those given. A level of 155 ppb was found in one individual with the highest and most recent consumption of fish from the contaminated lakes. This same individual showed 96 ppm of mercury in his hair.

In comparison with these figures, in Sweden and Finland, blood levels of up to 200 ppb have been reported for adults consuming mercury-contaminated fish, in whom no symptoms were present.

From the Lake St. Clair area, we have reports on three hair samples analyzed by Professor Jervis. One of these showed 4.4 ppm mercury, one showed 9.1 ppm and the third contained 49.9 ppm. The last sample was from a woman who ate fish three to five times per week. Hair samples from three Sarnia, Ontario, residents with a history of eating fish from Lake St. Clair, the St. Clair River, or the southern end of Lake Huron once or twice a week have recently been reported by the Radiation Protection Laboratory of the Department of Health as showing from 2 ppm to 3 ppm. Samples from two residents from Cornwall on the St. Lawrence River, who ate fish 3 to 4 times a week, showed 2 ppm and 5 ppm.

Increased Mercury Uptake

It is apparent from the foregoing that there has been an increased uptake of mercury among persons eating fish from contaminated lakes in Ontario. From the fish sampling program, evidence is accumulating that the problem is more widespread and more complex than we at first imagined. Within recent months, levels above 0.5 ppm but below 1 ppm have been found in some fish catches from lakes having no direct link with industry. In fact, in some instances the lakes are more than 100 miles away from built-up areas, and on different watersheds. It is believed that some of the mercury contamination may result from relatively high mercury levels in certain geological formations. Mercury levels of 1 ppm or slightly higher are believed to be common in rock formations in the Canadian shield. It is also possible that atmospheric transportation of mercury may have contributed to the unexpectedly high mercury residues in fish from these lakes.

The Occurrence of Mercury in the Environment and Man
Discussion Paper

Contributions by: J. Bails, T. W. Clarkson, H. M.
Cunningham, W. Fulkerson, L. Goldwater, D. I. Hammer,
R. E. Jervis, D. Klein, J. Konrad, L. T. Kurland,
D. G. Langley, D. J. Lisk, E. Mastromatteo, J. C.
Moran, D. B. Nelson, W. T. Sullivan, L. A. VanDenBerg

Many environmental components have been analyzed for mercury. It has been found in sediments throughout the major watersheds of the United States. In the tributaries to Lake Erie, more than 1 ppm mercury has been found in the sediments of the Black, Ashtabula, and Buffalo Rivers. All sediments from the Rouge, Huron, Maumee, Sandusky, Portage, Rocky, Cuyhahoga, Grande, and Raisin Rivers contained less than 1 ppm mercury. High levels of mercury were found in the sediments in the Niagara River area and in Lake Onondaga.

In some waste-treatment plant effluents, as much as 4 ppb mercury were found in places where no industrial sources were evident. In 1970, significant discharges of mercury were found in the Mississippi, Missouri, Ohio,

Columbia, Androscoggin, Penobscott, and Tennessee Rivers and the Houston Ship Channel, and in several other small tributaries in other river basins.

The diversity of sources of mercury is surprising. Coal and some crude oils have been found to contain significant amounts of mercury. Crude oils from the Cymric field in California have been reported to contain up to 21 ppm of mercury. However, this concentration of mercury in oils seems to be unusually high.

If the mercury released by power plants is all in the vapor form, which may not necessarily be true, then this source could easily be monitored using the sensitive airborne mercury analyzers commonly employed in geological surveys. However, there is some question as to the precision of available analytical techniques in assessing low levels of mercury contamination.

Since many materials have been analyzed for mercury, it may be possible to reassess the average mercury intake of people in the near future.

The first work on human dietary intakes of mercury was done by Stock in 1934,[1] in which he showed an average intake of about 5 micrograms of mercury a day in certain diets--other studies on diets that have been made since that time validate this to a certain extent, with intakes probably ranging up to 20 micrograms of mercury today in what might be considered an average diet.

With regard to the sources of this intake, fish appears to be the most important dietary source. Vegetables and fruits generally contain 20-50 ppb, and some components of the diet are well below 10 ppb.[2] Beef and pork tend to contain 50-140 ppb mercury; livers and kidneys may contain 100-200 ppb mercury. Milk powders contain about 140 ppb on a dry weight basis. To evaluate the actual mercury intake will require the consideration of any changes in mercury concentrations in food preparation. There is some evidence that normal cooking procedures do not reduce methylmercury concentrations.

Perkons and Jervis[3] reported the trace metal content of normal human hair. Mercury was one of the elements measured. These data indicated mercury levels from somewhat less than 1 ppm to approximately 3 ppm in a skewed distribution, with a statistical mode of about 1.5 ppm mercury in human hair from a "normal" North American population. Somewhat higher levels were reported occasionally during about 1965 from Sweden, Scotland, and Japan. According to Jervis, some European populations typically had about

5 ppm mercury in hair without any evidence of unusual mercury exposure.

Recent studies have used hair as an index for mercury exposure in fish eaters in Ontario.[2] There may also be a generalized increase in the average mercury concentration in human hair since 1962. Preliminary data indicate that hair concentrations of 3-6 ppm mercury may be more typical for 1970. However, until good correlations between intake, hair levels, and mercury levels in body organs can be made, these data will have to serve primarily as indicators. Trace metal levels in hair may also be affected by external influences, such as cosmetic ingredients.

Swedish workers have assumed a linear correlation factor indicating that mercury is approximately 250x concentrated in hair over blood. When the extremes of the available mercury data in hair and blood in North America are compared with levels which were considered to be the lower toxic limits in Sweden, there appears to be some overlap, and certainly not any great margin of safety. Since there is a dearth of epidemiological studies on the effects of environmental mercury exposures in the United States and Canada, this situation gives reasons for concern.

References

1. Stock, A. and F. Cucuel. "Die Quantitative Bestimmung Kleinster Quecksilbermengen," *Naturwiss.*, *22*, 390 (1934).
2. Jervis, R. E., D. Debrun, W. LePage, and B. Tiefenbach. *Mercury Residues in Canadian Foods, Fish, Wildlife.* Progress Report. National Hlth. Grant 605-7-510. University of Toronto, Canada. (1970) 39 pp.
3. Perkons, A. K., R. E. Jervis. "Trace Elements in Human Head Hair," *Forensic Sciences*, *11* (1):50 (1966).

PART II

METHODS OF ANALYSIS

CONTRIBUTORS TO PART II

Richard A. Copeland, Ph.D., Environmental Research Group, Inc., Ann Arbor, Michigan

H. M. Cunningham, Food and Drug Directorate, Department of National Health and Welfare, Ottawa, Ontario, Canada

J. T. Davis, Environmental Science and Engineering Corporation, 2100 West End Avenue, Nashville, Tennessee

J. C. Gage, Ph.D., Imperial Chemical Industries Ltd., Industrial Hygiene Research Laboratories, Alderley Park, Nr Macclesfield, Cheshire, England

Rolf Hartung, Ph.D., Department of Environmental and Industrial Health, University of Michigan, Ann Arbor

John D. Jones, Phoenix Memorial Laboratory, University of Michigan, Ann Arbor

Harry B. Mark, Jr., Ph.D., Department of Chemistry, University of Cincinnati, Cincinnati, Ohio

J. C. Méranger, Food and Drug Directorate, Department of National Health and Welfare, Ottawa, Ontario, Canada

D. G. Nicholson, Environmental Science and Engineering Corporation, 2100 West End Avenue, Nashville, Tennessee

K. K. S. Pillay, Western New York Nuclear Research Center, State University of New York at Buffalo, Buffalo, New York

J. Mark Rottschafer, Department of Chemistry, University of Michigan, Ann Arbor

A. R. Schulert, Environmental Science and Engineering Corporation, 2100 West End Avenue, Nashville, Tennessee

Ralph G. Smith, Ph.D., Department of Environmental and Industrial Health, School of Public Health, The University of Michigan, Ann Arbor

Methods of Analysis for Mercury and
Its Compounds: A Review

Ralph G. Smith

As long ago as 1917, a paper by Dr. J. A. Elliott entitled "A New and Delicate Method for the Detection of Mercury" appeared in the Journal of the American Medical Association. In this method, mercury was collected on copper dust from an acid solution, and was subsequently heated such that the distilled mercury was deposited on gold foil, which was then examined by eye with a hand lens. The author claimed that his method was "accurate" to one millionth of a grain per 500 cc of fluid, or, alternatively, one fifteen-thousandth of a milligram per 500 cc. (Expressed in more modern terms, this detection limit was about 0.1 ppb.) Most of the published methods which have appeared since 1917 could not equal the sensitivity Dr. Elliott claimed, but presumably all the effort expended in the 50 years has resulted in some advances in other aspects of analyzing samples for mercury.

There has been no shortage of interest in the subject since that time. This review includes a bibliography of about 460 papers concerned with mercury analysis, and doubtless more could be gathered with additional effort. It is not possible to discuss or even mention each method in this brief presentation, but a classification scheme may be useful. The most obvious basis for classification is the means ultimately used to determine the quantity of mercury present, but for some purposes, a classification based on the kinds of samples to be analyzed would be equally useful. The former scheme has been used, but a brief note is made of the more frequently analyzed kinds of samples to indicate the extent of the challenge presented to the analyst.

Substances Analyzed for Mercury Content

Traditionally, analyses of air have been made to evaluate occupational exposure to mercury and its compounds, and almost as frequently urine and blood analyses have been performed for the same purpose. Today there is also interest in analyzing ambient air as well as emissions from stacks and other potential sources of air pollution. Numerous biological samples in addition to blood and urine are also being submitted for analysis. Almost every possible tissue, human or animal, has been subjected to analysis, as have such differing samples as saliva, feces, amniotic fluid, hair, nails, etc., not to mention eggs, feathers and numerous other specimens more or less unique to some particular kind of domesticated animal or wildlife. All sorts of plants, grains, fruits, and foods in general must be analyzed, as well as the soils from which they originate, and many other mineral substances. Finally, the aquatic environment has presented us with some of our most difficult analytical challenges, consisting as it does of such diverse media as water and muds, or sediments, containing a number of plant and animal organisms, all potentially involved in complex biosynthetic schemes which may require the separation and quantitation of specific organic mercury compounds, rather than a relatively simple total mercury determination.

Separation of Mercury from Organic Matter

It is probably safe to say that any sample will be found to contain some mercury, given a method of suitable sensitivity and a sample of sufficient size. A sample of manageable size, however, will normally contain microgram or nanogram amounts of mercury, so trace methods are always required, and the usual problems peculiar to trace metal analyses must be solved. For biological samples, one of the major problems is the separation of the mercury from the large mass of organic matter with which it is associated. To make this separation, many procedures for total mercury require an ashing or digestion step which can be a source of considerable error in the subsequent determination. Ashing is most commonly achieved by digestion with any of numerous oxidizing substances or mixtures, or by combustion. The most frequently used oxidizing mixture is probably potassium permanganate in sulfuric acid solution, but other digestion mixtures employ nitric acid, perchloric acid, hydrogen peroxide, bromine, and numerous other acid and alkaline mixtures. It is probable that the failure of many methods to yield results comparable to apparently similar methods can be traced to incomplete ashing, or losses sustained during the ashing process. Falsely high results can likewise be traced to digestion mixtures which contain variable quantities of mercury as a contaminant, but such errors can generally be minimized by careful selection of reagents, and frequent analyses of blanks and standards.

Following the ashing step, if one is required, most procedures utilize one of a large variety of means to concentrate, isolate, or otherwise render the mercury suitable for final estimation. Some of the more popular choices for this purpose include extraction into an organic solvent, ion exchange separation, electrodeposition or amalgamation, precipitation, and reduction to elemental mercury, followed by aeration. Many procedures utilize additional rather complex schemes to improve further the separation of mercury from interfering substances, but, for the most part, these steps consist of conventional chemical manipulations of pH and addition of complexing agents or other reagents.

Classification of Analytical Methods

Analysis is ultimately carried out by any of a variety of means which can be classified somewhat arbitrarily as follows:

I. Elemental, Total and Inorganic Mercury Analysis Methods
   A. Activation Analysis (Neutron Activation)
   B. Atomic Absorption and Fluorescence
      1. Volatilization by Flame and by Heated, Non-Flame Methods, Direct Air Analysis by Ultraviolet Photometry, etc.
      2. "Cold-Vapor" Methods (Measurement After Reduction of Hg^{++} to Hg Vapor)
   C. Chromatographic Analysis (Paper, Thin Layer, Liquid and Ionophoresis)
   D. Colorimetric (Spectrophotometric)
      1. Dithizone
      2. Non-Dithizone Reagents (Also Fluorometric Methods)
   E. Electrometric (Polarographic, Amperometric, Coulometric, etc.)
   F. Gravimetric
   G. Micrometric
   H. Radiometric

This outline of the various analytical approaches that
have been used to analyze samples for total mercury and
the organic compounds of mercury makes it evident that almost every instrumental technique known to the analyst has
been applied to the problem. Several excellent reviews of
analytical methods have been published within the last
year, and there is no good purpose served by repeating the
details of the numerous analytical methods described. Instead, reference should be made to those papers or articles
in the bibliography under the heading "IV. Reviews," wherein the contributions by the U. S. Geological Survey (1970),
Wallace, et al., of the Oak Ridge National Laboratory
(1971), the Study Group on Mercury Hazards, Special Report
to the U. S. Department of Health, Education, and Welfare
Secretary's Pesticide Advisory Committee (1971), and the
Expert Group Report to the National Institute of Public
Health, Stockholm, Sweden (1971) will be found particularly
useful. All of these reviews describe the more popular
methods of mercury analysis, including several variations
of atomic absorption spectrophotometry.

If the bibliography is examined further, however, it is
apparent that certain analytical approaches have been much
more favored than others. Historically, one of the more
elegant methods used was that devised by Stock and his co-
workers and classified in the outline under "micrometric
methods." Determinations of mercury content by this method
were almost unique in the realm of trace metal analyses, in
that mercury compounds were actually reduced to elemental
mercury in the form of a small sphere of mercury, the diameter of which was then measured with considerable precision by means of a microscope. Although it is probable
that no analyses are conducted by this means today, it must
have been satisfying to have performed an analysis in which
the element was actually visualized, rather than detected
by means of some indirect physical or chemical phenomenon
as in most procedures.

Widely Used Methods for Determining Mercury

Until relatively recently, the most popular methods for determining mercury in almost any type of sample have been based on use of the reagent diphenylthiocarbozone, or dithizone. Since this color-forming reagent was introduced by Fischer in 1925, it has been widely used for determining a variety of trace metals, and mercury is perhaps second only to lead in the number of papers describing variations in dithizone procedures. A number of variables influence the manner in which dithizone behaves toward mercury and interfering elements, and the large number of published papers is ample evidence of the ingenuity of chemists in making these determinations even more specific, sensitive, accurate, and rapid. There is little need to review the chemistry of these procedures, for today it is likely that relatively few laboratories are continuing to perform analyses by means of dithizone procedures. The reason is the appearance on the analytical scene of methods which have proven to be much more sensitive and convenient, and which, for the most part, involve the determination of mercury by some variation of atomic absorption measurement. Agreement is almost unanimous that such procedures, and particularly the so-called "flameless" or "cold vapor" techniques, are the most useful for almost any kind of total mercury analysis. Mercury is unique among metals in that it has a very high vapor pressure at relatively low temperatures, and can be vaporized quantitatively with ease. Thus, the simple application of heat to many samples will drive off the mercury, so that it may thereafter be collected in some fashion and separated from the sample matrix of which it was a part. The isolated mercury may then be revolatilized by the application of heat, or may be placed in solution, reduced to elemental mercury and removed quantitatively by aeration. It is this latter approach that is generally designated "cold vapor" analysis, while those methods in which the mercury is volatilized by heat are usually referred to as "flameless" atomic absorption. Historically, once again, such methods are, in reality, quite old, for the ultraviolet photometers or mercury vapor meters developed first in the 1930's are a special kind of atomic absorption analyzer. Mercury is most frequently found in industrial or ambient air as a vapor, and these photometers are relatively simple devices for measuring the absorption by mercury of the resonant energy emitted by an excited mercury vapor source.

Methods of Analysis After Heat Application

As noted previously, mercury may be driven from most
samples by the application of heat, and many methods have
relied on the pyrolysis of samples or the application of
sufficient heat to volatilize mercury. The simplest
possible method of analysis, after such treatment, would
be the direct measurement of the vapor released upon heating,
but most methods have not elected to make this measurement
due to interfering substances resulting from the decomposi-
tion of the samples. In our laboratories at Wayne State
University, and subsequently at The University of Michigan,
we have devised an apparatus which successfully measures
mercury in most samples a few seconds after the introduction
of the sample into a furnace system. The original system
is described in the publication by Hermann and Smith (1968)
and is listed in the bibliography under "I.B. Atomic
Absorption Methods." Subsequently, the apparatus has been
refined to some extent. However, it has been demonstrated
by many thousands of analyses that the system is a reliable
means of analyzing any samples of biological origin, and
many other types of samples which have so far included air,
coal, fly ash, water, bottom sediments, etc. The amount of
sample required is very small, so that in the case of blood
and urine samples, for example, a sample of 50 to 100
microliters is entirely adequate, while in the case of most
solid samples, 5 to 10 milligrams is ample. The problem of
interfering substances which may also absorb ultraviolet
energy has been solved by placing a series of traps in the
gas stream, and it has been demonstrated that the interfering substances are removed without loss of mercury.
Although the method has not yet gained wide acceptance, it
would seem probable that its inherent simplicity and the
low probability of external contamination of samples should
result in gradually increasing usage. One principal dis-
advantage to the use of the method at present is the lack
of commercial suppliers of equipment suitable for the
analysis, so that each laboratory must fabricate its own
apparatus. For further discussion concerning the method,
reference should be made to the previously cited paper in
the bibliography.

Activation Analysis for Mercury

Another widely used method of analysis today is that
based on activation analysis; the bibliography contains an
extensive listing of papers describing the activation

analysis methods used. There are obvious advantages to this kind of analysis, of which the principal are the relatively small amount of operator time which may be required, the ability to perform non-destructive analyses in some cases, and the great sensitivity and accuracy of the procedure. However, the method is not available to most laboratories which do not have the intense neutron flux sources available. Fortunately, there are a number of laboratories which do have the necessary reactors or other sources of neutrons, and analysis can be made on a commercial basis for those desiring them. The publications listed in the bibliography under "I.A. Activation Analysis" should be consulted for details of procedural methods, and the reviews previously cited will be found particularly useful in assessing the general capabilities of this method of analysis.

The numerous other analytical approaches that have been used to determine mercury are distinctly secondary to those already mentioned, and no discussion of the underlying principles, limitations, etc., will be made. However, the bibliography does contain reference to a number of publications which are based on other instrumental analytical methods, and it should be consulted for details concerning them. It is certainly possible that some of these methods, which to date have not been widely used, will become of much greater interest in the future, when other laboratories have had occasion to confirm their general applicability.

Identification of Organic Mercury Compounds

All of the discussion thus far has related to the analysis of samples for total mercury, wherein no effort is made to discriminate between inorganic or organic forms of mercury. However, the much publicized concern with environmental mercury levels made it evident to all that such methods are often inadequate to evaluate properly the hazard of ingestion of foodstuffs containing elevated levels of mercury. Organic mercurials have long been used as such, of course, and, more recently, the ability of micro-organisms to convert inorganic to organic mercury has been shown to be a factor of importance in regard to environmental contamination. The identification of the numerous organic compounds of interest has proved to be a major analytical challenge and one requiring quite different analytical methodology than used in total mercury analyses. In general, the alkyl mercury compounds have been of greatest concern, and, in order to isolate and identify them, most procedures rely on either gas chromatographic separations or other solid phase chromatographic procedures. The bibliography contains a number of references to methods which have been arbitrarily classified as dealing either with alkyl mercury compounds, or with non-alkyl mercury compounds. In some instances, the individual methods are applicable to both kinds of compounds, but the classification was made based on the principal intent of the method. These references, and in particular the review paper by the "Expert Group Report" to the Swedish National Institute of Public Health (1971), should be consulted for details on the methods of determining organic forms of mercury.

Research related to the analysis of all types of samples for mercury has been greatly stimulated by the environmental mercury problem, and new procedures, as well as improvements in existing methodologies, are appearing with much greater frequency than in preceding years. Doubtlessly there will emerge from all of this research methods of great specificity and sensitivity, which will permit the rapid determination of mercury in all its forms, so that our understanding of the mechanisms of action of mercury compounds need not be hampered in the future by imperfect data, as it has in the past.

Reference Sources Used

I. Elemental, Inorganic, and Total Mercury Methods
   A. Activation Analysis (Neutron Activation)

Bate, L. C. "The Use of Activation Analysis in Procedures for the Removal and Characterization of the Surface Contaminants of Hair," J. Forensic Sci., *1*:60 (1965).

Brar, S. S., D. M. Nelson, E. D. Kanabrocki, C. E. Moore, C. D. Burnham, and D. M. Hattori. "Thermal Neutron Activation Analysis of Airborne Particulate Matter in Chicago Metropolitan Area," U. S. National Bureau of Standards Special Publication (1969), pp. 43-54.

Brar, S. S., D. M. Nelson, J. R. Kline, P. F. Gustafson, E. L. Kanabrocki, C. E. Moore, and D. M. Hattori. "Instrumental Analysis for Trace Elements Present in Chicago Area Surface Air," J. Geophys. Res., *75*:2939 (1970).

Brune, D. "Low Temperature Irradiation Applied to Neutron Activation Analysis of Mercury in Human Whole Blood," Acta Chem. Scand., *20*: 1200 (1966).

Brune, D. "Aspects of Low Temperature Irradiation in Neutron Activation Analysis," Anal. Chim. Acta, *44*: 15 (1969).

Brune, D. and K. Jirlow. "Determination of Mercury in Aqueous Samples by Means of Neutron Activation Analysis with an Account of Flux Disturbances," Radiochim. Acta 8: 161 (1967).

Christell, R., et al. "Methods of Activation Analysis for Mercury in the Biosphere and in Foods," in Proceedings of 1965 International Conference on Modern Trends in Activation Analysis (Texas A & M University Press, 1966), p. 380.

Comar, D., C. LePoec, M. Joly, and C. Kellershorhn. "Analysis by Radioactivation. Application to the Determination of Iodine, Mercury, Copper, Manganese, and Zinc in Biological Material," Bull. Soc. Chim. (France, 1962), p. 56.

Dams, R., J. A. Robbins, K. A. Rahn, and J. W. Winchester. "Nondestructive Neutron Activation Analysis of Air Pollution Particulates," Anal. Chem., 42:861 (1970).

Ehman, W. D. and J. R. Huizenga. "Bismuth, Thallium and Mercury in Stone Meteorites by Activation Analysis," Geochim. Cosmochim. Acta, 17:125 (1959).

Häsänen, E., "Determination of Mercury in Biological Material by Neutron Activation Analysis," Suomen. Kemistlehti, 43:251 (1970).

Hoshino, O., K. Tanzawa, T. Terao, T. Ukita, and A. Ohuchi. "Quantitative Determination of Mercury in Hair by Activation Analysis," J. Hyg. Soc. Japan, 12: 94 (1966).

Ishida, K., S. Kawamura, and M. Izawa. "Neutron Activation Analysis for Mercury," Anal. Chim. Acta, 50:351 (1970).

Johansen, O. and Steinnes. "A Simple Neutron Activation Method for Mercury in Biological Material," Int. J. Appl. Radiat. Isotopes, 20: 751 (1969).

Kellershohn, C., D. Comar, and C. LePoec. "Determination of the Hg Content of Human Blood by Activation Analysis," J. Lab. Clin. Med., 66: 168 (1965).

Kim, C. K. and J. Silverman. "Determination of Mercury in Wheat and Tobacco Leaf by Neutron Activation Analysis Using Mercury-197 and a Simple Exchange Separation," Anal. Chem., 37: 1616 (1965).

Kosta, L. and A. R. Byrne. "Activation Analysis for Mercury in Biological Samples at Nanogram Level," Talanta, 16: 1297 (1969).

Kusaka, Y., H. Tusji, I. Fujii, H. Muto, and K. Miyoshi. "X-Ray Spectrometry in Radioactivation Analysis with 14-Mev. Neutrons," Bull. Chem. Soc. Japan, 38: 616 (1965).

Montalvo, J. G., Jr., D. P. Thibodeaux, and E. Klein. "Sample Preparation for Neutron Activation Analysis. Deposition of Mercury on a Plastic Matrix," Anal. Chim. Acta, *52*: 160 (1970).

Pijck, J. "Determination of Mercury Traces in Histological Sections by Radioactivation," J. Pharm. Belg., *20*: 420 (1965).

Rayudu, G. V. S., B. Tiefenbach, and R. E. Jervis. "Neutron Activation Determination of Trace Mercury in Canadian Foods," in Transactions of the American Nuclear Society 14th Annual Meeting (1968), p. 54.

Rottschafer, J. M., J. D. Jones, and H. B. Hark, Jr. "A Simple, Rapid Method for Determining Trace Mercury in Fish via Neutron Activation Analysis," Environ. Sci. Technol., *5*: 336 (1971).

Samsahl, K. "Radiochemical Method for Determination of Arsenic, Bromine, Mercury, Antimony and Selenium in Neutron-Irradiated Biological Material," Anal. Chem., *39*: 1480 (1967).

Samsahl, K., D. Brune, and P. O. Webster. "Simultaneous Determination of 30 Trace Elements in Cancerous and Non-Cancerous Human Tissue Samples by Neutron Activation Analysis," Int. J. Appl. Radiat. Isotopes, *16*: 273 (1965).

Sion, H. "The Separation of Traces of Mercury and the Determination Thereof by Activation Analysis with Thermal Neutrons," Verhandel. Koninkl. Vlaam. Acad. Wetenschap., Belg., Kl. Wetenschap., *26*: 110 (1964).

Sion, H., J. Hoste, and J. Gillis. "Collection of Mercury from Urine and Determination by Neutron-Activation Analysis," Microchem. J. Symp. Ser., *2*: 959 (1962).

Sjostrand, B. "Simultaneous Determination of Mercury and Arsenic in Biological and Organic Materials by Activation Analysis," Anal. Chem., *36*: 814 (1964).

Smith, H. "Estimation of Mercury in Biological Material by Neutron Activation Analysis," Anal. Chem., *35*: 635 (1963).

Szkolnik, M., K. D. Hickey, E. J. Broderick, and D. J. Lisk. "Mercury Residue of Apple Fruit as Related to Application Schedules and to the Colorimetric and the Neutron Activation Analysis," Plant Disease Reporter, *49*: 568 (1965).

U. S. Geological Survey. "The Determination of Mercury in Water by Neutron Activation Analyisis," Unpublished (1970).

Westermark, T., and B. Sjostrand. "Activation Analyisis of Mercury," Int. J. Appl. Radiat. Isotopes, *9*: 1 (1960).

Westermark, T. and K. Ljunggren. "Development of Analytical Methods for Mercury and Studies on its Dissemination from Industrial Sources," in Report to the Swedish Technical Research Council, Isotope Technics Labs., S-114 28 (Stockholm, Sweden: 1968).

B. Atomic Absorption and Fluorescence
   1. Volatilization by Flame and by Heated, Non-Flame Methods, Direct Air Analysis by Ultraviolet Photometry, etc.

Azzaria, L. M., and G. R. Webber. "Mercury Analysis in Geochemical Exploration," Can. Inst. Mining Met. Bull. *62*: 521 (1969).

Ballard, A. E., L. W. Stewart, W. O. Kamm, and C. W. Zuehlke. "Photometric Mercury Analysis - Correction for Organic Substances," Anal. Chem., *26*: 921 (1954).

Ballard, A. E. and C. W. D. Thornton. "Photometric Method for Estimation of Minute Amounts of Mercury," Ind. Eng. Chem., Anal. Ed., *13*: 893 (1941).

Barakso, J. J. and C. Tarnocai. "Mercury Determination Method and its Use for Exploration in British Columbia," Can. Inst. Mining Met. Bull., *63*: 501 (1970).

Berman, E. "Determination of Cadmium, Thallium and Mercury in Biological Materials by Atomic Absorption," At. Absorption Newslett., *6*: 57 (1967).

Berman, E. "Applications of Atomic Absorption Spectrometry to Trace Metal Analyses of Toxicological Materials," Progr. Chem. Toxicol., *4*: 155 (1969).

Biggs, L. R. "Mercury Vapor Detection," J. Ind. Hyg. Toxicol., *20*: 161 (1938).

Brandenberger, H. and H. Bader. "Determination of Mercury by Flameless Atomic Absorption. II. A Static Vapor Method," At. Absorption Newslett., *7*: 53 (1968).

Brandenberger, H. and H. Bader. "Determination of Nanogram Levels of Mercury in Solution by a Flameless Atomic Absorption Technique," Helv. Chim. Acta, *50*: 1409 (1967).

Brandenberger, H. and H. Bader. "Determination of Nanogram Levels of Mercury in Solution by a Flameless Atomic Absorption Technique," At. Absorption Newslett., *6*: 101 (1967).

Delaughter, B. "Mercury Determination in Industrial Plant Atmospheres by Atomic Absorption Spectrophotometry," At. Absorption Newslett., *9*: 49 (1970).

Ely, T. S. "Improved Mercury Vapor Detector," WASH-744, Div. of Biology and Medicine. (U. S. Atomic Energy Commission: Health Protection Branch, October 1957).

Feldman, C. and R. Dhumwad. "An Atomic Absorption Tube for Use With an Atomizer Burner: Application to the Determination of Mercury," Proc. 6th Conf. Anal. Chem. in Nucl. React. Tech., Gatlinburg, AEC. TID 7655:379 (1962).

Fishman, M. J. "Determination of Mercury in Water," Anal. Chem., *42*: 1462 (1970).

Hasegawa, N., A. Hiral, and T. Kashiwagi. "Application of Atomic Absorption Analysis in the fields of Medicine, Biology and Hygienics," Annual Report of the Research Institute of Environmental Medicine, Nagoya University (Japan), *16*: 1 (1968).

Hemeon, W. C. and G. F. Haines. "Automatic Sampling and Determination of Microquantities of Mercury Vapor," Amer. Ind. Hyg. Assoc. J., *22*: 75 (1961).

Hermann, W. J., Jr., J. W. Butler, and R. G. Smith. "The Determination of Mercury in Biological Fluids," Manual of Procedures for the Applied Seminar on Laboratory Diagnosis of Diseases Caused by Toxic Agents (1968), p. XII-1.

Hingle, D. N., G. F. Kirkbright, and T. S. West. "Determination of Mercury by Atomic Absorption Spectroscopy in an Air-acetylene Flame," Analyst, *92*: 759 (1967).

Hinkle, M. E. and R. E. Learned. "Determination of Mercury in Natural Waters by Collection on Silver Screens," U. S. Geological Survey Professional Paper, 650-D D251-4 (1969).

Ipatov, V. A. and L. P. Pakhomov. "Photoelectric Apparatus for the Determination of Mercury Vapor in Air," Pribory i Tekh. Eksperimenta., *2*: 91 (1958).

Jacobs, M. B. "Microdetermination of Mercury in Tissue," Amer. Ind. Hyg. Assoc. Conf. Abstracts (Houston, Texas: 1965).

Jacobs, M. B., L. J. Goldwater, and H. Gilbert. "Ultramicrodetermination of Mercury in Blood," Amer. Ind. Hyg. Assoc. J., *22*: 276 (1961).

Jacobs, M. B. and R. Jacobs. "Photometric Determination of Mercury Vapor in Air of Mines and Plants," Amer. Ind. Hyg. Assoc. J., *26*: 261 (1965).

Jacobs, M. B., S. Managuchi, L. Goldwater, and H. Gilbert. "Determination of Mercury in Blood," Amer. Ind. Hyg. Assoc. J., *21*: 475 (1960).

James, C. H. and J. S. Webb. "Sensitive Hg Vapor Meter for Use in Geochemical Prospecting," Bull. Inst. Mining Met., *691*: 633 (1964).

Kalb, G. W. "Determination of Mercury in Water and Sediment Samples by Flameless Atomic Absorption," At. Absorption Newslett., *9*: 84 (1970).

Kudsk, F. N. "Determination of Hg in Dithizone Extracts by Ultra-violet Photometry," Scand. J. Clin. Lab. Invest., 17: 171 (1965).

Kuznetsov, Y. N. and L. P. Chabovskii. "Automatized Rapid Determination of Hg in Powders," Zavdosk. Lab.,31: 1085 (1965).

Lidums, V. and U. Ulfvarson. "Mercury Analysis in Biological Material by Direct Combustion in Oxygen and Photometric Determination of the Mercury Vapor," Acta Chem. Scand., 22: 2150 (1968).

Lidums, V. and U. Ulfvarson. "Preparation of Average Sample Solution of Heterogeneous Organic Materials for Determination of Microquantities of Mercury Using Purified Sodium Hydroxide," Acta Chem. Scand., 22: 2379 (1968).

Lindström, O. "Rapid Microdetermination of Mercury by Spectrophotometric Flame Combustion," Anal. Chem., 31: 461 (1959).

Ling, C. "Portable Atomic Absorption Photometer for Determining Nanogram Quantities of Mercury in the Presence of Interfering Substance," Anal. Chem., 40: 1876 (1968).

Ling, C. "Sensitive Simple Hg Photometer Using Hg Resonance Lamp as a Monochromatic Source," Anal. Chem., 39: 798 (1967).

Malenfant, E. M. "Mercury Pollution Monitoring by Atomic Absorption Utilizing a Gas Cell Technique," Presented at 12th Ann. Eastern Anal. Conf. (New York, 1970).

Manning, D. C. and F. Fernandez. "Cobalt Spectral Interference in the Determination of Mercury," At. Absorption Newslett., 7: 24 (1968).

Mansell, R. E. "Analytical Method for Industrial Application of Atomic Absorption Spectroscopy," 12th Anachem. Mtg. (Detroit, October 1964).

Mansell, R. and E. Hunemorder. "A Photometric Method for Trace Mercury Determination Using a Beckman DU Spectrophotometer," Anal. Chem., 35: 1981 (1963).

Mansfield, J. M., J. D. Winefordner, and C. Veillon. "High Sensitivity Determination of Zinc, Cadmium, Mercury, Thallium, Gallium and Indium by Atomic Fluorescence Flame Spectrometry," Anal. Chem., 37: 1049 (1965).

McBryde, W. T. and F. Williams. "A Rapid Determination of Micro Quantities of Mercury in Urine and Water Using the Mercurimenter," U. S. Atomic Energy Commission Report Y-1178 (1957).

Mesman, B. B. and B. S. Smith. "Determination of Mercury in Urine by Atomic Absorption, Utilizing the APDC/MIBK [Ammonium Pyrrolidine Dithiocarbamata/Methyl Isobutyl Ketone] Extraction System and Boat Technique," At. Absorption Newslett., *9*: 81 (1970).

Meyer, W. T. and D. S. Evans. "Determination of Trace Mercury in Soil and Rock Media. Comments," Econ. Geol., *65*: 357 (1970).

Moffitt, A. E. and R. E. Kupel. "A Rapid Method Employing Impregnated Charcoal for the Determination of Mercury," Submitted to Amer. Ind. Hyg. Assoc. J. (1971).

Monkman, J. L., P. A. Maffett, and T. F. Doherty, "The Determination of Mercury in Air Samples and Biological Materials," Ind. Hyg. Quart., *17*: 410 (1956).

Muller, K. "New Method to Determine the Content of Mercury in Air, "Z. Phys., *65*: 739 (1930).

Muller, K. and P. Pringsheim. "Optical Method for Measuring Mercury Content of Air.," Naturwissenschaften, *18*: 364 (1930).

Nakanishi, S. and K. Fukuda. "Determination of Mercury in Getter for Cathode Indicator Tubes by Atomic Absorption Spectrophotometry," Shin. Nippon Denki Giho, *5*: 26 (1970).

Novikov, V. M. and S. Ya Gol'dapel. "Atomic Absorption Determination of Mercury in Rocks," Ezheg. Inst. Geokhim. Sib. Otd. Akad. Nauk SSSR (1968), p. 297.

Poluektov, N. S. and R. A. Vitkun. "Determination of Hg by Absorption Flame Photometry," Zh. Anal. Khim., *18*: 37 (1963).

Pyrih, R. Z. and R. E. Bisque. "Determination of Trace Mercury in Soil and Rock Media. Reply to Comments," Econ. Geol., *65*: 358 (1970).

Razumov, V. A. and T. P. Utkina. "Device for the Rapid Atomic Absorption Determination of Trace Amounts of Mercury in Liquids, Powders, and Optical Coatings," Spektrosk. Tr. Sib. Soveshch., 4th (1969), p. 291.

Saltzman, R. S., E. S. Taylor, R. S. Crowder, and G. W. Reilly, Jr. "Multipoint Analyzer for Atomic Monitoring for Parts Per Billion Organic Mercury," Proc. Ann. Instr. Autom. Conf. Exhibit 17, Pt. 2:40-1-62, 1-8 (1962).

Shater, K. S., A. F. Eremina, A. I. Semeryakova, V. V. Smirnov, and A. V. Efremov. "Spectral Determination of Mercury in Waste Waters," Zavod. Lab., *36*: 1470 (1970).

Slavin, W. "Applications of Optical Absorption Spectroscopy to Analytical Biochemistry and Toxicology," Occup. Hlth. Rev., *17*: 9 (1965).

Smith, R. G., R. E. Barrow, and P. Roggenbaum. "The Determination of Mercury in Air," Abstract, Amer. Ind. Hyg. Assoc. Mtg. (Houston, Texas, 1965).

Stepanov, I. I., A. A. Rudkovskii, and V. Z. Fursov. "Metallic Gold Sorbent for Mercury Determination in Geochemical Samples by an Atomic Absorption Method," Izv. Akad. Nauk. Kaz. SSR, Ser. Geol., *26*: 84 (1969).

Szadkowski, D., G. Lehnert, and H. G. Essing. "Mercury Determination in Urine as the Medical Procedure to Detect Disease," Med. Welt., *28*: 1298 (1970).

Tindall, F. M. "Mercury Analysis by Atomic Absorption Spectrophotometry," At. Absorption Newslett., *6*: 104 (1967).

Toribara, T. Y. and C. P. Shields. "Analysis of Submicrogram Amounts of Mercury in Tissues," Amer. Ind. Hyg. Assoc. J., *29*: 87 (1968).

Troy, D. J. "Measurement of Atmospheric Pollution by Ultraviolet Photometry," Anal. Chem., *27*: 1217 (1955).

Ulfvarson, U. "Determination of Mercury in Small Quantities in Biologic Material by a Modified Photometric Mercury Vapor Procedure," Acta Chem. Scand., *21*: 641 (1967).

U. S. Geol. Survey. "Tentative Method for Determining Mercury in Water (Silver Wire AA Procedure)," U. S. Geological Survey, unpublished (1970).

Vaughn, W. W. "A Simple Hg Vapor Detector for Geochemical Prospecting," U. S. Geological Survey Report 540 (1967).

Vaughn, W. W. and J. H. McCarthy, Jr. "An Instrumental Technique for the Determination of Submicrogram Concentrations in Mercury in Soils, Rocks and Gas," U. S. Geological Survey Professional Papers 501-D D123 (1964).

Vickers, T. J. and S. P. Merrick. "Determination of Part-Per-Millard Concentrations of Mercury by Atomic Fluorescence Flame Spectrometry," Talanta *15*: 875 (1968).

Vitkun, R. A., N. S. Poluektov, and Yu. V. Zelyukova. "Atomic-Fluorescent Determination of Mercury," Zh. Anal. Khim., *25*: 474 (1970).

Wenninger, J. A. "Direct Microdetermination of Mercury in Color Additives by the Photometric-Mercury Vapor Procedure," J. Ass. Offic. Anal. Chem., *48*: 826 (1965).

Wenninger, J. A. and J. H. Jones. "Determination of Submicrogram Amounts of Mercury in Inorganic Pigments by the Photometric Mercury Vapor Procedure," J. Ass. Offic. Agr. Chemists, *46*: 1018 (1963).

Willis, J. B. "Determination of Pb and Other Heavy Metals in Urine by Atomic Absorption Spectroscopy," Anal. Chem., *34*: 614 (1962).

Williston, S. H. Method of Detecting Hg Vapor by Collecting the Hg and Thereafter Analyzing the Collected Hg by Ultraviolet Analysis. U. S. Patent 3,281,596. Cl. 250-435 (Oct. 25, 1966. Appl. Mar. 23, 1964), 6 pp.

Williston, S. H. "Mercury in the Atmosphere," J. Geophysical Res., 73: 7051 (1968).

Winefordner, J. D. and R. A. Staab. "Determination of Zinc, Cadmium, and Mercury by Atomic Fluorescence Flame Spectrometry," Anal. Chem., 36: 165 (1964).

Woodson, T. T. "Industrial Mercury Vapor Detector," Rev. Sci. Instrum., 10: 308 (1939).

Zuehlke, C. W. and A. E. Ballard. "Estimation of Minute Amounts of Mercury--Use of G. E. Germicidal Ultraviolet Intensity Meter," Anal. Chem., 22: 953 (1950).

B. 2. "Cold-Vapor" Methods (Measurement After Reduction of Hg^{++} to Hg Vapor)

Chau, Y. K. and H. Saitoh. "Determination of Submicrogram Quantities of Mercury in Lake Waters," Environ. Sci. Technol., 4: 839 (1970).

Dill, M. S. "Determination of Submicrogram Quantities of Mercury in Water and Lithium Hydroxide Solutions," AEC Res. & Dev. Rept. Y-1 (Oak Ridge, 1967).

Dow Chemical Company. Determination of Mercury by Atomic Absorption Spectrophotometer Method. (Midland, Michigan: The Dow Chemical Co., 1971).

Gage, J. C. and J. M. Warren. "Determination of Mercury and Organic Mercurials in Biological Samples," Ann. Occup. Hyg., 13:115 (1970).

Hatch, W. R. and L. O. Welland. "Determination of Sub-Microgram Quantities of Mercury by Atomic Absorption Spectrophotometry," Anal. Chem., 40: 2085 (1968).

Hoover, W. L., J. R. Melton, and P. A. Howard. "Determination of Trace Amounts of Mercury in Foods by Flameless Atomic Absorption," J. Ass. Offic. Anal. Chem., 54: 860 (1971).

Jeffus, M. T., J. S. Elkinds, and C. Kenner. "Determination of Mercury in Biological Materials," J. Ass. Offic. Anal. Chem., 53: 1172 (1970).

Lindstedt, G. "A Rapid Method for the Determination of Mercury in Urine," Analyst, 95: 264 (1970).

Lindstedt, G. and I. Skare. "Microdetermination of Mercury in Biological Samples. II. An Apparatus for Rapid Atomic Determination of Mercury in Digested Samples," Analyst, 96: 223 (1971).

Magos, L. and A. A. Chernik. "A Rapid Method for Estimating Mercury in Undigested Biological Samples," Brit. J. Ind. Med., 26: 144 (1969).

Manning, D. C. "Nonflame Methods for Mercury Determination by Atomic Absorption. A Review," At. Absorption Newslett., 9: 97 (1970).

Manning, D. C. "Compensation for Broad-Band Absorption Interference in the Flameless Atomic Absorption Determination of Mercury," At. Absorption Newslett., 9: 109 (1970).

Munns, R. K. and D. C. Holland. "Determination of Mercury in Fish by Flameless Atomic Absorption," J. Ass. Offic. Anal. Chem., 154: 202 (1971).

Omang, S. H. "Determination of Mercury in Natural Waters and Effluents by Flameless Atomic Absorption Spectrophotometry," Anal. Chim. Acta, 53: 415 (1971).

Pappas, E. G. and L. A. Rosenberg. "Determination of Submicrogram Quantities of Mercury in Fish and Eggs by Cold Vapor Atomic Absorption Photometry," J. Ass. Offic. Anal. Chem., 49: 792 (1966).

Pappas, E. G. and L. A. Rosenberg. "Determination of Submicrogram Quantities of Mercury by Cold Vapor Atomic Absorption Photometry," J. Ass. Offic. Anal. Chem., 49: 782 (1966).

Rathje, A. O. "A Rapid Ultraviolet Absorption Method for the Determination of Mercury in Urine," Amer. Ind. Hyg. Assoc. J., 30: 126 (1969).

Schachter, M. M. "Apparatus for Cold Vapor Atomic Absorption of Mercury," J. Ass. Offic. Anal. Chem., 49: 778 (1966).

Schutz, A. "Analytical Method for Small Amounts of Mercury in Blood, Urine, and Other Biological Materials," Rept. 691020 from Dept. of Occup. Med., Univ. Hosp., S-221 85 (Lund, Sweden, 1969).

Stainton, M. P. "Syringe Procedure for Transfer of Nanogram Quantities of Mercury Vapor for Flameless Atomic Absorption Spectrophotometry," Anal. Chem., 43: 625 (1971).

Thorpe, V. A. "Determination of Mercury in Food Products and Biological Fluids by Aeration and Flameless Atomic Absorption Spectrophotometry," J. Ass. Offic. Anal. Chem., 54: 206 (1971).

Uthe, J. F., F. A. J. Armstrong, and M. P. Stainton. "Mercury Determination in Fish Samples by Wet Digestion and Flameless Atomic Absorption Spectrophotometry," J. Fish Res. Bd. Can., 27: 805 (1970).

C. Chromatographic Analysis (Paper, Thin Layer, Liquid, and Ionopheresis)

Canic, V. D., S. M. Petrovic, and A. K. Bern. "Separation of Group II Cations by Using Thin-Layer Chromatography on Corn Starch," Z. Anal. Chem., 213: 251 (1965).

Hayek, E. and I. Haring. "Paper Chromatography of Inorganic Salts in a Completely Aqueous System," Mikrochim. Acta, 211 (1962).

Ivanov, St. A., D. Maneva, P. Toleva, and N. P. Mashev. "Separation of Mercury (I) and Mercury (II) by Means of Precipitation Chromatography," Nauch. Trudove, Visshiya Inst. Kranitelna i Vkusova Prom., 5: 353 (1959).

Johuri, K. N., H. C. Mehra, and N. K. Kaushik. "Determination of Germanium (IV), Tin (II), Lead (II), and Zinc (II), Cadmium (II),Mercury (II) by Ring Chlorimetry After Separation by Thin-Layer Chromatography," Chromatographia, 3: 347 (1970).

Lewandowski, A. and M. Owoc. "Application of Impregnation Method to Indirect Quantitative Determinations," Zeszyty Nauk. Uniw, Posnaniu, Mat., Fiz, Chem., 3: 9 (1960).

Mizak, Bogdan. "Laboratory Detection of Poisoning With Hg, As, Zn, Cu, Th, and Pb by Means of Paper Ionophoresis," Polskie Arch. Weterynar, 9: 595 (1966).

Seiler, H. "Thin-Layer Chromatography as an Aid in Radio-chemistry. 5. Separation of Mercury from a Mixture of Cations," Helv. Chim. Acta, 53: 1893 (1970).

Takitani, S., N. Fukuoka, Y. Iwasaki, and H. Hasegawa. "Inorganic Thin Layer Chromatography. VI. Total Analysis of Metallic Ions by Thin-Layer Chromatography. 3. Effect of Humidity," Bunseki Kagaku, 14: 652 (1965).

Tripathi, I. N. and S. N. Tewari. "Determination in Forensic Toxicology, of Metallic Poisons by Paper Chromatography," J. Prakt. Chem., 9: 1 (1959).

Wasicky, R. "Applications of Paper Chromatography as Additional Means of Characterizing Medical Substances and Other Compounds," Anales Fac. Farm. e Odontol., Univ. Sao Paulo, 17: 33 (1960).

D. Colorimetric (Spectrophotometric)
   1. Dithizone

Ackermann, G. and W. Angermann. "Scheme for the Simultaneous Photometric Determination of Traces of Copper, Mercury, Cadmium, and Thallium," Fresenius' Z. Anal. Chem., 250: 353 (1970), German.

Ajtai, I. R. "Determination of Mercury in Blood," Munkavedelem, 9: 56 (1963).

Ajtai, I. R. "Determination of Urinary Mercury Content by a Simplified Dithizone Method," Munkavedelem, *9*: 46 (1962).

Akiyama, T. and K. Shiokawa. "Circular Paper Chromatography of a Few Metals by the Dithizone Complex," Kyoto Yakka Daigaku Gakuho, *12*: 51 (1964).

American Industrial Hygiene Association. Analytical Guides. "Mercury and Inorganic Compounds," Amer. Ind. Hyg. Assoc. J., *30*: 326 (1969).

American Industrial Hygiene Association. Analytical Guides. "Mercury," Amer. Ind. Hyg. Assoc. J., *30*: 327 (1969).

Analytical Methods Committee, Society for Analytical Chemistry. "The Determination of Small Amounts of Mercury in Organic Matter," Analyst, *90*: 515 (1965).

Ashizawa, T. "Chromatographic Analysis of Traces of Metals with Dithizone. III. Determination of Traces of Mercury by Dithizone Chromatography," Bunseki Kagaku, *10*: 443 (1961).

Association of Official Agricultural Chemists. "Analysis of Mercury," Official Methods of Analysis, 10th ed., secs. 4.150-4.151, 4.152, 32.266-32.272 (Washington, D.C., 1965).

Awaya, H. "Determination of Small Quantities of Mercury by Dithizone and Some Discussions on Oxidation of Mercury," Bunseki Kagaku, *9*: 305 (1960).

Bache, C. A., C. McKone, and D. J. Lisk. "Rapid Determination of Mercury in Fish," J. Ass. Offic. Anal. Chem., *54*: 741 (1971).

Baeumler, J. and S. Rippstein. "Determination of Mercury," Mitt. Gebiete Lebensm. Hyg., *54*: 472 (1963).

Barnes, H. "Determination of Mercury and Copper in Antifouling Compositions: Potassium Cobalt Cyanide as Complex-Forming Agent in Dithizone Technique," Analyst, *71*: 578 (1946).

Barrett, F. R. "Determination of Mercury in Urine, With Results in Cases of Pink-Disease," Med. J. Australia, *42*: 411 (1955).

Barrett, F. R. "Micro-Determination of Mercury in Biological Materials," Analyst, *81*: 294 (1956).

Brookes, H. E. and L. E. Solomon. "The Determination of Mercury by Distillation from Its Compounds and Preparations," Analyst, *84*: 622 (1959).

Buckell, M. "The Rapid Estimation of Mercury in the Atmosphere of Workrooms," Brit. J. Industr. Med., *8*: 181 (1951).

Buis, D. M. and H. Jansen. "A Simplified Method for the Determination of Small Amounts of Mercury in Urine," Pharm. Weekblad., *86*: 359 (1951).

Buis, D. M. and H. Jansen. "Simplified Method for the Estimation of Small Quantities of Mercury in Urine," Pharm. Weekblad., *87*: 789 (1952).

Cafruny, E. J. "A Rapid Procedure for Determination of Mercury in Urine and Kidney," J. Lab. Clin. Med., *57*: 468 (1961).

Campbell, E. E. and B. M. Head. "The Determination of Mercury in Urine--Single Extraction Method," Amer. Ind. Hyg. Assoc. Quart., *16*: 275 (1955).

Cappellina, F. and S. Terlizzi. "Analytical Determination of Mercury in Liquids and Solids of a Chlorine-Soda Electrochemical Plant," Nuova Chim., *46*: 44 (1970).

Carlson, O. T. and P. O. Bethge. "Determination of Mercury in Pulp and Paper," Svensk Papperstidn., *57*: 405 (1954).

Central Industrial Toxicology Lab, Bucherest, Rumania. "Microdetermination of Mercury in Industrial Atmosphere," Rev. Chim., *17*: 368 (1966).

Chen, C. L. "Photometric Determination of Microamount of Mercury in Urine," Sheng Li Pao, *20*: 71 (1958).

Church, F. W. "Determination of Mercury in Air," Referee Std. Method. Am. Conf. Gov't Ind. Hygienists (Accepted Sept. 11, 1951).

Davis, D. E. and K. Linke. "Determination of Traces of Mercury in Paper Mill Products," Proc. Australian Pulp and Paper Ind. Tech. Assoc., *8*: 251 (1954).

Delperdange, G. R. "Control of Mercury Determinations in Biological Analyses," Arch. Int. Physiol. Biochim., *72*: 315 (1964).

Drew, R. G. and E. King. "Determination of Atmospheric Mercury Trapped in Permanganate Solutions: A Modified Method," Analyst, *82*: 461 (1957).

Epps, E. A. "Colorimetric Determination of Mercury Residues in Rice," J. Ass. Offic. Anal. Chem., *49*: 793 (1966).

Fabre, R., R. Truhaut, and C. Boudene. "Microdosage of Mercury in Urine," Ann. Biol. Clin., *16*: 286 (1958).

Falus, V. "Determination of Mercury in Air," Munkavedelem, *7*: 53 (1961).

Friedeberg, H. "Separation and Determination of Microgram Quantities of Silver, Mercury, and Copper with Dithizone," Anal. Chem., *27*: 305 (1955).

Gettler, A. O. and S. Kaye. "A Simple and Rapid Analytical Method for Mercury, Bismuth, Antimony, and Arsenic in Biological Material," J. Lab. Clin. Med., *35*: 146 (1950).

Gettler, A. O. and R. A. Lehman. "A Simplified Method for the Determination of Mercury in Urine," Am. J. Clin. Path., *8*: 161 (1938).

Gladysheva, K. F. "Determination of Small Amounts of Mercury," Sb. Nauchn. Tr. Vses. Nauchn.-Issled. Gorno-Met. Inst. Tsvetn. Metal., *7*: 325 (1962).

Goldberg, D. M. and A. D. Clarke. "Measurement of Mercury in Human Urine," J. Clin. Path., *23*: 178 (1970).

Griffini, G. M. and G. C. Gerosa. "Microdetermination of Mercury in the Air and in Biological Materials," LaMedicina del Lavoro, *12*: 69549 (1954).

Gutenmann, W. H. and D. J. Lisk. "Rapid Determination of Mercury in Apples by Modified Schöniger Combustion," J. Agr. Food Chem., *8*: 306 (1960).

Irving, H., G. Andrew, and E. J. Risdon. "Studies with Dithizone. I. Determination of Traces of Mercury," J. Chem. Soc., 541 (1949).

Irving, H. M. and A. M. Kiwan. "Dithizone. XV. Reactions with Organomercury Compounds," Anal. Chim. Acta, *45*: 255 (1969).

Irving, H. M. and A. M. Kiwan. "Dithizone. XVI. Water-Soluble Arylmercury (II) Dithiazonates and Secondary Arylmercury (II) Dithizonates," Anal. Chim. Acta, *45*: 271 (1969).

Irving, H. M. and A. M. Kiwan. "Studies with Dithizone. XVII. Extraction Constants of Organomercury (II) Dithizonates," Anal. Chim. Acta, *45*: 447 (1969).

Jacobs, M. B. and A. Singerman. "One Color Method for the Determination of Mercury in Urine," J. Lab. Clin. Med., *59*: 871 (1962).

Johansson, A. and H. Uhrnell. "Determination of Mercury in Urine," Acta Chem. Scand., *9*: 583 (1955).

Kanazawa, J. and R. Sato. "Determination of Mercury in Organic Mercury Fungicides by the Dithizone Method," Bunseki Kagaku, *8*: 440 (1959).

Kato, T., S. Takei, and A. Okagami. "Determination of Substances in Minute Quantity. XIII. The Determination of a Small Amount of Mercury in the Presence of Large Amounts of Cl Ion and an Equilibrium of Enolized Dithizone-Mercury (II) Compound," Technol. Repts. Tohoku Univ., *21*: 291 (1957).

Kimura, Y. and V. L. Miller. "Mercury Determination at the Microgram Level by a Reduction-Aeration Method of Concentration," Anal. Chim. Acta, *27*: 325 (1962).

Klein, A. K. "Report on Mercury," J. Ass. Offic. Agr. Chem., *32*: 351 (1949).

Klein, A. K. "Report on Mercury," J. Ass. Offic. Agr. Chem., *33*: 594 (1950).

Klein, A. K. "Report on (Determination of) Mercury," J. Ass. Offic. Agr. Chem., *34*: 529 (1951).

Klein, A. K. "Report on Mercury," J. Ass. Offic. Agr. Chem., 35: 537 (1952).

Kopp, J. F. and R. G. Keenan. "Determination of Submicrogram Quantities of Mercury in Urine by Ion Exchange Separation," Amer. Ind. Hyg. Assoc. J., 24: 1 (1963).

Kozelka, F. L. "Determination of Mercury in Biological Material," Ind. Eng. Chem. Anal. Ed., 19: 494 (1947).

Kudsk, F. N. "Specific Determination of Mercury in Urine," Scand. J. Clin. Lab. Invest., 16: 670 (1964).

Kudsk, F. N. "Determination of Mercury in Biological Materials. Specific and Sensitive Dithizone Method," Scand. J. Clin. Lab. Invest., 16: 575 (1964).

Kudsk, F. N. "Chemical Determination of Mercury in Air," Scand. J. Clin. Lab. Invest. 16, Suppl., 77: 1 (1964).

Laug, E. P. and K. W. Nelson. "Report on Mercury," J. Ass. Offic. Agr. Chem., 25: 399 (1942).

Loffler, A. and M. Putinaru. "Colorimetric Determination of Mercury with Dithizone," Rev. Chim. (Bucharest), 13: 374 (1962).

Mabmann, W. and D. Sprecher. "Toxicological Analysis for Mercury," Arch. Toxicol., 16: 264 (1957).

Majer, V. "Determination of Traces of Mercury," Chem. Listy, 28: 169 (1934).

Marecek, J. and E. Singer. "Determination of Cu, Hg, and Ag in Pure U Compounds," Z. Anal. Chem., 203: 336 (1964).

Maren, T. H. "A Simple and Accurate Method for the Determination of Mercury in Biological Material," J. Lab. Clin. Med., 28: 1511 (1943).

Mayer, J. "Digestion of Oysters for the Determination of Mercury," Bull. Environ. Contam. Toxicol., 5: 383 (1970).

Melles, J. L. and W. de Bree. "The Determination of Microgram Quantities of Mercury," Rec. Trav. Chem. Pays-Bas, 72: 576 (1953).

Merodio, J. C. "The Separation and Determination of Small Amounts of Mercury in Organic Compounds," Rev. Fac. Cienc. Quim., Univ. Nacl. La Plata, 33: 111 (1960-61).

Miller, V. L. and F. Swanberg, Jr. "Determination of Mercury in Urine," Anal. Chem., 29: 391 (1957).

Miller, W. L. and L. E. Wachter. "Determination of Traces of Mercury in Copper Alloys," Anal. Chem., 22: 1312 (1950).

Milton, R. F. and J. L. Hoskins. "The Estimation of Traces of Mercury in Urine," Analyst, 72: 6 (1947).

Nagai, H. "Paper Chromatography of Inorganic Cations with Dithizone," Nippon Kagaku Zasshi, 80: 617 (1959).

Nagai, H. "Paper Chromatography of Inorganic Ions by Using Organic Analytical Reagents. VIII. Paper Chromatography of Cations with Dithizone," Kumamoto J. Sci. Ser. A4: 265 (1960).

Nardini, F. and S. Pasquini. "Mercury Determination in Biological Material," Med. D. Lavoro, 47: 13 (1956).

Nishimura, M. and H. Aoki. "A Simplified Method of Determining Mercury in Urine," Med. Biol. (Tokyo), 70: 167 (1965).

Nobel, S. and D. Nobel. "Determination of Mercury in Urine," Clin. Chem., 4: 150 (1958).

Ohta, N., M. Terai, and M. Isokawa. "Photometric Determination of Mercury in Natural Waters," Nippon Kagaku Zasshi, 91: 351 (1970).

Oliver, W. T. and H. S. Funnell, "A Quantitative Determination of Mercury in Animal Tissues," Am. J. Vet. Research, 19: 999 (1958).

Pedrero, P. S. and M. D. Hermoso. "Spectrophotometric Determination of Mercury in Urine and Other Biological Samples," Med. y Seguridad Trabajo, 9: 23 (1961).

Pickard, J. A. and J. T. Martin. "Determination of Mercury in Soil," J. Sci. Food Agr., 24: 706 (1963).

Polley, D. and V. L. Miller. "Rapid Microprocedure for Determination of Mercury in Biological and Mineral Materials," Anal. Chem., 27: 1162 (1955).

Rolfe, A. C., F. R. Russell, and N. T. Wilkinson. "The Absorptiometric Determination of Mercury in Urine," Analyst, 80: 523 (1955).

Sandell, E. B. Colorimetric Determination of Traces of Metals. 3rd Ed. (New York: Interscience Publishers, Inc., 1959), p. 635.

Sandell, E. B. Colorimetric Determination of Traces of Metals. 4th Ed. (New York: Interscience Publishers Inc., 1965).

Saredo, J. F. and N. S. Arrechea. "Causes of Losses of Mercury in Destruction of Organic Matter With Nitric and Sulfuric Acids," Anales Fac. Quim. Univ. Rep. Oriental Uruguay, 6: 99 (1960).

Saredo, J. F. and N. S. Arreddiea. "Determination of Mercury in Urine," Anales Fac. Quim. Y. Farm., Univ. Rep. Oriental Uruguay, 6: 81 (1960).

Sheyanova, F. R. and G. Ya Kozhokina. "Dependence of Extraction of Dithizonates of Mercury, Cobalt, and Thallium on Several Factors," Trudy po Khim. i Khim. Tekhnol., 3: 70 (1960).

Simonsen, D. G. "Determination of Mercury in Biologic Materials," Am. J. Clin. Path., 23: 789 (1953).

Smart, N. A. and A. R. C. Hill. "Determination of Mercury
    Residues in Potatoes, Grain, and Animal Tissues Using
    Perchloric Acid Digestion," Analyst, *94*: 143 (1969).
Sorby, D. L. and E. M. Plein. "A Simplified Colorimetric
    Method for Determination of Mercury in Biologic
    Materials," J. Amer. Pharm. Ass., *49*: 160 (1960).
Tomitaro, F., M. Yamada, and S. Masuda. "A Simplified
    Method for the Determination of Mercury in the Urine,"
    Koshu Eiseiin Kenkyu Hokoku, *11*: 56 (1962).
Tsuchiya, K., T. Suzuku, and M. Mishimura. "A Joint Study
    of Microdetermination of Urinary Mercury by Investigators
    from Three Different Institutes, in Order to Establish
    a Standard Method," Jap. J. Hyg., *18*: 229 (1963).
Ujihira, Y. "Separation and Concentration of Traces of
    Elements by Carrier Precipitation with Dithizone,"
    Bunseki Kagaku, *14*: 399 (1965).
United Kingdom Atomic Energy Authority. "The Determination
    of Mercury in Human Urine (Analytical Method)," IGO-
    Am/CA-174 UKAEA. Industr. Group. (Capenhurst, England:
    Capenhurst Works, 1958).
Vasak, V. and V. Sedivec. "Application of Complexone in
    Colorimetry-Determination of Mercury," Collection
    Czechoslav. Chem. Communs., *15*: 1076 (1951).
Vasilevska, A. E., V. P. Shcherbakov, and E. V. Karadazova.
    "Determination of Mercury in Coals," Zh. Anal. Khim.,
    19: 1200 (1964).
Vasilevska, A. E., V. P. Shcherbakov, and V. I. Klimenchuk.
    "Determination of Mercury in Coal by Dithizone," Zavod.
    Lab., *28*: 415 (1962).
Vasilevskaya, A. E. and V. P. Shcherbakov. "Determination
    of Mercury in Soils," Pochvovedenie, *10*: 96 (1963).
Vasilevskaya, A. E., V. P. Shcherbakov, and A. V. Levchenko.
    "Determination of Small Amounts of Mercury in Water,"
    Zh. Anal. Khim., *18*: 811 (1963).
Vesterberg, R. and O. Sjoholm. "On the Determination of
    Mercury and Copper in Biological Material," Ark. Kemi
    Mineral Geol., *22* (1946).
Ward, F. N. and E. H. Bailey. "Camp and Sample-Site
    Determination of Traces of Mercury in Soils and Rocks,"
    Am. Inst. Mining, Metall., and Petroleum Engineers,
    Trans., *217*: 343 (1960).
Ward, F. N. and J. B. McHugh. "A Determination of Mercury
    in Vegetation with Dithizone - A Single Extraction
    Procedure," U. S. Geol. Survey Prof. Paper 501D, 128
    (1964).
Weber, A. O. and K. Voloder. "The Determination of Small
    Amounts of Mercury in Biological Material," Arhin. Za.
    Higijenu. Rada., *1*: 235 (1957).

Weiner, I. M. and O. H. Muller. "Interference of Sulfhydryl Groups in Analysis of Urinary Mercury and Its Elimination," Anal. Chem., *27*: 149 (1955).
White, M. N. and D. J. Lisk. "Note on the Determination of Mercury in Soil by Oxygen Flash," J. Ass. Offic. Anal. Chem., *53*: 530 (1970).
Winkler, W. O. "Report on Mercury," J. Ass. Offic. Agr. Chem., *21*: 220 (1938).
Winkler, W. O. "Report on Mercury," J. Ass. Offic. Agr. Chem., *23*: 310 (1940).
Yamamura, S. "Simplified Colorimetric Determination of Mercury," Anal. Chem., *32*: 1896 (1960).

D. 2. Non-Dithizone Reagents (Also Fluorometric Methods)

Aleksandrov, A. and P. Vasileva-Aleksandrova. "Identification of Mercury(I) and Mercury(II), and Mo.," Mikrochim. Ichoanal. Acta, *23*: 5 (1963).
Asperger, S. and I. Murati. "Determination of Mercury in the Atmosphere. Sub-Microanalytical Determination of Mercuric Ion in Bromine and Chlorine Water Based on its Catalytic Action," Anal. Chem., *26*: 543 (1954).
Asperger, S., I. Murati, and I. O. Cupahin. "Spectrophotometric Determination of Traces of Mercuric Ions in Distilled Water," Acta Pharm. Jugoslav., *3*: 20 (1953).
Auergesellschaft, G. mbH (by Wolfgang Fleischer). Detecting Mercury Vapors in Air. Patent. Ger. 1,145,829, (Cl. 421, Mar. 21, 1963, Appl. Aug 9, 1961).
Barnes, E. C. "The Determination of Mercury in Air," J. Ind. Hyg. Toxicol., *28*: 257 (1946).
Barni, B. and I. Barni. "The Application of Polley and Miller's Method to the Determination of Mercury in Biological Fluids," Lav Umano, *18*: 462 (1966).
Blazsek, A. and M. Gyorgy. "The Complexometric Determination of Mercury in Certain Inorganic and Organic Drugs," Farm. Aikakauslehti, *71*: 89 (1962).
Bregvadze, U. D. and M. N. Mirianashvili. "Linear-Colorimetric Method for Determining Mercury Vapors in Air," Sb. Nauchn. Rabot Inst. Okhrany Truda, Vses. Tsentr. Sov. Prof. Soyuzov, No. 4: 120 (1961).
Bregvadza, V. D. and M. N. Mirianashvili. "Determination of Small Amounts of Mercury in Dust," Sb. Nauchn. Rabot Inst. Okhrany Truda Vses. Tsentr. Soveta Prof. Soyuzov, No. 3: 103 (1961).
Bukowska, A. and W. Wawrzyczek. "Titration of Mercurous Ions with Sodium Molybdate," Chem. Anal. (Warsaw), *9*: 625 (1964).

Busev, A. I. and L. Khintibidze. "Antipyrene Dyes as Reagents for the Photometric Determination of Mercury (II)," Zh. Analit. Khim., 22: 857 (1967).

Cholak, J., and D. Hubbard. "Micro-Determination of Mercury in Biological Material," Ind. Eng. Chem., Anal. Ed., 18: 149 (1946).

Deguchi, M. and K. Sakai. "Colorimetric Determination of Mercury(II) With Methylxylenol Blue," Bunseki Kagaku, 19: 241 (1970).

Dutkiewicz, T. "Determination of Mercury in the Air and Urine and Critical Evaluation of the Risks of Mercury Poisoning," Med. Pracy, 3: 257 (1953).

Efremov, G. V. and V. V. Dyatlova. "Use of Schoeniger's Method in Paper Chromatography," Vestn. Leningrad. Univ. 17: Ser. Fiz. i Khim. 2: 159 (1962).

Fabiani, P. and A. Queuille. "A Problem of Research and of the Estimation of Mercury in Urine," Ann. Biol. Clin. (Paris), 8: 199 (1950).

Gershkovich, E. E. "Catalytic Method for the Determination of Mercury in the Atmosphere," Gigiena Truda i Prof. Zabolevaniya, 6: 57 (1962).

Grigorescu, I., V. Marinescu, and G. Toba. "Contributions to the Microdetermination of Mercury in the Industrial Atmosphere," Revised De Chimie, 17: 368 (1966).

Gross, W. "Detection of Mercury in Urine," Klin. Wochenschr., 40: 979 (1962).

Grosskopf, K. "Detection of Small Quantities of Mercury in Air," Draegerheft, 191: 3589 (1937).

Gurvits, B. I.,and G. P. Chuklenkova. "Rapid Method for Determining Mercury Vapors in the Air," Metod. Materialy i Nauchn. Soobshch. Vses. Nauchn Issled. Inst. Zheleznodor. Gigieny, 2: 21 (1962).

Hakkila, E. and G. R. Watterbury. "Separation and Spectrophotometric Determination of Microgram Quantities of Mercury Using Diethyldithiocarbonate," Anal. Chem., 32: 1340 (1960).

Hamamoto, Y. and M. Kotakemori. "Colorimetric Determination of Mercury with Cu-Diethyldithiocarbonate and Estimation of the Solubility of Some Organic Mercury Compounds," Nippon Nogei Kagaku Kaishi, 34: 885 (1960).

Hashitani, H. and K. Katsuyama. "Spectrophotometric Determination of Microquantities of Mercury with Thiothenoyltrifluoroacetone," Bunseki Kagaku, 19: 355 (1970).

Hinkle, M., K. W. Leong, and F. N. Ward. "Field Determination of Nanogram Quantities of Mercury in Soils and Rocks," in Geol. Survey Research, U. S. Geol. Survey Prof. Paper 650-D (1966), p. D251.

Ho, L-S, C-N Kuo, C-S, Shih, and W. Chiang. "Extraction-Colorimetric Determination of Traces of Mercury with 1-(2-Pyridylazo)-2-Naphthol," Hua Hsueh Tung Pao, 4: 250 (1965).

Ho, L-S, C-S Shih, and W. Chiang. "Direct Colorimetric Determination of Mercury with 1-(2-Pyridylazo)-2-Naphthol (PAN)," Hua Hsueh Tung Pao, 4: 253 (1965).

Hubbard, D. M. "Determination of Mercury in Urine," Ind. Eng. Chem. Anal. Ed., 12: 768 (1940).

Hubbard, D. M. and E. W. Scott. "Synthesis of di-B-Naphthylthiocarbazone and Some of its Analogs," J. Amer. Chem. Soc., 65: 2390 (1943).

Iritani, N. and T. Miyahara. "Colorimetric Determination of Mercury with Methylthymol Blue," Bunseki Kagaku, 12: 1183 (1963).

Johar, G. S. "Qualitative Reactions of 5-Chloro-7-Iodo-8-Quinolinol (Iodochlor-Hydroxyquin) with Metal Ions," Labdev. Part A, 8: 150 (1970).

Kato, K. and H. Kakihana. "Microchemical Detection of Mercury(II) with Ion-Exchange Resin Particles," Nippon Kaguku Zasshi, 84: 405 (1963).

Komatsu, S. and S. Kuwano. "Indirect Spectrophotometric Determination of Mercury Ion with Copper Diethyl-dithiocarbamate," Nippon Kagaku Zasshi, 83: 1262 (1962).

Kothny, E. L. "Micromethod for Mercury," Amer. Ind. Hyg. Ass. J., 31: 466 (1970).

Leach, H., E. G. Evans, and W. C. R. Grimmin. "The Estimation of Mercury in Urine Di-B-Naphtylthiocarbazone," Clin. Chim. Acta, 1: 80 (1956).

Malkov, I. I. and N. A. Glebov. "Determination of Small Amounts of Mercury in Mineral Material Using Sample Pulverization," Soobshch. Dal'nevost. Fil. Sibirsk. Otd. Akad. Nauk SSSR, 17: 43 (1963).

Milton, R. F. and W. D. Duffield. "The Estimation of Mercury Compounds in the Atmosphere," Analyst, 72: 11 (1947).

Negoiu, D. and A. Kriza. "Colorimetric Determination of Hg^{++} with Titan Yellow," Analele Univ. "C.I. Parhon" Bucuresti, Ser. Stiint. Nat. Chim., 11: 117 (1962).

Nikolaev, A. V. "Rapid Method for the Determination of Metal Poisons in the Organism of Animals Dead from Poisoning," Veterinariya, 36: 63 (1959).

Nikolaev, A. V. "Mercury Estimation with Na Hydrosulfite," Tr. Vses. Inst. Eksperim. Vet., Vses. Akad. Sel'skokhoz. Nauk, 26: 209 (1962).

Nikolcheva, Y. "A Microquantitative Method for the Determination of Mercury in the Urine by Means of Impregnated Chromatographic Paper," Hig. Zdraveop, *9*: 591 (1966).

Oshima, G. and K. Nagasawa. "Fluorometric Method for Determination of Mercury(II) with Rhodamine B.," Chem. Pharm. Bull., *18*: 687 (1970).

Pavlovic, D. and S. Asperger. "Determination of Traces of Mercury in Biological Material of Catalytic Action of Mercuric Ions. Microelectrolysis of Mercury," Anal. Chem., *31*: 939 (1959).

Pavlovskaya, N. A. "Isolation of Small Quantities of Mercury from Biologic Materials," Aptechnoe Delo, *5*: 25 (1956).

Ploezhaev, N. G. "A Technique for Determination of Mercury in the Air," Gigiena i Sanit., *21*: 74 (1956).

Prasal, Z. "Amino Acid Complexes With Mercury and Copper," Ann. Univ. Mariae Curie-Sklodowska, Lubin-Polonia Sect. D, *17*: 1 (1962).

Protopopova, V. P. "Quantitative Determination of Manganese, Lead, and Mercury in Biological Material," Novoe v Oblasti Sanit.-Khim. Analiza (Raboth po Prom.-Sanit. Khim.), 248 (1962).

Romanowski, H., K. Izdebska, and Z. Przezdziek. "Hydrazine Sulfate and Hydroxylamine HCl as Specific Reagents for the Detection of Mercury and Silver in Toxicological Analysis by a Paper Chromatographic Method," Farm. Polska, *10*: 452 (1961).

Sergeant, G. A., B. E. Dixon, and R. G. Lidzey. "Determination of Mercury in Air," Analyst, *82*: 27 (1957).

Spacu, G. and G. Suciu. "A New and Rapid Method for the Determination of Mercury," Bull. Soc. Stiinte Cluj, *4*: 403 (1929).

Stitt, F. and Y. Tomimatsu. "Analysis: Mercury Vapor Detection," Chem. Eng. (April, 1949).

Stitt, F. and Y. Tomimatsu. "Sensitized Paper for the Estimation of Mercury Vapor," Anal. Chem., *23*: 1098 (1951).

Stock, A. and E. Pohland. "Colorimetric Determination of Very Small Quantities of Mercury," Z. Angew Chem., *39*: 791 (1926).

Stock, A. and W. Zimmerman. "Determination of Minute Amounts of Mercury," Z. Angew. Chem., *41*: 546 (1928).

Stock, A. and W. Zimmerman. "Determination of Minute Quantities of Mercury," Z. Angew. Chem., *42*: 429 (1929).

Taimni, I. K. and R. Paksphal. "Application of Selenium Salts in Inorganic Analysis," Anal. Chim. Acta, *25*: 438 (1961).

Tertoolen, J. W. F., C. Buijze, and G. J. vanKolmeschate. "Photometric Diethyldithiocarbamate Determination of Hg(II) and Ag in the Presence of Large Amounts of Cu and Cu- Alloying Minerals," Chemist-Analyst, *52*: 100 (1963).

Thabet, S. K., N. E. Salibi, and P. W. West. "Redox Reactions on the Ring-Oven. I. Microdetermination of Mercury," Anal. Chim. Acta, *49*: 575 (1970).

Thilenius, R. and R. Winzer. "The Determination of Minute Quantities of Mercury," Z. Angew Chem., *42*: 284 (1929).

Troitskii, A. A. "Determination of Mercury in Urine," Gigiena i Sanit, *4*: 51 (1953).

Truhaut, R. and C. Bondene. "Microdetermination of Mercury in Biologic Material of Animal Origin," Bull. Soc. Chim. Fr., *286*: 1850 (1959).

Truhaut, R. and C. Boudene. "Microdetermination of Mercury in Plants and Foodstuffs," Phytiat.-Phytopharm., *10*: 175 (1961).

Truhaut, R. and C. Boudene. "Microdetermination of Mercury in Air," Arch. des Maladies Professionnelles, Paris, *12*: 694 (1961).

Truhaut, R. and C. Boudene. "Microdetermination of Mercury in Urine and Biological Materials," Occup. Health Rev., *15*: 4 (1963).

Tsubouchi, M. "Spectrophotometric Determination of Trace Amounts of Mercury(II) by Extraction with Bindschedler's Green," Anal. Chem., *42*: 1087 (1970).

Vavoulis, A. "A Spot Test Scheme for the Identification of Metal Ions," J. Chem. Educ., *39*: 395 (1962).

Vol'berg, N. Sh. and E. E. Gershkovich. "Determination of Mercury Present in the Air," Izobiet. Prom. Obaztsy, Tovarnye Znaki, *43*: 100 (1966).

Weyers, J. "Colorimetric Method for the Determination of Mercury in Pharmaceutical Preparations," Dissertationes Pharm., *12*: 29 (1960).

Wronski, M. "Volumetric Determination of Mercury(II) with Thiofluorescein as Indicator," Zh. Anal. Chim., *169*: 351 (1959).

Zhivopistsev, V. P. and A. P. Lipchina. "Pyrazolone Dyes as Analytical Reagents. 2. Extraction-Photometric Determination of Mercury," Uch. Zap., Perm. Gos. Univ. No. *178*, 174 (1969).

E. Electrometric (Polarographic, Amperometric, Coulometric, etc.)

Druzhinin, I. G. and P. S. Kislitsyn. "Inner Electrolysis as an Analytical Method for Determination of Small

Amounts of Some Metals," Trudy Inst. Khim., Akad. Nauk Kirgiz. SSR No. 6, 139 (1955).

Ehrlich, , S. Rogozinsky, and R. Sperling. "Amperometric Determination of Mercury in Organomercurials and Proteins," Anal. Chem., 42: 1089 (1970).

Grandi, F. and L. Salvagnini. "Polarographic Determination of Mercury in Brines and Industrial Waters," Chim. e ind., 41: 430 (1959).

Israel, Y. "Rapid Polarographic Determination of Low Concentrations of Mercuric Ion," Anal. Chem., 31: 1473 (1959).

Kadowaki, H., K. Okamoto, and M. Nakajima. "Organic Mercurial Diuretics. I. Polarographic Determination of Mercury in Urine," J. Pharm. Soc. Japan, 75: 485 (1955).

Merkle, F. H. and C. A. Discher. "Coulometric Titration of Various Organomercurials and Mercury-Containing Compounds," J. Pharm. Sci., 51: 117 (1962).

Mukhamedzhanova, D., Sh. T. Talipov. and V. A. Khadeev. "Amperometric Extractive Titration of Some Cations by Sodium Diethyldithiocarbamate," Uzb. Khim. Zh., 14: 8 (1970).

Overman, R. F. "Potentiometric Titration of Mercury Using the Iodide-Selective Electrode as Indicator," Anal. Chem., 43: 617 (1971).

Usatenko, Yu. I. and A. I. Shumskaya. "Amperometric Titration of Silver and Mercury with Thiourea Solution," Zavod. Lab., 26: 149 (1960).

F. Gravimetric

Donner, R. "Rapid Determination of Mercury in Organic Compounds," Z. Chem., 5: 466 (1965).

Dutt, N. K. and B. K. Bhattacharyya. "Monoallyldithiocarbamidohydrazine as an Analytical Reagent. II. Determination of Zinc and Mercury," Sci. Cult. (Calcutta), 29: 257 (1963).

Elliot, J. A. "A New and Delicate Method for the Detection of Mercury," J. A. M. A., 68: 1693 (1917)

Fabre, R. and R. Moreau. "Mercury in Urine," Bull. Soc. Chim. Biol., 26: 202 (1944).

Goldman, F. H. "Determination of Mercury in Carroted Fur," Public Health Reports, 52: 221 (1937).

Jerie, H. "Microdetermination of Mercury and Halogens in Organic and Inorganic Substances," Mikrochim. Acta, 5: 1089 (1970).

Krylova, A. N. "Detecting 'Metallic' Poisons by a Fractional Method. Main Points," Sud. Med. Ekspertiza, 13: 33 (1970).

Newcomb, C., S. R. Naidu, and K. S. Varadachar. "Mercury in Viscera," Analyst, 60: 732 (1935).

Pechanec, V. "A Universal Method for Determination of Mercury in Inorganic Substances Containing 100-0.001% of Mercury," Collect. Czech. Chem. Commun., 29: 716 (1964).

Soloniewicz, R. "Thiourea as a Reagent for Precipitating Metal Sulfides. II. Determination of Mercury as Mercuric Sulfide," Chem. Anal. (Warsaw), 7: 965 (1962).

Stock, A. and R. Heller. "Determination of Small Quantities of Mercury," Z. Angew. Chem., 39: 466 (1926).

Todorova, Tz. "Microdetermination of Mercuric and Cupric Ions," Compt. Rend. Acad. Bulgare Sci., 16: 509 (1963).

Vernon, F. "Determination of Mercury in Mercurial and Organo-Mercurial Pesticides," Anal. Chem., 33: 1435 (1961).

Willard, H. H. and A. W. Boldyreff. "Determination of Mercury as Metal by Reduction with Hydrazine or Stannous Chloride," J. Amer. Chem. Soc., 52: 569 (1930).

Yoshimura, J., Y. Takashima, Y. Murakami, and T. Kusaba. "The Determination of Some Metal Ions by Precipitation with Hexaminecobalt(III) Chloride and Sodium Thiosulfate," Bull. Chem. Soc. Japan, 35: 1433 (1962).

G. Micrometric

Bodnar, J. and E. Szep. "Ultramicromethods for the Determination of Mercury," Biochem. Z., 205: 219 (1929).

Booth, H. S. and N. E. Schreiber. "The Determination of Traces of Mercury. I. The Sensitivity of the Qualitative Tests for Mercury. A New Method for the Dtection of Mercury Sensitive to 1 Part in a Billion," J. Amer. Chem. Soc., 47: 2625 (1925).

Booth, H. S., N. E. Schreiber and K. C. Zwick. "The Determination of Traces of Mercury. II. The Quantitative Determination of Mercury in the Presence of Organic Matter," J. Amer. Chem. Soc., 48: 1815 (1926).

Fraser, A. M. "The Determination of Mercury in Air and in Urine," J. Indust. Hyg., 16: 67 (1934).

Majer, V. "Mercury Determination in Air and Absorption of Mercury Vapors by Metallic Gold," Chem. Listy, 28: 228 (1934).

Raeder, M. G. and E. Snekvik. "Mercury Determinations in Fish and Other Aquatic Organisms," Kongelige Norske Videnskabers Selskabs, Forhandlinger, 21: 102 (1949).

Raeder, M. G. and E. Snekvik. "Mercury Contents of Fish and Other Aquatic Organisms," Kgl. Norske Videnskab. Selskab, Forh., 21: 105 (1949).

Schreiber, N. E., T. Sollman, and H. S. Booth "The Determination of Traces of Mercury. III. The Quantitative Determination of Mercury in Urine and Feces and the Influence of Medication," J. Amer. Chem. Soc., *50*: 1620 (1928).

Stock, A. "Determination of Traces of Mercury and Its Significance," Naturwissenschaften, *19*: 499 (1931).

Stock, A. "Microanalytical Determination of Mercury and Its Application to Hygienic and Medical Problems," Svensk. Kem. Tidskr., *50*: 342 (1938).

Stock, A. "Microchemical Determination of Mercury," Mikrochemie ver. Mikrochim. Acta, *30*: 128 (1941).

Stock, A. and F. Cucuel. "Determination of the Mercury Content in Air," Ber. Bunsenges. Phys. Chem., *67B*: 122 (1934).

Stock, A., H. Lux, F. Cucuel, and F. Gerstner. "Determination of Traces of Mercury," Z. Angew. Chem., *44*: 200 (1931).

Stock, A., H. Lux, F. Cucuel, and H. Köhle. "Micrometric Determination of Minute Quantities of Mercury," Z. Angew. Chem., *46*: 62 (1933).

Stock, A. and N. Neuenschwander-Lemmer. "Action and Distribution of Mercury. XXVII. The Microanalytical Determination of Mercury," Ber. Bunsenges. Phys. Chem., *71B*: 550 (1938).

Storlazzi, E. E. and H. B. Elkins. "The Significance of Urinary Mercury. I. Occupational Mercury Exposure," J. Industr. Hyg. and Toxicol., *23*: 459 (1941).

H. Radiometric

Clarkson, T. W. and M. R. Greenwood. "Simple and Rapid Determination of Mercury in Urine and Tissues by Isotope Exchange," Talanta, *15*: 547 (1968).

Davis, S. and A. Arnold. "Applicability of an Isotope Exchange Method for the Determination of Milligram and Microgram Quantities of Organic Mercurials. I. Pharmaceutical and Agricultural Mercurials," J. Ass. Offic. Anal. Chem., *48*: 1134 (1965).

Goodman, C., J. W. Irvine, and C. F. Horan. "Mercury Vapor Measurement. A Radioactive Measurement," J. Indust. Hyg. and Toxicol., *25*: 275 (1943).

Kamada, H., Y. Ujihira, and K. Fukuda. "Separation and Concentration of Trace Amounts of Metals by the Use of Copper Sulfide as a Collector," Radioisotopes (Tokyo), *14*: 206 (1965).

Magos, L. "Radiochemical Determination of Metallic Mercury Vapour in Air," Brit. J. Ind. Med., *23*: 230 (1966).

Ruzicka, J. and C. G. Lamm. "Automated Trace Analysis by Substoichiometric Radioisotope Dilution," Technicon Symposium, 2: 315 (1967).

Ruzicka, J. and C. G. Lamm. "Automated Trace Analyses by Substoichiometric Radioisotope Dilution," Nord. Hyg. T. 50: 89 (1969).

Ruzicka, J. and C. G. Lamm. "Automated Determination of Traces of Mercury in Biological Materials by Substoichiometric Radioisotope Dilution," Talanta, 16: 157 (1969).

I. Spectrographic (Emission)

April, R. W. and D. N. Hume. "Environmental Mercury: Rapid Determination in Water at Nanogram Levels," Science, 170: 849 (1970).

Dal Cortivo, L. A., S. B. Weinberg, P. Giaquinta, and M. B. Jacobs. "Mercury Levels in Normal Human Tissue. I. Spectrographic Determination of Mercury in Tissue," J. Forensic Sci., 9: 501 (1964).

Matusiak, W., M. Cefola, L. Dal Cortivo, and C. J. Umberger. "Determination of Mercury in Biological Substances," Anal. Biochem., 8: 463 (1964).

Mavrodineanu, R. and R. C. Hughes. "Radio Frequency Discharge at Atmospheric Pressure and its use as an Excitation Source in Analytical Spectroscopy," Develop. Appl. Spectry., 3: 305 (1963).

Razimov, Z. A. and T. K. Aidarov. "Chemical Spectral Microdetermination of Pb and Hg in Air of Industrial Buildings and in Some Billogical Objects," Tr. po Khim. i Khim. Teknol., 3: 397 (1964).

Rudnevskii, N. K., A. N. Tumanova, and V. T. Demarin. "Determination of Small Amounts of Mercury in Sulfuric and Acetic Acids by a Spectrographic Method," Tr. Khim. Khim. Tekhnol., 1: 95 (1969).

Veres, G. I. and A. P. Perfil'ev. "Accessory Device for a Spectrograph for Determining Trace Amounts of Mercury," Zavod. Lab., 36: 248 (1970).

J. Titrimetric

Belikov, V. V. and M. S. Shraiber. "Complexometric Titration in the Analysis of Complex Medicinal Preparations. III. Direct Titration of Lead and Mercury," Farmatsevt. Zh. (Kiev), 17: 7 (1962).

Coulter, B. and D. G. Bush. "Titrimetric Determination of Mercury (II) with Thioacetamide," Anal. Chim. Acta, 51: 431 (1970).

De'Anil, K. and S. K. Majumdar. "Separation of Ag, Pb, and Hg(II) by Ion-Exchange Chromatography," Talanta, 10: 201 (1963).

Dugandzic, M. and V. Medenica. "Diphenylcarbazone as an Indicator During Direct Complexometric Titration of Mercury," Arh. Farm., *20*: 145 (1970).

Elmore, J. W. "Determination of Mercury in Paints and Toxicological Material," J. Ass. Offic. Anal. Chem., *29*: 387 (1946).

Fritz, J. S. and S. A. Sutton. "Titration of Mercury with Bis(2-Hydroxyethyl) Dithiocarbamate," Anal. Chem., *28*: 1300 (1956).

Ghosh, N. N. and M. N. Majumder. "Semimicro and Macro Titrimetric Method for Determination of Mercury(II) and the Associated Free Acid Using N-(Benzene-Sulfonyl) Glycine," J. Indian Chem. Soc., *41*: 286 (1964).

Kai, F. "Reaction Between Mercury(II) and Organic Compounds. VIII. Titrimetric Determination of Mercury(II) with 6-(2-Thiazolylazo)-2-4-Dichlorophenol as a Metallochromic Indicator," Bull. Chem. Soc. Jap., *43*: 759 (1970).

Kinoshita, S. and K. Hozumi. "Microdetermination of Organic Mercury with a Simple Wet Combustion Method," Microchem. J., *8*: 79 (1964).

Komatsu, S., C. Kitazawa, and S. Nasu. "Indirect Chelatometric Determination of Mercury(II) Using a Suspension of Copper Diethyldithiocarbamate," Nippon Kagaku Zasshi, *85*: 598 (1964).

Martin, F. and A. Floret. "Determination of Mercury in Organomercurials and Some Mineral Compounds," Bull. Soc. Chim. Fr., 610 (1960).

Seal, D. C. "Quantitative Study of Oxidation Products of Iodine at the End Points of the Titrations of Mercuric and Silver Salts with Iodide-Iodine Solutions," J. Indian Chem. Soc., *38*: 811 (1961).

Shishkov, A. N. "Titrimetric Determination of Mercury(II) by Potassium Diphenyl Dithiophosphate," Nauch. Tr. Vissh. Pedagog. Inst., Plovdiv., Mat., Fiz., Khim., Biol., *8*: 133 (1970).

Southworth, B. C., J. H. Hodecker, and K. D. Fleischer. "Determination of Mercury in Organic Compounds, a Micro and Semimicro Method," Anal. Chem., *30*: 1152 (1958).

Ueno, K. "Simultaneous Complexometric Determination of Copper and Mercury," Anal. Chem., *29*: 1668 (1957).

Wawrzyczek, W. and W. Wisniewski. "Titrimetric Determination of Mercury(II) Ions with Potassium Iodide Using Iodine-Starch as Indicator," Fresenius' Z. Anal. Chem., *249*: 366 (1970).

Young, A. G. and F. H. L. Taylor. "Electrolytic Method for Determination of Small Amounts of Mercury in Body Fluids and Tissue," J. Biol. Chem., *84*: 377 (1929).

K. X-Ray (Fluorescence)

Berdichevskii, G. V., V. I. Vasil'ev, and Yu. G. Lavrent'ey. "Application of X-Ray Spectral Microanalysis for Diagnostics and Determination the Composition of Mineral Ores of Mercury Deposits," App. Metody Rentgenovskogo Anal. No. 5, 245 (1969).

Beyermann, K. and K. Cretius. "The X-Ray Fluorimetric Determination of Inorganic Constituents in Biologic Materials. I. Basis, Technique, and Limitations of the Method," Klin. Wochenschr., *40*: 86 (1962).

Brooks, E. J., O. R. Gates, and M. Nottingham. "The Determinations of Mercury in Urine by Means of X-Ray Spectroscopy," Am. J. Clin. Path., *41*: 154 (1964).

Leroux, J., P. A. Maffett, and J. L. Monkman. "Microdetermination of Heavy Elements Such as Mercury and Iodine in Solution, by X-Ray Absorption," Anal. Chem., *29*: 1089 (1957).

Link, W. B., K. S. Heine, J. H. Jones, and P. Wattlington. "Ion-Exchange Paper--X-Ray Emission Procedure for Determination of Microgram Quantities of Mercury," J. Ass. Offic. Anal. Chem., *47*: 391 (1964).

Rhodes, J. R. "Radioisotope X-Ray Spectrometry. A Review," Analyst, *91*: 683 (1966).

L. Miscellaneous Methods

Bell, C. F. and M. A. Quddus. "Nephelometric Determination of Silver and Mercury with Bis(1,3-Di(2-Pyridyl)-1,2-Diaza-2-Propenato) Cobalt (III) Perchlorate," Anal. Chim. Acta, *52*: 313 (1970).

Celap, M. B., T. J. Janjic, and Z. Spanovic. "Determination of Small Amounts of Metallic Ions on Impregnated Filter Papers. II. Determination of Hg, Ag, Au, Platinum and Palladium on Filter Paper Impregnated with CdS," Glas. Hem. Drus. Beograd, *25*: 531 (1960-61).

Gettler, A. O. "Simple Tests for Mercury in Body Fluids and Tissues," Am. J. Clin. Path. (Tech. Supp.), *7*: 13 (1937).

Krestovinikov, A. N. and L. G. Scheinfinkel. "Argon Detector for the Determination of Mercury in Gases," Gaz. Khromatogr., Sb., Moscow, *2*: 53 (1964).

Murphy, C. B. "Low-Level Gas Analysis by Condensation Nuclei Techniques," Instr. Control Systems, *38*: 101 (1965).

Norlander, B. W. "Quantitative Methods for the Determination of Mercury Vapor," J. Industr. and Eng. Chem., *19*: 522 (1927).

Ratzka, E. and G. Nowak. "Small Tube to Detect Mercury Vapor in Air or Other Gases," Ger. (East), *34*: 315 (Cl. G. Oln) (1964).

Tong, S. S. C., W. H. Gutenmann, and D. J. Lisk. "Determination of Mercury in Apples by Spark Source Mass Spectrometry," Anal. Chem., *41*: 1872 (1969).

Townshend, A. and A. Vaughan. "Applications of Enzyme-Catalyzed Reactions in Trace Analysis. VI. Determination of Mercury and Silver by Their Inhibition of Yeast Alcohol Dehydrogenase," Talanta, *17*: 299 (1970).

II. Methods for Analysis of Organic Mercury Compounds
   A. Alkyl Mercury Compounds

Izotov, B. N. "Isolation, Detection, and Quantitative Determination of Ethylmercuric Chloride in Biological Material," Farm. Zh. (Kiev), *24*: 70 (1969).

Jensen, S. "Sources of Error and Confirmation in the Determination of Methylmercury Radicals," Nord. Hyg. Tidskr., *50*: 85 (1969).

Johansson, F., R. Rykage, and G. Westöö. "Identification and Determination of Methylmercury Compounds in Fish Using Combination Gas Chromatograph Mass Spectrometer," Acta Chem. Scand., *24*: 2349 (1970).

Kimura, Y. and V. L. Miller. "Vapor-Phase Separation of Methyl- or Ethyl-Mercury Compounds and Metallic Mercury," Anal. Chem., *32*: 420 (1960).

Kitamura, S., T. Tsukamoto, D. Hayakawa, K. Sumino, and T. Shibata. "Gas-Chromatographic Determination of Alkylmercury Compounds," Igaku to Seibutsugaku, *72*: 274 (1966).

Linch, A. L., R. F. Stalzer, and D. T. Lefferts. "Methyl and Ethyl Mercury--Recovery from Air and Analysis," Amer. Ind. Hyg. Assoc. J., *29*: 79 (1968).

Nishi, S. and Y. Horimoto. "Gas-Chromatographic Behavior of Traces of Alkylmercury Compounds," Bunseki Kagaku, *17*: 75 (1968).

Nishi, S. and Y. Horimoto. "Determination of Trace Amounts of Organic Mercury Compounds in Aqueous Solutions," Bunseki Kagaku, *17*: 1247 (1968).

Rissanen, K. and J. K. Miettinen. "Thin-Layer Chromatography of Alkyl and Alkoxy Mercury Derivatives and Location of Mercury in the Yolk of Hen Eggs," Ann. Agr. Fenn. Suppl. *7*: 22 (1968).

Sumino, K. "Analysis of Organic Mercury Compounds by Gas Chromatography. Part I. Analytical and Extraction Method of Organic Mercury Compounds," Kobe J. Med. Sci., *14*: 115 (1968).

Sumino, K. "Analysis of Organic Mercury Compounds by Gas Chromatography. Part II. Determination of Organic Mercury Compounds in Various Samples," Kobe J. Med. Sci., *14*: 131 (1968).

Swedish Institute for Water and Air P llution Research (IVL). Gas Liquid Chromatography of Methyl Mercury. Stencils, Drottuing Kristinas Väg 47 S-114 28 (Stockholm, Sweden, 1958).

Tatton, J. O'D. and P. J. Wagstaffe. "Identification and Determination of Organomercurial Fungicide Residues by Thin-Layer and Gas Chromatography," J. Chromatogr., *44*: 284 (1969).

Teramoto, K. et al. "Chemical Analysis of Methylmercury Compounds in Mercury Phenylacetate, by Gas Chromatography," Kogyo Kagaku Zasshi, *70*: 1601 (1967), Fisheries Research Board of Canada Translation Series No. 1407.

Westermark, T., D. Hagman, A. Vestermark, and K. Ljunggren. "Concentration Electrophoresis Method for the Separation and Demonstration of Charged Mercury Compounds in Aqueous Solution," Nord. Hyg. Tidskr., *50*: 79 (1969).

Westöö, G. "Determination of Methylmercury Compounds in Foodstuffs. I. Methylmercury Compounds in Fish, Identification and Determination," Acta Chem. Scand., *20*: 2131 (1966).

Westöö, G. "Determination of Methylmercury Compounds in Foodstuffs. II. Determination of Methylmercury in Fish, Egg, Meat, and Liver," Acta Chem. Scand., *21*: 1790 (1967).

Westöö, G. "Determination of Methylmercury Salts in Various Kinds of Biological Material," Acta Chem. Scand., *22*: 2277 (1968).

Westöö, G. and K. Noren. "Mercury and Methylmercury in Fish. The Amount of Mercury and Methylmercury in Fish Caught or Brought from September 1966 to November 1967," Var Foda, *19*: 138 (1967).

Yamaguchi, S. and H. Matsumoto. "Ultramicro Determination of Alkylmercury Compounds by Gas Chromatography," Kurume Med. J., *16*: 33 (1969).

Yamaguchi, S. et al. "Microdetermination of Organic Mercurials by Thin-Layer Chromatography," Kurume Med. J., *16*: 53 (1969).

Zamyslova, S. D. and N. P. Ashmarina. "Determination of Ethylmercuric Chloride and Diethylmercury in Water," Vop. Gig. Vody Sanit. Okhr. Vodoemov, 138 (1968).

B. Non-Alkyl Organic Mercury Compounds

Beuesch, R. and R. C. Beuesch. "Polarographic Studies of Organic Mercury Compounds," J. A. C. S., *73*: 3391 (1951).

Beyer, E. B. "Polarographic Determination of Thimerosal Tincture and Solution NF," J. Ass. Offic. Anal. Chem., *52*: 844 (1969).

Gage, J. C. "The Trace Determination of Phenyl- and Methyl Mercury Salts in Biological Material," Analyst, *86*: 457 (1961).

Hopes, T. M. "Polarographic Determination of Organomercury Drugs," J. Ass. Offic. Anal. Chem., *48*: 840 (1966).

Kitamura, S., K. Sumino, and K. Hayakawa. "Gas-Chromatographic Determination of Phenylmercuric Compounds," Igaku to Seibutsugaku, *73*: 276 (1966).

Levedeva, A. L. and K. Sh. Kramer. "Simultaneous Microdetermination of Carbon, Hydrogen and Mercury in Organomercury Compounds," Izv. Akad. Nauk. SSR, Otd. Khim. Nauk., *1962*: 1305 (1962).

Miller, V. L., D. Lillis, and E. Dsonka. "Microestimation of Intact Phenyl-Mercury Compounds in Animal Tissue," Anal. Chem., *30*: 1705 (1958).

Miller, V. L. and D. Polley. "Determination of Diphenylmercury Alone or in Presence of Phenylmercuric Compounds," Anal. Chem., *26*: 1333 (1954).

Ostlund, K. "Thin-Layer Chromatographic Separation of Organic Mercury Compounds," Nord. Hyg. Tidskr., *50*: 82 (1969).

Polley, D. and V. L. Miller. "Direct Determination of Methyl Mercuric Dicyandiamide," J. Agr. Food Chem., *2*: 1030 (1954).

Sera, K. et al. "Detection of Organomercury Pesticide," Kumamoto Med. J., *15*: 38 (1962).

III. Analytical Considerations, Errors, Calibration Procedures, Ashing Problems

Berg, E. and J. Truemper. "Ion Exchange Separation of Zinc, Cadmium, and Mercury in Aqueous and Partial Nanaqueous Media," Anal. Chem., *30*: 1827 (1958).

Casini, A. "Loss of Mercury in Toxicological Analyses," Ann. Chim. (Rome), *40*: 677 (1950).

Gage, J. C. "A Hi-Speed Absorber for the Determination of Toxic Substances in Air," J. Sci. Instrum., *29*: 409 (1952).

Gorsuch, T. T. "Radiochemical Investigation on the Recovery for Analysis of Trace Elements in Organic and Biological Materials," Analyst, *84*: 135 (1959).

Greenwood, M. R. and T. W. Clarkson. "Storage of Mercury at Submolar Concentrations," Amer. Ind. Hyg. Ass. J., *31*: 250 (1970).

Magos, L., A. A. Tuffery, and T. W. Clarkson. "Volatilization of Mercury by Bacteria," Brit. J. Industr. Med., *21*: 294 (1964).

Nakagawa, G. "Ion Exchange Extraction with High Molecular Weight Amines. VII. Extraction of Cu(II), Ag, Cd, Hg(II), Ga(III), and In from HCl Solutions," Nippon Kagaku Zasshi, *81*: 1533 (1960).

Nelson, G. O. "Generating Known Concentrations of Mercury Vapor in Air," Rev. Sci. Instrum., *41*: 776 (1970).

Nelson, G. O., W. vanSandt, and P. E. Barry. "A Dynamic Method for Mercury Vapor Detector Calibration," Amer. Ind. Hyg. Assoc. J., *26*: 388 (1965).

P'yankov, V. A. "Oxodation and Vaporizationoof Mercury and Absorption of Mercury Vapor," Novosti Med., *26*: 68 (1952).

Stock, A. "Effects and Distribution of Mercury. Film Phenomena and the Determination of Mercury," Ber. Bunsenges Phys. Chem., *72B:* 1844 (1939).

Toribara, T. Y., C. P. Shields, and L. Koval. "Behavior of Dilute Solutions of Mercury," Talanta, *17*: 1025 (1970).

Vasileva, A. and M. Shaikova. "Losses of Mercury in Forensic Analysis," Aptechnoe Delo, *2*: 46 (1953).

Vasileva, A. A. and M. D. Shvaikova. "Certain Problems Connected with Isolation of Mercury Compounds from Biological Material," Aptechnoe Delo, *4*: 23 (1955).

Wall, H. and C. Rhodes. "Effect of Bacterial Contamination and Aging on the Volatility of Mercury in Urine Specimens," Clin. Chem., *12*: 837 (1966).

IV. Reviews

Association of Official Analytical Chemists. Official Methods of Analysis of the AOAC (Washington, D. C., 1970), p. 418.

Browett, E. V. "Analytical Methods," Ann. Occup. Hyg., *8*: 21 (1965).

Chlorine Institute, Inc., New York. "Analytical Methods for Determination of Total Mercury (Dow Method CAS-Am 70.13)." Chlorine Institute Pamphlet No. MIR-104 (September 18, 1970).

Coetzee, J. F. in Treatise on Analytical Chemistry, Part II, Vol. 3. Edited by I. M. Kolthoff and P. J. Elving (New York: Interscience Publishers, 1961), p. 231.

Gainullina, E. T. and R. N. Nurmukhametov. "Luminescent Analysis of Industrial Air Pollution," Zh. Vses. Khim. Obshchest., *15*: 506 (1970).

Kolthoff, L. M., P. D. Elving, and E. B. Sandell. "Treatise on Analytical Chemistry," in Analytical Chemistry of Elements, Part II, Vol. 3. (New York: Interscience Publishers, 1961), p. 391.

Kryukov, G. I. and S. L. Simkina. "Photoelectric Gas Analyzers," Zh. Vses. Khim. Obshchest., *15*: 495 (1970).

Launer, J. E. "Review of Methods for Mercury in Pesticide Formulations," J. Ass. Offic. Anal. Chem., *52*: 764 (1969).

National Institute of Public Health, Sweden. Report from an Expert Group. "Methyl Mercury in Fish." Chap. 3, Nordisk Hygienisk Tidskrift, Suppl. 4 (1971), p. 36.

Oda, N. "Mercury Analysis in Electrolytic Soda Industry," Soda to Enso, *21*: 123 (1970).

Quentin, K. E. and A. Rosopulo. "Presence and Determination of Mercury in Caustic Soda Solution with Regard to Deacidification of Drinking Water," Gas-Wasserfach, Wasser-Abwasser, *111*: 380 (1970).

Snell, F. D. and C. T. Snell. Colorimetric Methods of Analysis, 3rd ed., Vol. II. (New York: Von Nostrand Co., 1949), p. 63.

U. S. Department of Health, Education and Welfare, Study Group on Mercury Hazards. "Hazards of Mercury, Special Report to the Secretary's Pesticide Advisory Committee. Chap. 7," Environ. Res., *4*: 53 (1971).

Uthe, J. F., F. A. J. Armstrong, and K. C. Tam. "Determination of Trace Amounts of Mercury in Fish Tissues: Results of a North American Check Sample Study," J. Ass. Offic. Anal. Chem., *54*: 866 (1971).

Vignoli, L., R. Badre, M. Morel, and J. Ardorino. "A Comparative Study of Modern Techniques for the Micro Determination of Mercury," Chim. Anal. (Paris), *45*: 53 (1963).

Wallace, R. A., W. D. Shults, W. Fulkerson, and W. S. Lyon. "Analytical Methodology for Environmental Mercury. Mercury in the Environment - The Human Element," Oak Ridge National Laboratory (1971), p. 31.

Ward, F. N. "Analytical Methods for the Determination of Mercury in Rocks and Soils," U. S. Geological Survey, Mercury in the Environment, Prof. Paper 713 (1970), p. 46.

Widmark, Gunnar, et al. "Analytical Problems: Mercury in the General Environment," Oikos Supp., *9*: 9 (1967).

Preparation of Biological Samples
For Neutron Activation Analysis of Mercury

K. K. S. Pillay

Introduction

Mercury in the biota is found to exist in a variety of
organic and inorganic forms.[1] Many of these compounds are
known to be highly volatile and can readily elude detection
during analyses unless adequate precautions are taken.[2]
In activation analysis procedures involving chemical
isolation of mercury by carrier techniques, these precautions
have to be observed rigorously until an isotope exchange
between radioactive mercury and inactive carrier is achieved.
A subsequent chemical yield determination, which is an
essential part of radiochemical separation procedures, will
account for the actual losses after the isotope exchange
between active and inactive mercury.

Experimental Methods

In developing accurate and reliable neutron activation
analysis procedures for the determination of mercury in
both biological and environmental samples, it was realized
that several problems arising out of improper sample handling
cause significant losses of mercury from the samples. The
initial findings of an investigation of cold ashing techniques and/or freeze-drying methods to prepare convenient
analytical samples for neutron activation analysis of
mercury are presented here.

In neutron activation analyses using reactor neutrons,
it is highly desirable to have the sample compacted and
free from excessive amounts of moisture. Since biological
samples usually are not too dense and contain a significant
amount of moisture, processes such as oven-drying, freeze-
drying and ashing are often used to prepare samples suitable
for reactor irradiation and subsequent handling. During
this investigation, a low-temperature asher using oxygen
plasma for oxidizing tissues and a freeze-dryer (without
McLeod gauge) were used. Three fish homogenate samples
containing varying concentrations of mercury and several
human brain tissues were used to investigate the possible
losses of mercury during freeze-drying and cold ashing.
These samples were first analyzed for their mercury content
without any pre-processing, using neutron activation followed

by chemical separation and gamma ray spectrometry. Repeat analyses of the samples showed excellent precision for the mercury analysis by this procedure. The accuracy of this procedure was confirmed by several analyses involving spiked samples. Also, the analytical results of the three fish samples showed good agreement with the results obtained by cold atomic absorption analysis.

Several tissue homogenates were mixed with radioactive mercury (Hg^{++} form) and were stirred in the form of a slurry for several hours. These samples were aliquoted into standard freeze-drying flasks and the mercury content measured by gamma ray spectrometry using a 4" x 4" well-type scintillation detector and a multichannel pulse height analyzer. The samples were then quickly frozen, using a mixture of crushed dry ice, liquid nitrogen and ethyl alcohol. The freeze-drying continued, using a similar cold trap in a VirTis freeze-dryer. The radioactivity from the mercury was again measured and compared with standards used prior to freeze-drying. The results, shown in Table 17, indicate that there are no significant losses of radioactive mercury (Hg^{++} form) from the fish homogenates.

Table 17

Loss of Mercury (Hg^{++} form) in Biological Tissues During Freeze-Drying with VirTis Manifold-Type Freeze-Dryer

Sample identification	*No. of hours of freeze-drying*	*Per cent loss of mercury (Hg^{++} form)*
Fish G-20	6.5	0.02
Fish G-30	6.5	0.01
Fish G-40	6.5	0.01
Fish G-50	16.0	0.19
Fish G-60	16.0	0.05
Fish G-70	16.0	0.02

The freeze-drying procedures described above were repeated, using a set of fish homogenates and human brain tissue samples previously analyzed for their mercury content. The residual samples from the freeze-drying processes were again analyzed for their mercury content by neutron activation analysis. The results of these analyses are presented in Table 18. It is obvious that

Table 18

Loss of Mercury (Natural Form) from Biological Tissues
During Freeze-Drying with VirTis Manifold-Type Freeze-Dryer

Sample identification	No. of hours of freeze-drying	Initial levels of mercury (ppm)	Per cent loss of mercury
A. Fish Homogenates			
Fish D-21	4.0	1.77	16.4
Fish D-22	4.0	1.77	14.1
Fish E-21	4.0	0.12	18.3
Fish E-22	4.0	0.12	16.7
Fish G-21	4.0	4.56	38.8
Fish G-22	4.0	4.56	32.9
B. Human Brain Tissues			
Pons	6.5	0.43	56.5
Corona Radiata	6.5	0.15	24.3
Cerebral Cortex	2.0	0.25	15.8
Cerebellar Cortex	2.0	0.72	18.0

there is mercury lost during the freeze-drying of these tissues. Since earlier experiments showed that there was no significant loss of Hg^{++} mercury during freeze-drying, the losses observed here may be attributed to volatile forms of mercury present in biological tissues. A sample of fish G was subjected to prolonged ether extraction for about 48 hours and the residue was analyzed for mercury. This showed a 37.7% loss of mercury during ether extraction. The similarity between the amounts of mercury lost during freeze-drying and the loss of mercury during ether extraction needs further investigation.

The investigation of the use of a low-temperature asher (Tracerlab Model 505) for preparing analytical samples for neutron activation involved the use of fish homogenates spiked with radioactive mercury (in Hg^{++} form) as described earlier. The mercury content of the aliquots used was measured by gamma ray spectrometry before and after ashing. The results, shown in Table 19, clearly demonstrate that this technique is highly undesirable for preparation of ashed samples for neutron irradiation.

Table 19

Loss of Mercury (Hg^{++} form) from Biological Tissues
During Low Temperature Ashing*

Sample identification	No. of hours of Ashing	Per cent loss of mercury (Hg^{++} form)
Fish 1	3.5	81.4
Fish 2	3.5	81.9
Fish 3	3.5	91.8
Fish 4	7.0	98.0
Fish 5	7.0	98.0
Fish 6	7.0	98.0

*Tracerlab Low Temperature Asher Model No. 505
Radiofrequency power level - 200 watts (Maximum)
Oxygen flow rate - 100 cc/minute
Sample temperature - 110° C (Maximum)

Discussion

It seems apparent that both the freeze-drying and cold ashing procedures described here are not satisfactory for the preparation of analytical samples of biological tissues for neutron irradiation. Although the loss of mercury was significant during freeze-drying processes, it should be mentioned that the method still offers potential application, if a satisfactory method of converting all mercury in biological tissues to Hg^{++} form can be applied. High flux gamma irradiation could well serve this purpose.

Recognizing that this investigation was limited only to biological tissues, it should be pointed out that similar losses of mercury could result from plant tissues as well as other environmental samples containing mercury. The pre-irradiation handling of these samples, as well as plankton/algae, sediments, water, and aquatic fauna is presently being investigated.

The biological tissues for neutron irradiation, which are not subjected to any pre-processing, are handled as follows: They are encapsulated in heavy-duty polyethylene bags. These bags have a free volume of five to six times the volume of the sample. Prior to heat-sealing, the air from the bag is squeezed out to allow expansion during reactor irradiation. Since neutron and gamma irradiation from the reactor readily converts organic mercury compounds to Hg°, Hg$^+$ and/or Hg^{++} form, the mercury in the tissues is in a much less volatile form after reactor irradiation. The samples are extracted with nitric acid, wet-ashed with mercury carrier, chemically isolated, and determined by the gamma ray spectrometry of Hg^{197m}, Hg^{197} and Hg^{203} produced. Such an irradiation procedure can withstand up to 4 hours of reactor irradiation at a thermal and fast neutron flux of 10^3 neutrons cm^{-2} sec^{-1} and a gamma flux of about 10^7 R/hour.

Acknowledgment

This investigation is part of a long range program to study the mercury levels of Lake Erie and its aquatic life, supported by the Bureau of Sport Fisheries and Wildlife, U. S. Department of the Interior. The author wishes gratefully to acknowledge the assistance of his colleagues Mr. Charles C. Thomas, Jr., Mr. James A. Sondel and Dr. John Y. Yang.

References

1. Jernelöv, A. "Conversion of Mercury Compounds," in Chemical Fallout, Ed. by M. W. Miller and G. G. Berg. (Springfield, Illinois: Charles C. Thomas, 1969), pp. 68-74.
2. Gorsuch, T. T. "Radiochemical Investigations on the Recovery for Analysis of Trace Elements in Organic and Biological Materials," Analyst, 84, 135-173 (1959).

Mercury Content of Canadian Foods and Cereals Determined by Different Methods

H. M. Cunningham and J. C. Méranger

Every three months, mixed diet samples representing the 12 major classes of foods consumed by Canadians are obtained from stores and markets and analyzed for trace minerals and other constituents. Table 20 shows the analysis of these foods for mercury by the Association of Official Analytical

Table 20

Mercury Determination by Dithizone Colorimetric Procedure

Sample Type	Number of Samples Analyzed	Mercury Content (p.p.m.)
Enriched White Flour	10	<0.02
Skim Milk Powder	10	<0.02
Enriched White Bread	10	<0.01
Fresh Eggs	10	<0.01
Potatoes	10	<0.01
Cabbage	10	<0.01
Apples	10	<0.01
Whole Milk	10	<0.01
Pork Liver	10	<0.01
Beefsteak	10	<0.01
Beef Liver	2	<0.01
Chicken Liver	2	<0.01

Table 21

Recovery of Mercury from Various Mercury Compounds Using
Chemical Digestion with Vanadium Catalyst and
Atomic Absorption Spectrometer

Compound*	% Recovery
Mercurous Chloride	99.8
Phenylmercury Chloride	95.6
Methylmercury Chloride	81.4
Methoxyethyl Mercuric Chloride	89.1
Ethoxyethyl Mercuric Chloride	84.2
O-Chlormercuriphenol	94.5

*0.2 micrograms of mercury equivalent was added to 5 g
of flour sample. The organo-mercury compounds were reagent
grade laboratory chemicals.

Chemists (A.O.A.C.) dithiazone technique which, although tedious and time—consuming, was sensitive to 0.01 ppm mercury. Ten samples of most classes of foods were analyzed, and none of these samples showed more than 0.02 ppm mercury.

Like many other laboratories, the Food and Drug Directorate has recently changed over to flameless atomic absorption techniques. One of the most satisfactory techniques that we have used is chemical digestion with H_2SO_4 and HNO_3, with a vanadium pentoxide catalyst and a dry ice "cold finger" condenser as used by Dr. Malaiyandi of the Canada Department of Agriculture (described in the Proceedings A.O.A.C. Meetings, Washington, October, 1970). We first tried to see if this technique could detect and recover the mercury in a number of inorganic and organic mercury compounds when added as a "spike" to flour. The recoveries shown in Table 21 were quite acceptable, considering that these were only laboratory reagent-grade chemicals which had not been subjected to any purification after they were purchased, and that the chemicals were added at a level of 0.04 ppm or 0.2 µg/5 g of flour.

We next used this technique to check the mercury content of 10 different commercial flour products and of 2 samples of wheat. One of the wheat samples was collected from the bin of a farmer near Brandon, Manitoba, who had not used mercury seed treatment. The other sample was obtained from a carload of wheat shipped from an elevator at Killarney, Manitoba, about 50 miles away. As shown in Table 22, none of the wheat or flour samples contained above 0.013 ppm mercury. We were, however, able to confirm the analysis of a sample of contaminated barley supplied to us by Dr. Malaiyandi, which contained 0.18 ppm mercury.

Last spring our Food and Drug Directorate obtained samples of wheat and flour from widely separated areas in Canada; these were analyzed for mercury by neutron activation analysis by Dr. R. Jervis and colleagues at the University of Toronto (Table 23). Analysis of these samples by chemical digestion and flameless atomic absorption analysis showed much lower levels of mercury. Four of these samples were analyzed by Dr. Malaiyandi and showed similar values. In case the chemical digestion of the flour was not releasing the mercury so that it could be detected, samples were combusted in the Schöniger apparatus and analyzed by flameless atomic absorption analysis. They also showed only negligible amounts of mercury.

We do not know the reason why the analysis for mercury in wheat and flour by chemical techniques does not agree with the results obtained by neutron activation analysis

Table 22

Mercury Content of Wheat and Flour Samples, Using
Chemical Digestion with Vanadium Catalyst and
Atomic Absorption Spectrometer

Code	Mercury (ppm Fresh Weight	Average
Wheat		
1 Brandon, Manitoba	0.002, 0.0035	0.003
2 Killarney, Manitoba	0.012, 0.0135	0.013
Flour		
1	0.012, 0.005	0.009
2	0.004, 0.003	0.004
3	0.004, 0.001	0.003
4	0.004, 0.002	0.003
5	0.003, 0.003	0.003
6	0.004, 0.003	0.004
7	0.007, 0.001	0.004
8	0.005, 0.001	0.003
9	0.008, 0.003	0.006
10	0.007, 0.004	0.006

since in an earlier collaborative study on the analysis
of fish for mercury, the results with these techniques
were in fairly good agreement. However, since many laboratories are now using chemical techniques with flameless
atomic absorption analysis to determine the mercury content
of cereals and flour, it is quite important to know the
reasons for this variation.

Table 23

Comparison of Mercury Analysis of Wheat and Flour Analyzed by
Different Techniques (ppm)

FDD Sample No.	Neutron Activation[1]	Chemical Digestion and Atomic Absorption	Schöniger Combustion and Atomic Absorption
18464 Wheat	0.079	0.002, 0.005, (0.008)[2]	(.006)
20445 Wheat	0.30	0.007, 0.008	
18465 Wheat	0.40	0.003, 0.004, (0.013)	(.008)
20389 Wheat	0.34	0.006, 0.010	0.01, 0.01
32573 Flour	0.38, 0.29	0.007, 0.007, (0.007)	(.007)
32574 Flour	0.26, 0.14	0.007, 0.007, (0.007)	0.01, 0.01, (.007)
32575 Flour	0.22	0.006, 0.004	

1. R. E. Jervis, D. Debrun, W. Lepage and B. Tiefenbach. Mercury Residues in Canadian Foods, Fish, and Wildlife. University of Toronto.
2. Results in parentheses obtained by Dr. Malaiyandi of the Canada Department of Agriculture.

A Simple, Rapid Method for the Determination of
Trace Mercury in Fish via Neutron Activation Analysis

J. Mark Rottschafter, John D. Jones,
and Harry B. Mark, Jr.

As a consequence of the recent concern over mercury
pollution in the environment, the development of simple,
rapid, analytical methods for the accurate determination
of trace amounts of mercury has become very important.
This paper describes the application and results of a
modified version of a neutron activation analysis (NAA)
method[1] which has been conveniently employed for the
determination of mercury in fish tissue.

The method of Bowen and Gibbons,[1] which is based on a
technique originated by Ehman and Huizinga,[2] employs
(after irradiation, dissolution of the sample and dilution
with HCl) an anion-exchanging column on which the mercury
as a $HgCl_4$ complex, is absorbed. Other interfering cations,
$^{24}Na^+$ in particular, are not absorbed, and pass through the
column. The $HgCl_4$ complex of the Bowen and Gibbons method
is subsequently eluted with HNO_3, and then precipitated as
HgS from solution for counting. We have found, in this
study, that quantitative and/or reproducible elution of
the mercury from the exchange resin was difficult, and
required large amounts of the HNO_3 solution for optimum
results. Thus, the method was modified to count the exchange resin directly, thereby eliminating the subsequent
chemical steps which seemed to result in losses and/or
irreproducibility. It is also shown that the standard
radiochemical technique of adding a holdback carrier pre-
vents large losses of the sample mercury during the digestion
and the chemical steps preceeding the ion exchange step, and,
thus, has great advantage over other techniques not employing
NAA for the determination.

Experimental Methods

Weighed fish tissue samples of 0.8 g to 1.0 g are individually sealed in quartz tubes (4" x 1/4"). Also,
tissue from the same specimen, plus an exactly known amount
of $HgNO_3$ as an internal standard, are individually sealed
in individual quartz tubes. Both the quartz ampules, containing the unknown and the internal standard, are then
irradiated together in the Ford Nuclear Reactor of the
Michigan Memorial-Phoenix Project (neutron flux of 10^{13}

neutrons/cm^2/sec) for 36 hours.   Then, after a delay of
2 to 3 days to allow the gross activity to decay to a level
where the samples can be safely handled, each ampule is
broken open after freezing in liquid N_2, the contents are
placed in a 125 ml Erlenmeyer flask, and 1.0 ml of the
mercury holdback carrier (20 mg Hg^{++}/ml) is added.

The samples are then covered with a watch glass and
digested with just sufficient 1:1 concentrated HNO_3:H_2SO_4
to bring the samples into solution. (This typically requires about 5 ml of the acid mixture.) After cooling,
the solutions are diluted to 25 ml with 1M HCl. This
solution is then passed at a flow rate of about 5 ml/min
through an ion exchange column containing 10 cc of Dowex,
2x8 (50 to 100 mesh) ion exchange resin, that has been
previously equilibrated with 1M HCl. The flask is rinsed
several times with 1M HCl and the rinsings passed through
the column. In order to remove all the Na^{24} from the
column, a total of about 100 ml of the 1M HCl, in 10 ml
aliquots, is passed through the column. The resin is then
removed from the column, placed in a glass vial, and
counted for 400 sec by means of a Camberra 25 cc coaxial
Ge(Li)detector and a Nuclear Data 4096 Channel Analyzer.
The area under the 77.3 Kev gamma photopeak of ^{197}Hg
(half-life = 65 hr) is used to determine the amount of
mercury present in the sample and internal standard. The
additional activity present in the internal standard over
that in the sample is used to calculate the activity per
microgram of mercury present, and this is used to calculate
the amount of mercury originally present in the sample.

Experiments were also carried out to determine if it was
necessary to use a replicate fish tissue sample in the tube
employed as a reference mercury standard in the procedure.
If not, the time needed for preparation of the tissue
sample for irradiation could be shortened, as the standards
could be prepared in quantity in advance. These standards
were prepared simply by pipetting 100λ aliquots of standard
mercury solution (10 µg Hg^{++}/ml) into individual quartz
ampules and sealing them. One standard ampule and two
samples were then tied together with aluminum wire for
irradiation. The standard received the same chemical
treatment as the sample. Extensive comparisons between
"external" and "internal" standard tests showed no significant difference in the amounts of mercury found, and it
appears that either method can be used with success.
However, it should be mentioned that in both cases the
amount of standard mercury should be of the same order of
magnitude as that expected in the samples, so that dead

time losses in the analyzer are comparable.   Also, it should be understood that unsuspected interferences (not present in any sample tested here) might lead to error when "internal" standards are not used.

Fish samples supplied by the U. S. Bureau of Commercial Fisheries, Ann Arbor, Michigan, and others obtained independently, were analyzed directly. As the amounts of mercury actually present in the samples were unknown, comparisons were made between our results and those obtained by other laboratories using a variety of methods, such as atomic absorption, standard neutron activation analysis (NAA), and X-ray fluorescence. Table 24 shows a comparison of analytical results obtained for the same fish tissue samples.

Table 24

Representative Results of Mercury Analyses
in Fish Edible Tissue

	Method	*Results (ppm)*
Sample 1.	Atomic Absorption[a]	0.60
	Atomic Absorption[a]	1.0
	Atomic Absorption	0.85[b]
	X-ray Fluorescence	0.40
	Destructive Neutron Activation Analysis (NAA)	0.87
	This Method	0.86 (10% standard deviation)
Sample 2.	This Method	0.58 (10% standard deviation
	NBS (non-destructive NAA)[c]	0.54
	Average results of 15 laboratories (various methods)	0.51 (Values ranged from 0.19 to 1.2)

[a]Atomic absorption results of three different laboratories.
[b]Results supplied by Grieg.[3]
[c]Results supplied by LaFleur.[4]

Results and Discussion

In all cases, the results compared favorably for the same samples, and replicate results using the method described here showed less scatter than the results reported by the other laboratories. It should be pointed out that the fish tissue showed very large inhomogeneity of mercury content. Thus, all samples were ground and mixed carefully before analysis. The mercury content reported represents total concentration in the whole tissue sample, as provided.

As a further test of the method, a whole Coho Salmon, caught in Lake Erie, was obtained from the U. S. Bureau of Commercial Fisheries for the purpose of comparing mercury content in various organs with that in the edible tissue. The results obtained are shown in Table 25. It is

Table 25

Mercury Content in Various Fish Organs and Tissue

Sample Source	*Mercury Found (ppm)*
Edible tissue	0.48
Brain	0.23
Stomach	0.17
Kidney	0.36
Liver	0.87
Heart	0.44

interesting to note that the mercury concentration varies significantly in the various organs of the fish.

In an attempt to obtain mercury-free blank tissue samples (zero mercury content fish tissues) for use as a "zero" blank in the determination, fish from several bodies of water remote from known sources of mercury pollution were tested. It is interesting to note that all samples showed significant amounts of mercury (Table 26) and samples containing "no mercury" were unobtainable.

As a result of numerous analyses, the lower limit of detection is estimated to be 10 ppb ± 20%, based on counting statistics. This limit could easily be lowered by

Table 26

Mercury Content in Fish from Various Geographical Locations

Type of Fish	Source	Mercury Found (ppm)
Large Mouth Bass	Bonham State Park Lake, Texas	0.14
White Fish	Northern Lake Huron	0.05 to 0.15[a]
Blue Gill	Sandy Bottom Lake, Mich.	0.40
Rock Bass	Sandy Bottom Lake, Mich.	0.42
Coho Salmon	Southwestern Lake Erie	0.48
White Bass	Western Lake Erie	0.60
Yellow Perch	Western Lake Erie	0.17
Yellow Perch	Eastern Lake Erie	0.34
Walleyed Pike	Lake St. Clair, Mich.	1.56

[a]Several different fish

using a higher neutron flux, longer irradiation time, and/or longer counting time. In the concentration range of mercury found in fish tissue, 0.05 ppm to 10 ppm, the standard deviation of results was found to be ± 10%.

It was found that bromide ion in the sample was the only observable interference in this method. The bromide ion is retained on the ion exchange resin, and the ^{82}Br (half-life = 35 hr) spectrum is a major component of the total gamma spectrum of the sample. However, it was found that, with the high resolution of the Ge (Li) detector, concentrations of bromide ion in the levels found in the samples examined could easily be tolerated without causing any measurable error in the mercury determination. No interference was found for any other metal ion in the fish tissue studied. Furthermore, with the volume of 1M HCl used in the rinse and sodium elution, no detectable mercury (as a loss) was found in these solutions after passing through the column, and only trace Na-24 remained on the column.

In conclusion, it appears that this technique has advantages over other methods of trace mercury analysis. Especially with the addition of "carrier" mercury after irradiation, the per cent losses of sample mercury during chemical separation are lowered significantly compared to other methods. The elimination of the chemical steps in the Bowen and Gibbons method shortens the time per sample in the analyses. In addition, several samples can be run simultaneously by one technician so that the total time for preparation and counting of each unknown can be lowered to about 10 to 15 minutes per sample.

References

1. Bowen, H. J. M. and D. Gibbons. Radio Activation Analysis (Oxford: The Clarendon Press, 1963), p. 264-5.
2. Ehman, W. D. and J. R. Huizenga. "Bismuth, Thallium, and Mercury in Stone Meteorites by Activation Analysis," Geochim. Cosmochim. Acta, *17*: 125 (1959).
3. Grieg, R. Bureau of Commercial Fisheries, Department of the Interior, Ann Arbor, Michigan. Personal Communication (1970).
4. LaFleur, P. D. National Bureau of Standards, Washington, D. C. Personal Communication (1970).

Determination of Mercury by Non-Destructive Neutron Activation Analysis

Richard A. Copeland

Mercury can be analyzed nondestructively by neutron activation, by measurement of the 279 KeV gamma ray produced by decay of 47-day mercury-203. At the Great Lakes Research Division of the University of Michigan, we employ this method of mercury determination because of the multiple elemental analyses we make on limited quantities of organic and sediment samples.

In general, we follow the analytical method outlined by Gordon et al.[1] The samples, along with a standard solution containing mercury, are packaged in aluminum foil and irradiated for 50 hours at a thermal neutron flux of 10^{13} neutrons/cm^2-sec. The samples (usually about 0.5 grams dry weight) are allowed to decay for 30 days, and are then removed from the aluminum foil and placed in non-irradiated plastic vials. The samples and standards are counted, using a 4% Ge(Li) detector and a 4096 channel analyzer. Data is stored on magnetic tape, and pulse height analyses are performed by computer.

Correction for Selenium Interference

One hundred and twenty day selenium-75, which is present in all the biological samples, also has a gamma ray of 279 KeV energy.[2] This contribution must be removed from the mercury peak before mercury can be determined.[3] Selenium 75 also has a gamma ray of 264 KeV. With our equipment, using pure selenium, we established that the 279 KeV gamma ray has 40% of the intensity of the 264 KeV gamma ray. We thus subtract 40% of the area of the 264 KeV peak from the 279 KeV peak to obtain the mercury contribution alone. For mercury concentrations greater than 0.5 ppm, this correction produces less than 20% change in most organic samples.

We are unable to analyze nondestructively for mercury by using 65-hour mercury-197. The half-life is so short and the gamma ray energy so low (77 KeV) that the peak is lost under the noise produced by beta decay of 14-day phosphorus-32. We are presently attempting to develop a Ge-Ge coincidence method to analyze nondestructively for mercury-197 using the 77 KeV gamma ray and the coincident gold X-ray at 66 KeV.

Why Nondestructive Mercury Analysis is Used

There are several disadvantages and several advantages to nondestructive mercury analysis. First, it is very slow. About 30 days, including 8 hours of instrument time, are required to complete one analysis. In addition, irradiation times are relatively long (50 hours) and sensitivity rather poor, being about 0.1 ppm mercury for a 0.5 gram sample. The advantages are twofold. First, the sample is not destroyed. For most environmental work this is usually not very important, but in forensic work and archaeology it may be imperative. Second, the 50-hour irradiation and 8 hours of instrument time gives us measurements of approximately 20 elements in addition to mercury with no extra effort required on our part. To summarize this method is not the method of choice for rapid routine measurement of mercury alone. However, when sample quantity is small, or too valuable to destroy, or when a number of elements in addition to mercury must be measured, this analytical method may be best.

Acknowledgments

The author would like to thank Consumers Power Company, American Electric Power Service Corporation, Commonwealth

Edison Company, Wisconsin Public Service Corporation, Northern Indiana Public Service Company, and Wisconsin Electric Power Company for their financial assistance in making this work possible.

References

1. Gordon, G. E., K. Randle, G. G. Goles, J. B. Corciss, M. H. Beeson, and S. S. Oxley. "Instrumental Activation Analysis of Standard Rocks With High Resolution γ-ray Detectors," Geochem. Cosmochem. Acta, *32*: 369 (1968).
2. Adams, F. and R. Dams. "A Compilation of Precisely Determined Gamma-transition Energies of Radionuclides Produced by Reactor Irradiation," Journal of Radioanalytical Chemistry, *3*: 99-125 (1969).
3. Rancitelli, L. A., J. A. Cooper, and R. W. Perkins. "The Multi-element Analysis of Biological Material by Neutron Activation and Direct Instrumental Techniques," Modern Trends in Activation Analysis, NBS Spec. Pub. 312, Vol. 1 (1969), p. 101-109.

Determination of Mercury in Biological Tissues

A. R. Schulert, J. T. Davis, and D. G. Nicholson

The recent intense interest in mercury contamination has underscored the surprising inadequacy of some of the analytical methods in the literature, at least when applied to the specific problem of total mercury in fish muscle. Environmental Science and Engineering Corporation has tried four assay procedures, two of which are standard published procedures that do not work.

The procedure presented in the Perkin-Elmer Atomic Absorption Manual involves the deproteinization of the homogenized sample with TCA (trichloracetic acid), and then extraction of the mercury from the filtrate (after pH adjustment and addition of a chelator) into methyl isobutyl ketone. However, inorganic radiotracer added to the system is removed only to the extent of 2 to 10%, and about 75% of the added radiotracers never leave the initial TCA precipitate. Recovery from liver and kidney tissue appears somewhat higher than for muscle.

The Association of Official Analytical Chemists procedure, in which the sample is acid-digested and the mercury extracted from the digested homogeneous solution, works satisfactorily with inorganic standards but not with mercury in fish. Approximately 100% of the inorganic tracer added to the fish muscle sample is lost.

We then decided to take advantage of the extreme volatility of mercury by merely condensing the evolved vapor in a "cold finger." This works with about 100% recovery of the mercury in a "cold finger" condenser immersed in liquid nitrogen, but with a dry ice-acetone mixture, the recovery was incomplete. While workable, the procedure is expensive and tedious and subject to other logistic problems. For example, there was frequently a problem of clogging the line in the "cold finger," due to frozen CO and water evolved from the digested sample.

Finally, we had the good fortune to visit a research group at Wayne State University and observe their procedure, which involves the combustion of the sample in a 1,000° C furnace under a flow of oxygen, absorbing out water and oxides of carbon and nitrogen, and then measuring the atomic absorption of the mercury vapor.

We have found that the system works very adequately, is reproducible, and, once the sample is prepared for loading, the actual run takes only 3 minutes. We have employed some minor modifications; one is the incorporation of aluminum oxide as an additional filter in the line, following combustion before passage of the vapor through the atomic absorption detector. This is not necessary as long as one is sure of complete combustion of the sample, but we have found that, depending on sample size and oxygen flow, combustion is occasionally incomplete, and the resultant hydrocarbons will give a signal. These hydrocarbons are removed by the aluminum oxide.

The Determination of Ethylmercury in Blood

J. C. Gage

Most methods currently in use for the determination of trace amounts of mercury measure only total mercury. In the Industrial Hygiene Research Laboratories of Imperial Chemical Industries Limited, we have for some years been interested in the separate determination of inorganic and organic mercury, in connection with a study of the metabolism of organic mercurials in experimental animals. The first analytical technique used[1] separated the organic mercury by means of solvent extraction, a procedure which was subsequently much improved by Westöö.[2] In a later study of the metabolism of methoxyethylmercury, the differential method of Gage and Warren[3] was used. This method makes use of the varying lability of different organic mercurials in the presence of an acid-cysteine reagent,[4] which enables organic mercurials to be distinguished from inorganic mercury and, to some extent, from each other. In this method, alkaline stannous chloride solution was added to release mercury vapor, which was then measured in a mercury vapor meter.[5] Alkaline stannous chloride provides advantages over acidic stannous chloride, because some organic mercurials are rapidly degraded under acidic conditions, and also because alkaline conditions inhibit the frothing of blood solutions.

We have recently become interested in the measurement of organic mercury in the blood of workmen exposed to mercurial seed dressings containing a small proportion of an ethylmercury salt. Some difficulties were encountered in applying the method of Gage and Warren to the low concentrations likely to be present in blood, partly due to the mercury content of the acid-cysteine reagent.

Separate Determination of Inorganic and Organic Mercury

During the course of this investigation, it was discovered that ethylmercury is fairly rapidly broken down to release mercury vapor by a strong solution of stannous chloride in alkali, provided that an air current was used to blow off the vapor. With nitrogen there was no measurable release of mercury; conversely, the rate of mercury release could be increased by using oxygen. As mercuric salts release mercury vapor with this reagent in the absence of oxygen, the separate determination of inorganic and organic mercury may be effected by first blowing off the mercury from inorganic salts with nigrogen, then changing to air or oxygen to break down the ethylmercury.

Satisfactory results have been obtained by adding 1 ml blood to 10 ml water with a little silicone antifoam emulsion in a glass bubbler. Nitrogen is passed through the bubbler and then to the mercury vapor meter via a spray trap. The meter is connected to a pen recorder. While nitrogen is passing, 2 ml 0.2M stannous chloride in 5N NaOH is added; after the release of mercury from any mercuric salts is complete, air is passed through the system. The area of the tracing obtained with known amounts of ethylmercury chloride indicates that conversion is complete. At the highest sensitivity of the instrument, there is some interference from organic vapors liberated from blood in the presence of the reagent; this can be avoided by passing the air through a furnace before it enters the meter.

A limited number of experiments have indicated that methylmercury is much more stable than ethylmercury under the conditions of this method, and so far, attempts to modify the method to deal with methylmercury have not been very successful.

References

1. Gage, J. C.   Brit. J. Ind. Med., *21*: 197 (1964).
2. Westöö, G. "Determination of Methylmercury Compounds in Foodstuffs. I. Methylmercury Compounds in Fish, Identification and Determination," Acta Chem. Scand., *20*: 2131 (1966).
3. Gage, J. C. and J. M. Warren. "Determination of Mercury and Organic Mercurials in Biological Samples," Ann. Occup. Hyg., *13*: 115 (1970).
4. Weiner, I. M., R. I. Levy, and G. H. Mudge. J. Pharmacol., *138*: 96 (1962).
5. Magos, L. and A. A. Chernik. "A Rapid Method for Estimating Mercury in Undigested Biological Samples," Brit. J. Ind. Med., *26*: 144 (1969).

The Determination of Mono- and Dimethylmercury Compounds By Gas Chromatography

Rolf Hartung

Since it has been shown that inorganic mercury can be converted to monomethylmercury and dimethylmercury in anaerobic sediments,[1] we have developed a method which will analyze both of these species of mercury in a single sample.

Dimethylmercury, if present, would be labile under the acidic conditions specified by Westöö[2] for the extraction of methylmercury. Since the dimethylmercury dissociates to monomethylmercury under those conditions, that method may produce somewhat elevated values for environmental samples which also contain dimethylmercury.

The essential step of this new method for the analysis of both monomethyl- and dimethylmercury is the initial addition of a cysteine-borate buffer at pH 8.2 to the sample. The purpose of this buffer is to stabilize the dimethylmercury, and to combine with any free monomethylmercury to form the water-soluble cysteine adduct. At this time, only the dimethylmercury is available for extraction by toluene. Once it has been extracted, it is analyzed by a procedure modified from that of Jensen and Jernelöv,[1] with the optional addition of an additional purification step. The method consists of saponifying the extract with 4-6 M KOH under reflux, washing, and subsequent conversion of the dimethylmercury to monomethylmercury according to:

$$CH_3HgCH_3 + HgBr_2 \xrightarrow[\Delta]{} 2\ CH_3HgBr$$

This step has a twofold purpose. First, it improves the specificity of the test by producing a specific derivative. Second, it greatly improves the sensitivity of the test because the dimethylmercury is not very readily detected by electron-capture gas chromatography, while methylmercuric bromide has a strong electron affinity.

The sample which has been extracted for dimethylmercury can now be processed according to a modification of the method of Westöö,[2] by acidifying it strongly with HCl to displace the methylmercury from its sulfhydryl binding sites so that it can then become available for extraction with toluene.

The method readily distinguishes between $CH_3Hg\ X$ and $(CH_3)_2Hg$ which have been added to samples, giving recoveries between 80% and 95%.

Toluene must be purified by fractional distillation to be suitable for the procedure. The degree of purity can be readily tested by GLC. The hydrochloric acid must be of the highest available degree of purity.

During the analysis of dimethylmercury, there is a remote possibility that, in some samples, there may be substances capable of acting as methyl donors under the analytical conditions of synthesizing the CH_3HgBr derivation from $(CH_3)_2Hg$. While this possibility, as yet, has not been proven, it has also not been excluded. A way to circumvent that difficulty would be to analyze the toluene from the first extraction for its mercury content. This step would, however, have the shortcoming of also determining any other R-Hg-R compounds which are relatively nonpolar in nature.

Cross-checks on the identity of dimethylmercury can also be made by subjecting the supernatant containing $(CH_3)_2Hg$ to acid hydrolysis, which would result in one mole of CH_3HgCl for every mole of $(CH_3)_2Hg$.

The gas chromatographic analysis is normally conducted at an oven temperature of 100° C. Periodically, the column is programmed to 210° C, in order to clear interfering compounds with longer retention times out of the column. Since the CH_3Hg X peak is analyzed for both monomethyl and dimethylmercury, the only differences seen are those caused by materials which were not removed during the clean-up (see Figures 20 and 21).

Laboratory Procedure

Homogenize a 10 gm to 20 gm sample with an equal volume of cysteine-borate buffer (1 gm $Na_2B_4O_7 \cdot 10H_2O$ + 0.4 gm cysteine $\cdot$ HCl in 20 ml H_2O).

Extract with 5 to 10 ml toluene; repeat 3 times. Separate by centrifugation.

To the residue, containing CH_3Hg-S-R and other R-Hg-cysteines, add an equal volume of concentrated HCl and 5-10 ml toluene. Extract and separate by centrifugation. Repeat this procedure once. Save the supernatant; the residue contains inorganic Hg. To the supernatant, add 10 ml 2% cysteine-borate. Stir 15 minutes, and save the lower layer. Add concentrated HCl and toluene as described above. After the centrifugation, save the toluene layer and dry over Na_2SO_4. Perform the gas chromatographic analysis according to the conditions described in Table 28.

To the supernatant of the original centrifugations, containing $(CH_3)_2Hg$ and other nonpolar R-Hg-R, saponify with 20 ml of 4-6M KOH. Separate the toluene layer, and

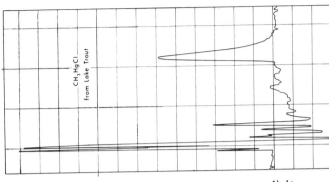

Figure 20: Gas Chromatographic
Tracing—Standard Solution

Figure 21: Gas Chromatographic
Tracing—Fish Sample After
Clean-Up

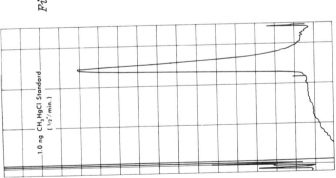

Table 27

Analysis of Alkyl Mercury Compounds in Birds,
Mainly from the Lake St. Clair Area,
Using the Method Described in This Paper

Species	Total Hg (ppm)	CH_3HgCl (ppm)	Contribution of CH_3HgCl to total Hg (%)
Pheasant	0.64	<0.002	–
Pheasant	0.31	0.05	13
Pheasant	0.28	<0.002	–
Pheasant	0.29	<0.002	–
Pheasant	0.64	0.08	10
Lesser Scaup	1.27	0.828	51
Lesser Scaup	1.27	0.490	30
Lesser Scaup	1.08	0.113	8
Lesser Scaup	1.27	1.10	68
Lesser Scaup	1.76	0.304	14
Lesser Scaup	1.20	0.318	21
Lesser Scaup	1.27	0.634	39
Lesser Scaup	0.84	0.359	34
Greater Scaup	0.94	0.235	20
Black Duck	0.70	<0.002	–
Mallard	0.83	<0.002	–
Mallard	0.18	0.02	9
Green-winged Teal	0.28	<0.002	–
Green-winged Teal	0.18	0.023	10

wash it twice with H_2O, using NaCl to break emulsions. Dry over Na_2SO_4. Prepare the monomethyl derivative by adding 0.15 gm $HgBr_2$ and 1 gm KBr in 10 ml H_2O. Reflux and stir one-half hour. If desired, perform a clean-up procedure-- add 10 ml 2% cysteine-borate, stir 15 minutes, and save the lower layer. Then add HCl and toluene as described in the previous paragraph, and save the toluene layer. Dry over Na_2SO_4, and perform the gas chromatographic analysis according to the conditions described in Table 28.

Table 28

Gas Chromatography Apparatus and Conditions for
Monomethylmercury and Dimethylmercury Determination

Column: 5 foot Pyrex column 1/4" diameter
Liquid Phase: 11% (QF-1 + OV-17)*
Support: 80/100 Gas-chrom Q*
Injector Temperature: 180° C
Oven Temperature: 100° C - program to 210° C
Detector Temperature: 220° C
Gas Flow: 60 ml N_2/min
Detector: tritium electron capture

*Available from Applied Science Laboratories, Inc.,
P.O. Box 440, College Park, Pa.

References

1. Jensen, S. and A. Jernelov. "Biological Methylation of
   Mercury in Aquatic Organisms," Nature, *223*: 753 (1969).
2. Westöö, G. "Determination of Methyl Mercury Salts in
   Various Kinds of Biological Material,"
   Scand., *21*: 2277 (1968).

Analytical Methodology for Mercury

Discussion Paper

Contributions by: H. M. Benedict, J. N. Bishop,
C. A. Burns, W. S. Ferguson, J. C. Gage, W. S.
Lyon, B. B. Mesman, J. F. Shea, and R. G. Smith

Sample preparation and sample storage presents unusual
problems for mercury and its compounds. When water samples
are stored in plastic containers at ordinary temperatures,
mercury losses can be up to 10% within two days, and up to
50% after one month. The storage of frozen fish samples
in plastic bags seems to be satisfactory, resulting in less
than 10% losses after nine months of freezer storage.
Analyses of 200 year old museum specimens indicate that

mercury in fish is quite stable, as long as the specimens have been kept properly preserved in nonplastic containers. Mercury-containing pigments have persisted for at least 3000 years in Egyptian mummies, indicating a high stability for some mercury compounds.

In addition to the analytical methods mentioned in the previous papers, the chelation of mercury from urine,and water with ammoniumpyrolidinedithiocarbamate (APDC), and subsequent extraction into methylisobutylketone (MIBK) has been successful. When 0.2 ml of this extract is analyzed in a tantalum boat by routine atomic absorption techniques, sensitivities of 0.01 ppm to 0.005 ppm were reported.

PART III

ENVIRONMENTAL DYNAMICS OF MERCURY

CONTRIBUTORS TO PART III

Ramon E. Bisque, Department of Chemistry, Colorado School
   of Mines, Golden, Colorado.
Rolf Hartung, Ph.D., Department of Environmental and
   Industrial Health, University of Michigan, Ann Arbor,
   Michigan.
Årne Jernelöv, PhD., Institute of Water and Air Pollution
   Research, Stockholm, Sweden.
Paul B. Trost, Department of Chemistry, Colorado School
   of Mines, Golden, Colorado.

Factors in the Transformation of Mercury
to Methylmercury

Årne Jernelöv

In Sweden the three main compounds of mercury that are
released into the aquatic environment are the bivalent
inorganic mercury, elementary mercury, and phenylmercury.
All three of these compounds tend to move into the sediments
first, for a variety of reasons. Phenylmercury, as it is
used in Sweden in the wood pulp industry, mainly sticks
to the fibers and will sediment with those.   Elementary
mercury is not very soluble in water, and it is well known
that it is a very heavy element and will sediment quite
close to the outlets. The bivalent mercury forms very
strong complexes with many organic and inorganic substances
and particles in the water and will settle down with them.
Of course, the mercury attached to particles might also
stay in suspension in the water for some time.
    In the next step, the different compounds are converted
into inorganic bivalent mercury, which means that the elemental mercury is oxidized and phenylmercury is broken
down.   From then on the biological part of the process
becomes important.   The mercuric ion is methylated to
monomethyl- or dimethylmercury. The monomethylmercury
will leach into the water and then further accumulate in
fish, algae, and other living water organisms, while
dimethylmercury will have more of a tendency to move with
gas bubbles through the water up to the atmosphere. It
is, however, not very stable in the atmosphere. Under
acidic conditions or ultraviolet light, dimethylmercury
will break down and form monomethylmercury that might fall
with precipitation in some nearby body of water or over
land. If it is converted to elementary mercury it might
also fall with precipitation, or take part in the global
circulation of elementary mercury vapor. The rate with

which these processes occur is dependent on different
physical, chemical and biological conditions in the waters
where the transformations take place.

Oxidation of Elementary to Bivalent Mercury

If we examine the oxidation of elementary mercury to
bivalent mercury, we find that this, like all oxidation
processes, is dependent on the redox potential in the
system. The redox potential that is necessary for this
oxidation can be calculated from the formula below[1]

$$E = 850 + 30 \log \frac{(Hg^{++})}{\alpha}$$

where E is the redox potential necessary. It is proportional to the total concentration of bivalent mercury in
the system, and it is negatively proportional to the alpha
coefficient, which is an estimation of the strength of the
binding between bivalent mercury and the available complex-
forming substances. As stated earlier, the complexes
between some organic substances and bivalent mercury are
very strong, which means that alpha coefficients for these
complexes are very high. If we estimate the alpha coefficients by comparison with other mercury complexes of known
strength, and substitute for the concentration of total
bivalent mercury in the equation a number which seems
reasonable in our aquatic environment, then we will find
that this oxidation takes place as soon as we have both
organic substances and oxygen present in the aquatic
system. Thus, this oxidation will occur in most of our
fresh waters.

$$Hg^{\circ} \rightleftarrows Hg^{++} \rightleftarrows CH_3Hg^+ \rightleftarrows (CH_3)_2Hg$$

Methylation of Mercuric Sulfide

Previously I discussed three types of mercury compounds
that are discharged into water. However, there is a special
form of bivalent mercury, mercuric sulfide, which also has
to be oxidized before methylation can take place, but which
does not act in quite the same way as elementary mercury.
Mercuric sulfide has a very low solubility product (it is
almost insoluble in water). Even if the theoretical
solubility product of 10^{-53} is just theoretical, and even
if it does not apply to the conditions in natural waters
where oxygen and competing complex forms are present, this
is still an extremely low solubility.

In order for the bivalent mercury to be available for methylation, an oxidation of the sulphur group from sulfide to sulfate has to take place. This might be a purely chemical process, but it can also be a biological process. With both elementary mercury and mercuric sulfide, we begin with an oxidation step and continue with the biological methylation. So, whether we begin with elementary mercury or with mercuric sulfide, the biological methylation will be a two-step process. The two cases provide different answers to the question about which part of this process is the rate-determining step.

$$HgS \rightleftarrows Hg^{++} \rightleftarrows CH_3Hg^+$$

In many experiments where elementary mercury has been added to aquaria or other systems, we obtained the same methylation rate whether elementary mercury or inorganic bivalent mercury was added. This indicates that for elementary mercury the last step in the reaction, the biological methylation, is the rate-determining one. When mercuric sulfide is added, a much smaller amount of methylmercury is formed within the same period than if we add inorganic bivalent mercury.

From laboratory tests, the ratio between methylation rates for ionic bivalent mercury and mercuric sulfide seems to be approximately $1:10^{-3}$. In this case, the first oxidation step is the rate-determining one.

Effects of Sediment on the Conversion of Mercury

It appears that the sediment, or perhaps the suspended particles, play a very important role for the conversion of mercury. We have, therefore, investigated the effects of depth of sediment on the formation and release of methylmercury. Mercury-rich sediment was placed at various depths in test containers and covered with different depths of sediments which contained little mercury. When there were only microorganisms present, methylmercury was found and released only when the mercury-rich layer was on the surface. When we added macroorganisms (tubificids) to the system, we found that mercury-rich layers down to a depth of 2 cm contributed to the formation and release of methylmercury. When we added some freshwater mussels (Anodonta), methylated mercury was released from a depth of 9 cm.

We can generally say that the ability to methylate mercury is not a unique thing among microorganisms. We have identified several different bacteria from different genera and also fungi with this ability, and have a very strong impression that the methylation rates are very well correlated with the general microbiological activity in the sediment. This means that the factors which promote and increase the general microbiological activity, such as a good supply of nutrients and moderately high water temperature, also effect the methylation rate in a similar manner.

Effects of pH on Methylation

It is clear from both laboratory tests and field studies that a lower water pH will result in a comparatively higher amount of mercury in the fish. One possible explanation would be that the total methylation rate is dependent upon pH. Another explanation is that of the two net products, mono- and dimethylmercury, monomethylmercury would be favored by a lower pH. Thus, at a higher pH, more of the methylating mercury is converted to dimethylmercury, of which part might leave that body of water and be released into the air and consequently not accumulate in the fish. From laboratory experiments, we have come to the conclusion that the latter of these hypotheses is the correct one. At the higher pH more dimethylmercury is formed, and at the low pH, which rarely occurs in natural water, dimethyl-mercury will not be stable at all; but long before this, the conditions seem to favor organisms that produce monomethylmercury rather than dimethylmercury. Thus the general conclusion is that, at a low pH, more of the methylated mercury will be monomethylmercury and stay within the system.

Anaerobic and Aerobic Conditions

The importance of anaerobic and aerobic conditions on the methylation of mercury is another much discussed factor.
The first system that was described for the methylation of mercury was the methylation from methyl cobalamine (methyl Vitamin B_{12}) as described by Wood and his collaborators.[2]   This is a strictly anaerobic process that will occur only in the absence of oxygen. Another possible method for the methylation of mercury within the cell is from a complex between inorganic bivalent mercury and homocysteine. When mercury is bound to homocysteine, the mercury appears to be methylated instead, thus forming methylmercuric monocysteine. This second process, described by Landner, is not a strict anaerobic one. From lab tests, we can easily show that the methylation activity very often

is higher under anaerobic conditions than under aerobic conditions. But, if we examine the situation in a lake or a river, hydrogen sulfide will be formed when oxygen disappears, and the result will be the formation of mercuric sulfide. Under the anaerobic conditions, no methylation will occur from mercuric sulfide as far as we can determine. Therefore, in fresh water we are more likely to have a high methylation rate under aerobic than under anaerobic conditions because of the occurrence of hydrogen sulfide and subsequent formation of mercuric sulfide.

Long-term Effects of Mercury in Water

If we look at the long-term effect of mercury in a body of water, we have some discouraging results in Sweden. We have a chloralkali industry that was closed down in 1925 (more than 45 years ago), and when we measure the amount of mercury in the upper part of the sediment and in the organisms today, we still find high concentrations. If we wish to wait for the lakes to recover by themselves, perhaps 45 years is an unacceptably long period. On the other hand, this is an oligotrophic lake. It has a very low sedimentation rate, so the mercury-rich sediment is only covered very slowly, and we also have permanently oxygenated sediments. There are other areas where mercury releases were stopped 25 to 30 years ago, in which at present the mercury is located some decimeters down in the sediment, and where the fish have relatively low concentrations of mercury. Consequently, the time it will take for a lake to recover is evidently dependent to a high degree on the local conditions. Generally it can be concluded that in an oligotrophic lake a much longer time will elapse before the decrease in mercury content in fish becomes evident than in an eutrophic lake.

In Sweden, we have studied the possibilities of increasing the speed of recovery from mercury contamination in lakes by four alternative methods. One of these is to cover the mercury-rich sediment with some inert material, like clay, or with some mercury-absorbing material like freshly ground silica. Another possibility is to try to form mercuric sulfide, which could be done simply by polluting the lake with sulfides. We could add hydrogen sulfide, which is very detrimental to the organisms living in the lake and would kill most of the fish as well, or some other sulfide like ferrous sulfide. A fourth method is to try to change the methylation process in such a way that more dimethylmercury would be produced, which is basically to raise the pH, and perhaps also to add some nitrogen in certain situations. This last method would mean, however, that we would spread the pollution over larger areas by dispersing the released dimethylmercury into the atmosphere.

References

1. Jernelöv, A. "Conversion of Mercury Compounds," Chapt. 4 in <u>Chemical Fallout</u> (C. C. Thomas Publ., 1969).
2. Wood, J. M., F. S. Kennedy, and C. G. Rosen. "Synthesis of Methylmercury Compounds by Extracts of a Methanogenic Bacterium," <u>Nature</u>, *220*: 173-174 (1968).

The Role of Food Chains in Environmental Mercury Contamination

Rolf Hartung

Our interest in food chains, especially as they interact with toxic substances, has been increasing steadily. Research on the role of food chains in the transport and magnification of chlorinated hydrocarbon pesticides has done a great deal to enlarge our knowledge in this important area. To what extent this knowledge can be applied to the study of the environmental and biological behavior of mercury is, as yet, not entirely clear.

In the case of mercury, our main concern is that those species which occupy the peak of the food chain, such as predatory animals or perhaps man, can under certain conditions receive inordinately high exposures when compared with those levels which one would find in the environment in general.

A critical analysis of food chains and their role in the biological dynamics of mercury is unusually complex, because of the number of mercury compounds which occur in the environment and which can be transformed into other compounds of mercury under appropriate naturally-occurring conditions.

The basic conceptual components of a food chain that may be able to concentrate a toxicant can be viewed in the following fashion:

Absorption: identification of routes of absorption and efficiency of absorption, contribution of toxicants in food intake to total body burden.

Concentration Factor: the ratio of the body burden
of the toxicant in the organism under study with
respect to the toxicant loadings in its food supply
(assuming that the entire body burden is derived
from that source alone), or with respect to its
surrounding medium (air, water, or soil), assuming
again that the entire body burden is derived directly
from that source.

Biological Half-Life: an empirically-derived description of the rates of excretion and metabolism of a
toxicant in an organism (an extended definition).

Ecological Community Structure: identification of
food webs and degree of dependence between different
trophic levels.

The general outline of such a food chain can be illustrated in simple terms in Figure 22. An important point

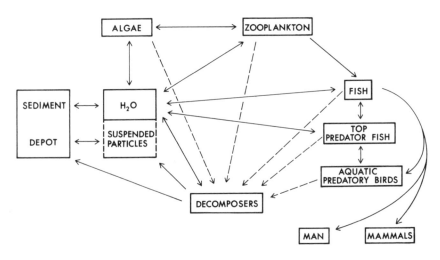

Figure 22: Environmental Dynamics of Hg in Aquatic
   Communities: The Role of Food Chains

to consider is that most organisms in the aquatic environment may derive their mercury burdens from more than just
a single source.
The major complexities in the consideration of the
environmental transport of mercury arise out of the presence

of the variety of mercury compounds known to occur in the environment. The most important classes of compounds in this respect appear to be HgS, Hg^{++}, $RSHg^+$, RHg^+, and $RHgR^+$. All of these groups of compounds have different solubilities, stabilities, and lipid-water partition coefficients. Therefore, they should also behave very differently in environmental transport and food chains.

To date, the vast majority of studies have restricted themselves to total mercury, which is obviously an oversimplification engendered by analytical convenience. Only a few studies have sought to define the mercury compounds present in environmental samples.

In spite of the complexity of the environmental dynamics of mercury and its compounds, this subject merits a great deal of practical and theoretical consideration because of its obvious implications to human health and the survival of predatory animals.

Mercury and Food Chains

Årne Jernelöv

One of the most obvious examples of the operation of food chains in the distribution of mercury can be illustrated by the connections between the uses of mercury as a seed dressing and the resulting levels of mercury in the feathers of birds. This work was done by Johnels and Westermark[1] in Sweden, using museum specimens.

If we plot the concentrations of mercury in feathers of terrestrial birds annually from 1840 to the present, for seed-eating birds and for birds of prey which consume seed-eating birds, we find a low constant mercury level in the feathers from 1840 to about 1946. After that, the concentrations of mercury increase very rapidly. This coincides with the introduction and increased use of methylmercury as a seed-dressing agent. In 1965, when these connections became clearly known, methylmercury was banned as a seed-dressing agent. In the following years the concentrations of mercury in seed-eating birds started to decrease again. We can see today that the mercury content in these birds is well on the way back towards prior levels. The relationship between mercury content in the feathers of these birds and the use of one specific mercury compound is very simple, but if we look at the aquatic food chains, the relationship is somewhat more complicated.

If we plot the mercury concentration in feathers of fish-eating birds in the same manner, starting at about 1840, we find a low basic level until 1880-1890, when the industrial revolution started in Sweden. From that time on, there is a constant increase in the mercury content in the feathers of fish-eating birds. The shape of this figure indicates that mercury contributions came from many sources. There is also a fair correlation between the mercury levels in the feathers of the birds and the mercury levels in fish in this environment. The birds accumulate mercury by eating fish and the fish accumulate it from their food, or perhaps directly from the water.

Mercury Levels in Fish and Fish Stomachs

In connection with another experiment, our laboratory caught about 1,500 kilograms of Northern pike from one of the heavily contaminated waters in Sweden, analyzed the mercury content of the fish found in their stomachs, and compared the mercury levels of these fish to that of the pikes which preyed upon them. Then we continued further and took the stomachs of the fish found within the stomachs of the pikes; these stomachs mainly contained different kinds of bottom fauna. There were some difficulties in making reliable mercury analyses on these organisms but, once we were able to identify what these fish had fed on, we could go back and catch the bottom fauna and analyze the mercury in them in relation to the quantities found in the fish stomachs.

The mercury concentrations of the pike were around 5.8 ppm. The fish found in their stomachs, largely Swedish whitefish, contained about 3.1 ppm of mercury, and in the bottom fauna we found 0.3 ppm mercury. A similar comparison from relatively uncontaminated water gives pike, 1.2 ppm; whitefish, 0.6 ppm; and bottom fauna, 0.05 ppm. This was all reported on a fresh weight basis. Then the question is, can we learn something from these figures about how the fish accumulate the mercury? I think we can, if we consider a small experiment in which we fed whitefish containing about 3 ppm mercury to pike in the laboratory and then analyzed the amount of that mercury which the pike accumulated. To our surprise, the pike accumulated only 10-15%.

Let us examine this level of absorption and then compare it with the normal standard figure for the relationship between food intake and growth (10 times), which means that in order to increase one kg in weight, a pike will consume approximately 10 kg of fish. If we now examine the mercury burdens, starting with the pike at about 5.8 ppm and the whitefish with 3.1 ppm, it is quite evident that if the pike did absorb all the mercury from the whitefish, their resulting body burdens should have been much higher. From these data, we could calculate a maximum uptake of 20% under environmental conditions.

If we extended this type of calculation to the whitefish and the bottom fauna which they were feeding on, we can account for all of the accumulations in that step. That is, if the whitefish consumed 10 kg of bottom fauna for every kg of weight gain, they would contain about the amount they do without taking up any mercury from the water directly. It is not very likely that there should be such a difference in absorption between the whitefish and the northern pike. If we use the laboratory datum of 10–15% mercury accumulation from dietary sources in pike and extend these to whitefish, then the whitefish would have accumulated only 0.3 ppm mercury out of 3.1 ppm mercury from dietary sources, and the northern pike would have accumulated only 3.1 ppm out of 5.8 ppm from its dietary sources. That means that the mercury uptake from the water for both the whitefish and the pike should be quite similar, roughly 3 ppm. Of course, there are differences between whitefish and pike, but it seems reasonable to assume that the uptake of mercury from water should be in the same range.

The picture which we get from this case is that food will contribute to the concentration of mercury in fish in such a way that it provides a basic level above which the fish then continues to accumulate mercury from the water directly. By looking at the percentage of the total body burden that different fish accumulate from food and from water, we find that the northern pike derives about 50% from food and the remaining 50% from water, while the whitefish derives about 10% from food and the remaining 90% from water. If we make similar calculations for the data from fish in waters that have a relatively low level of mercury pollution, the result is very similar.

Methylation by Microorganisms in Fish Slime

In relation to the mechanisms of mercury uptake by fish, I would like to discuss another experiment where we examined the ability of microorganisms in the slime on the surface of the fish to methylate mercury. The purpose of this experiment was to see whether the fish, or what might be called the system of the fish, could methylate mercury. There were some indications that this could happen, and we wanted to differentiate between the fish itself, the microorganisms in the intestine, and the microorganisms in the slime on the surface of the fish.

We injected inorganic mercury into the liver and muscles of the pike. The intestine was removed and inorganic mercury was added to it; mercury was also added to the slime from the surface of the fish. In the first two cases we could not show any methylation in the fish itself, either in the muscles or in the liver; but we could show a very low rate of methylation by the microorganisms in the intestine. With the slime we obtained a very high methylation rate during the first experiment. In this case, more than 90% of the added inorganic mercury was converted to methylmercury within a few hours. At the time, we thought that this was a very important finding, but, since it was just one experiment, we wanted to repeat it. I should mention that this experiment was started in early spring (March).

We caught fresh pikes, removed the slime, added inorganic mercury, and repeated the entire process. This time about 30% of the total amount of mercury was converted to methylmercury, which was still a very high conversion rate. However, as the results differed considerably, we caught new pikes and repeated the process again to determine the real value. This time the conversion rate turned out to be 10%. We continued repeating the experiment throughout the spring and into the beginning of summer. By the middle of July, we were down to a very small methylation rate which was perhaps insignificant.

After much investigation, we found that certain microorganisms which are predominant in fish slime during the late winter and early spring in Sweden have a high capacity to methylate mercury, while those living there the rest of the year do not have the same capacity. We also found that those microorganisms which methylated mercury, or which did so at a very high rate, only methylated mercury when kept on a fish extract substrate but not when kept on a meat extract substrate.

References

1. Johnels, A. G., and T. Westermark. "Mercury Contamination in the Environment in Sweden," Chapter 10 in Chemical Fallout. (C. C. Thomas Publ., 1969), pp. 221-239.

Distribution of Mercury in Residual Soils

Paul B. Trost and Ramon E. Bisque

Introduction

Secondary dispersion is largely controlled by the behavior of the chemical elements in the aqueous environment.[1] Gruner[2] and Graham[3] observed that humic acids were involved in the chemical weathering of certain minerals, resulting in solubilities far above values for pure water. Schnitzer[4] observed the formation of stable complexes between a fulvic acid (extracted from a soil) and numerous cations such as Cu, Pb, Fe, Ni, and Zn. As a result of this fulvic acid-cation complex, various cations may be mobilized in the soil profile. Dvornikov, and others, proposed that a humic acid-mercury complex occurs in the humus-rich fraction of a soil to explain its relatively high concentration of mercury.

Understanding factors that control the distribution of mercury in a soil may aid in the interpretation of soil geochemical programs which employ mercury as a pathfinder element, and may also provide a basis for sampling procedures in pollution studies.

Trost and Bisque[5] have suggested a method for the differentiation of vaporous soil mercury (usually associated with mineralization) and nonvaporous soil mercury (often of an ionic, transported origin) by the comparison of the mercury content in the organic-rich and clay-rich soil horizons.

Field sampling of soils in and adjacent to known mercury mineralization was conducted in southwest Oregon. Each soil horizon was analyzed for its mercury and humic acid* content. The relative distribution of the clay fraction in each soil horizon was determined by X-ray analysis.

Similar studies were made in central Colorado to determine any variations in the observed mercury distribution within a totally different geologic and climatic environment.

Laboratory studies were conducted to determine the effect of humic-acid-type organics on (1) the solubility of several mercury compounds, (2) the mercuric ion sorption capacities

---

*In this manuscript, the term "humic acid" will represent the total alkali soluble extract of the sample, i.e., both the humic and fulvic acid fractions.

of organic-rich and clay-rich horizons, and (3) the vaporous mercury sorption capacities of these same organic-rich and clay-rich samples.

Part I of this manuscript discusses certain variables that affect the distribution of mercuric ion, Hg^{++}, in residual soils, whereas Part II deals with variables affecting distribution of mercury vapor in residual soils.

Distribution of Mercury Ion (Hg^{++}) in Soils

Laboratory Studies

The potential effect of humic acids on the chemical weathering of cinnabar was investigated by comparing the aqueous mercury concentrations in humic acid solutions and distilled water, each in contact with 0.200 gm of crystalline HgS (<200 mesh).

Humic acid solutions were obtained by extracting with 0.1N NaOH the A_1 and A_2 soil horizons of a chernozem soil developed under coniferous and deciduous vegetation. The extract, which contained both the fulvic and humic acid fractions, was centrifuged, filtered, dialyzed, and passed through ion exchange columns. After the above purification techniques, an ash content of 20% still remained. Samples were characterized by infrared spectra, potentiometric titrations, absolute C,H,N analysis, visible spectrophotometry, and emission spectrophotometry, and found to be similar to humic and fulvic extracts obtained by other investigators.[4,6] Oxidizable carbon content in parts per million carbon (ppm C) was determined by the Walkley-Black method[7] and used as an index of concentration.

Aliquots, containing 850 ppm C humic acid, were adjusted to pH 5.0, 6,0, 7.0, with either dilute NaOH or HNO3 solutions, and placed in loosely-capped polyethylene bottles. Blanks, containing 150 ml of distilled water at similar pH values, also in contact with solid HgS, were prepared. Every three to four days, the pH of the solution was checked and, if necessary, adjusted with a few drops of dilute NaOH or HNO3. After three months equilibration, the solutions were centrifuged and filtered to remove any suspended HgS. Mercury analysis of the filtered solutions was accomplished using the Pyrih-Bisque technique.[8,9]

Additional solubility experiments were conducted over a two-month period with 250 ml of 166 ppm C humic acid and distilled water blanks, each in contact with 0.200 gm of HgO and 0.200 gm of Hg_2Cl_2 (<200 mesh). Polyethylene bottles were loosely stoppered to allow equilibration with the atmosphere and thus allow the pH to reach equilibrium (pH≈6.0).

Two approaches were used to contrast empirically mercuric sorption capacities of clay-rich and organic-rich fractions of soil samples. In the first set of experiments, 2.00 gm samples of dried <150 mesh peat, pine mull, illite, montmorillonite, and kaolinite were agitated for three hours in 100 ml of a solution containing 10 ppm Hg^{++} at 25 ± 1.0° C. The solid-liquid suspension was adjusted to pH 6.0 with dilute HNO_3 or NaOH. After equilibration, samples were centrifuged, filtered, washed with demineralized water, recentrifuged, and dried. Mercury concentration in the dried, homogenized, solid phase was determined by the Pyrih-Bisque technique. Similar experiments were repeated employing A and B soil horizons developed under coniferous, deciduous, and grass vegetations.

A second set of experiments was conducted to determine the effect of humic acids on mercuric sorption from aqueous solution by illite and montmorillonite at pH 6.0. This procedure consisted of shaking 1.00 gm of <100 mesh clay with 100 ml aliquots containing 10, 20, 30, 40, and 50 ppm Hg^{++} for two hours at room temperature (25 ± 1.0° C). The experiment was repeated with the aqueous solution containing 100 ppm C humic acid in addition to the mercury ions. Atomic absorption was used to analyze the filtered aqueous solution, noting any decrease in the aqueous Hg^{++} concentration. Experimental results were graphed as adsorption isotherms, i.e., amount of Hg^{++} sorbed per gram of clay vs. the equilibrium concentration of Hg^{++}.

In an effort to represent more closely the natural environment, the clays were not converted into a Na^+ or H^+ form or other uni-cationic form. Laser spectrographic analyses of the clays showed a wide variety of cations within each (Table 29).

Experimental Results

Experimental results of the effect of 850 ppm C humic acids (HA) on the solubility of <200 mesh, crystalline, red HgS are shown on Table 30.

In the pH range 5-7, humic acid at a concentration of 850 ppm C significantly increased the solubility of the HgS. The experimentally determined solubility of HgS in demineralized water (15 ppb) agrees quite well with published values.[10]

Table 29

Laser Spectrographic Analyses of
Illite (Wards #35) and Montmorillonite (Wards #26)

Sample	Element												
	Ti	Zn	Mn	Ni	Cu	Pb	B	Sn	Co	As	Sb	Ba	Sr
Illite	3000	70	500	30	50	50	100	<20	<50	<100	100	100	100
Mont-morillonite	500	85	70	7	20	150	20	20	<10	<100	<50	<100	260

Table 30

Increase in HgS Solubility by the Presence of
Humic Acid Solutions (HA) After 90 Days

Sample	pH	E_h (mv)	Hg (pbb)
HA + HgS	5.0	+185	450.0
	6.0	+155	48.0
	7.0	+145	10.0
Distilled H$_2$O + HgS	5.0	+150	15.0
	6.0	+140	0.0
	7.0	+130	0.0

Results of static solubility experiments using HgO and
Hg$_2$Cl$_2$, each in contact with demineralized water, and also
in 166 ppm C humic acid solutions, are shown in Table 31.

Table 31

Solubilities of Mercury Compounds in Humic Acid
Solutions (HA) and in Demineralized Water (H$_2$O)
After 60 Days

Sample	Solubility in HA (ppm)	Solubility in H$_2$O	Solubility in Handbook (ppm)
HgO	200	68.0	52.0
Hg$_2$Cl$_2$	12.5	2.50	2.0

Again, the presence of soluble humic acids (166 ppm C)
increased the solubility of the mercury compounds. Based
on the above experimental data, it appears that humic acid
solutions are therefore capable of increasing the solubility
of certain mercury compounds.

Schnitzer[4] observed that an interaction occurred between the carboxyl groups of fulvic acid and certain metal cations. To determine if a similar interaction occurs involving Hg^{++}, an infrared spectra of an evaporated humic acid solution containing Hg^{++} was run. This was compared to an evaporated humic acid solution containing no Hg^{++}. A shift was observed in the 1600 cm^{-1} region of the spectra, where the carboxyl group absorbs.

A schematic equation for this increase in mercury solubility by the humic acid may be written as

$$3RCOO^- + 2HgS \rightarrow (RCOO)_3 Hg_2^+ + 2S^=$$

where $RCOO^-$ represents the functional group of a humic acid molecule. The molar ratios for the mercuric-humate interaction were determined similarly to a method previously described by Schnitzer and Skinner.[11]

A Tyndal effect was not observed in any of the solutions, indicating that the humic acids were in true solution and apparently were not interacting as colloids.

Laboratory studies, therefore, suggest that the solubility of cinnabar in the organic-rich soil horizon may far surpass its solubility in the organic-poor soil horizons.

Clays may also affect mercuric ion distributions in soils through their cation exchange capabilities. Results of empirical laboratory experiments contrasting the mercuric ion sorption capacities of organic-rich and clay-rich samples are shown in Table 32 as the amount of Hg^{++} sorbed from a solution initially containing 1000γ Hg^{++} by a 2.00 gm sample.

Table 32

Mercuric Ion Sorption on Humic-rich vs. Clay-rich
Samples at pH 6.0

Sample	Hg^{++} sorbed γ
Peat	1000
Pine Mull	750
Kaolinite (API #4)	100
Illite (Beaver Bend)	350
Montmorillonite (Wards #26)	300

Humic-rich samples (peat, pine mull) appear to possess much higher mercuric sorption capacities than do the fairly pure clays. No significant variations in the amount of mercuric ion sorbed by the samples was observed when the concentrations of Hg^{++} ranged from 1000 to 10,000Y.

The experiments summarized in Table 32 were repeated employing samples from A and B soil horizons developed under coniferous, deciduous, and grass vegetations. Results are shown in Table 33.

Table 33

Mercuric Ion Sorption by A and B Horizons

Coniferous	Hg Sorbed Y	Deciduous	Hg Sorbed Y	Grass	Hg Sorbed Y
A Horizon	940	A Horizon	840	A Horizon	800
B Horizon	720	B Horizon	1000	B Horizon	660

(all values represent an average of three determinations)

Except for the deciduous samples, the humic-rich A horizons appear slightly enriched in sorbed Hg^{++} as compared to the clay-rich B horizons. Variations in the amount sorbed suggest a vegetative control over soil mercury distribution. Waksman[12] has stressed the chemical differences in humus developing beneath coniferous and deciduous vegetations.

To ascertain the effect of a mixture of solid clay and aqueous humic acid, as would occur in a soil, Hg^{++} sorption on clays, in the presence of aqueous 100 ppm C humic acids, was determined. Experimental results of mercuric ion sorption on illite were graphed as adsorption isotherms. These curves, shown in Figure 23, were interpreted as follows. Mercuric ion sorption on illite results in a "double break" adsorption isotherm, possibly suggesting two different kinds of sorption, but which result in a total exchange capacity of 7.5 mEq Hg^{++}/100 gm illite. The presence of aqueous 100 ppm C humic acid reduces Hg^{++} sorption on illite by approximately 35%.

This decrease in the Hg^{++}-illite adsorption isotherm in the presence of humic acids could result from mercuric complexation by the humic acids and/or formation of a humic

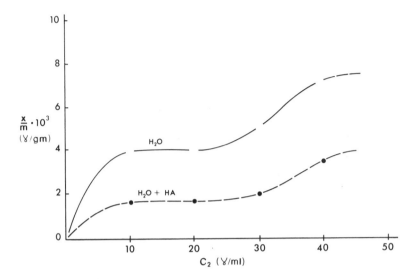

Figure 23: Adsorption Isotherm of Hg^{++} on Illite at pH
6.0. The adsorption isotherms display a decrease in
mercuric ion sorption from aqueous solution by 100 mesh
illite in the presence of aqueous humic acid (100 ppm C).

acid-clay complex. Formation of an organo-clay complex
(humic acid-illite) could occur on the edges of illite
crystals, effectively blocking the active cation exchange
sites.   This was considered unlikely however, because
of the following considerations:
  (1) The humic acid concentration determined spectro-
      photometrically before and after shaking with
      illite was found constant.
  (2) Retention of the shape of the adsorption isotherm
      suggests the same active sites--and cation exchange
      processes--were operative, even in the presence of
      the humic acid solution.
In a soil the formation of a mercuric-humate would
effectively decrease the mercuric ion activity in the
capillary water, decreasing the amount of Hg^{++} available
for illite sorption. A similar decrease in the mercuric
ion activity would be expected in a moist humus-illite soil
where humus concentrations would generally be much greater
than the experimental humic acid concentrations. In addition solid soil humus would possess the capability of
physical sorption (see Table 32).

   Adsorption isotherms of mercuric sorption on a sample
of Wards #26 montmorillonite are shown in Figure 24.   In

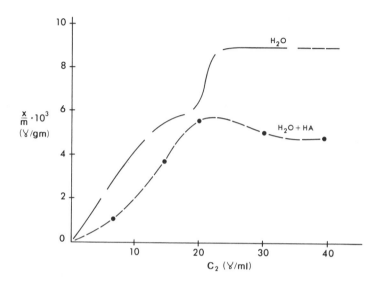

Figure 24:   Adsorption Isotherm of Hg^{++} on Montmorillonite
   at pH 6.0.   The adsorption isotherms display a decrease
   in mercuric ion sorption from aqueous solution by 100
   mesh montmorillonite in the presence of aqueous humic
   acid (100 ppm C).

the absence of humic acids, the mercuric-montmorillonite
adsorption isotherm (solid line) displayed a similarity to
the mercuric-illite adsorption isotherm, possibly indicating
similar types of sorption.   A total exchange capacity of
9.25 mEq Hg^{++}/100 gm montmorillonite was observed in the
absence of humic acid.

   For many cations, monotmorillonite displays an exchange
capacity three times the exchange capacity of illite.[11]
However, in the case of Hg^{++} sorption as determined under
these conditions, exchange capacities were not significantly
different (9.25 mEq Hg^{++}/100 gm for montmorillonite and 7.50
mEq Hg^{++}/100 gm for illite).   This suggests that variation
of clay type in soils may have a very minor effect on mercuric
content and distribution.

   Alteration of the mercuric-montmorillonite adsorption
isotherm's shape in the presence of humic acid may indicate

interlayer sorption of humic acid by the montmorillonite.
Schnitzer[4] observed an increase of interlamellar spacing
with the adsorption of 33.2 mg fulvic acid on 40.0 mg of
Na-montmorillonite. Thus it appears that the 40% decrease
in the mercuric-montmorillonite adsorption probably results
from the blocking of active exchange sites on the montmorillonite together with mercuric complexation by the
humic acid. In either case, the net result of the presence
of humic acids is to decrease the amount of mercuric ion
sorbed.

Field Studies

To determine the distribution of mercuric ion soils,
samples of each distinguishable soil horizon were taken
from both residual and transported (valley) soils developed
in nonmineralized areas (to decrease the possibility of a
vaporous mercury source). Nonmineralized areas adjacent
to the Bonanza, Palmer Cr., and War Eagle mines were
selected as sample sites. The Palmer Cr. mercury mine in
Sec. 3, T. 40 S., R. 4 W., and the War Eagle mine in Sec.
16, T. 34 S., R. 2 W., are located in Jackson County,
Oregon. The Bonanza Mercury mine is located in Sec. 16,
T. 25 S., R. 4 W., Douglas County, Oregon. Lithologies
ranged from Tertiary sandstones (Bonanza mine) to Triassic
metavolcanics (Palmer Cr. and War Eagle mines); vegetation
was both deciduous and coniferous, and soil depths ranged
from 12-48 in depth. Average precipitation in the areas
sampled generally exceeded 30 in./yr.

All samples were placed in sealed polyethylene bags.
After air drying, samples were sieved to <150 mesh,
homogenized, coned, quartered, and one gram digested and
analyzed for mercury following the Pyrih-Bisque technique.

A second 5.00 gm portion of each sample was weighed and
treated with 0.5 N NaOH to extract humic and fulvic acids.
After centrifugation and filtration, the carbon content
(reported in ppm C) was determined spectrophotometrically
at 650 mu, employing the 840 ppm C humic acid as a standard.

A near-linear, log-log correlation between the mercury
and humic acid content was observed in the three areas
sampled, as shown by the correlation diagram, Figure 25.
This correlation appeared to be independent of mercury
content, soil depth, lithology, and topography. The mull
or A horizon, which contained the highest humic acid concentration, also consistently contained the highest mercury
concentration.

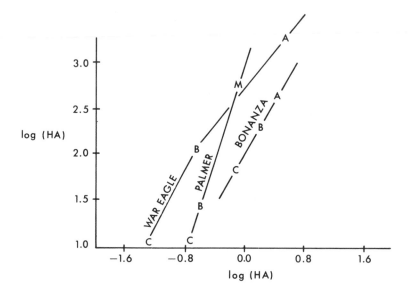

Figure 25:   Mercury and Humic Acid Content in Soils.   The
correlation diagram demonstrates a nearly linear log–log
relationship between the organic matter (humic acid) and
the mercury content in the Mull (M), A, B, and C, soil
horizon.

X-ray diffraction patterns were run on the Palmer Cr.
soil horizons to determine the relationship between mercury
and clay content.   Kaolinite was the main recognizable clay
type in the X-ray patterns.   Relative kaolinite content of
each soil horizon was estimated from the X-ray data.   Matrix
effects were neglected since matrix correction factors
calculated for a nearby soil horizon were found to have
little effect on the determination of relative keolinite
content.

Figure 26, a correlation diagram between mercury and
kaolinite content, in each of the Palmer Cr. soil horizons,
is shown below.   No correlation between the mercury and
kaolinite content was observed; and in certain horizons,
an inverse relationship existed between the mercury and
clay contents.

Additional soil samples were taken in Central Colorado
to determine if a change in climatic or geologic environment
affected this observed mercury distribution.

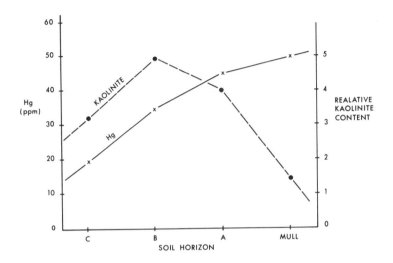

Figure 26: Mercury and Kaolinite Content in the Palmer Cr. Soil. No apparent correlation exists between the kaolinite and mercury content of a soil developed over non-mineralized rock.

The sample sites were located in Sec. 19, T. 4 S., R. 74 W., Clear Creek County, Colorado. Steep, sparsely-vegetated slopes, with an average elevation of 10,000 feet and with an annual precipitation of 30 in. are in marked contrast to the environment of southwestern Oregon.

Distribution of mercury in soil horizons sampled near a valley bottom was determined. Previous independent work had shown that a mercury anomaly up to 5 times background was present in this area.[14] This anomaly appeared to be of an ionic, transported origin however, based on the following:

(1) Drilling of the anomaly did not intersect any sulfide mineralization or faults.

(2) The stream passing near the sample site drains approximately 16 sq miles that include at least six inactive mines.

Mercury content appeared to be directly related to the degree of soil horizon development, as seen in Table 34.

The depth of soil development, which generally bears a direct relationship to the amount of organic matter present,

Table 34

Mercury Content of Soil Horizons from Valley Samples

Soil Horizon	Depth, inches	Hg content, ppm
A Horizon	0.5	0.31
B Horizon	12	0.37
A Horizon	12	0.48
B Horizon	15	0.20
A Horizon	1	0.43
B Horizon	12	0.58

appears to control the distribution of ionic mercury, corroborating conclusions based on observations in southwestern Oregon.

Conclusions

Both field and experimental data are compatible with the conclusion that ionic soil mercury distributions are controlled primarily by the humus matter. This was evidenced by the obvious correlation between the mercury and humic acid content of soil horizons developed in nonmineralized areas.

Soil samples displayed a near-linear, log-log correlation between their mercury and humic acid contents. The humic-rich soil horizon consistently contained the highest mercury (ionic) content. No correlation was observed between the mercury and clay contents in these same residual soil horizons.

Experimental data demonstrated that humus-rich portions of soils (Mull A) sorbed up to two times as much Hg^{++} as did the clay-rich (B) soil horizons.[5] Aqueous humic acid solutions were also found capable of increasing the solubility of certain mercuric compounds (HgS, HgO, and Hg_2Cl_2) far above their normal solubilities in demineralized water.

Relationship of Vaporous Mercury to Humic-Rich Materials

Laboratory Studies

Laboratory experiments were designed to contrast the
sorption capacities of peat, pine mull, illite (Beaver
Bend), montmorillonite (Wards #26), and kaolinite (API #4)
for vaporous mercury. All samples were sieved to <150
mesh, and dried at 50° C for 24 hours. After cooling, 1-
gm samples of each material were placed on Whatman #5, 5.5
cm filter paper in a sealed dessicator containing liquid
mercury in equilibrium with its vapor. Temperature was
maintained at 30 ± 0.5° C for five days. Experiments were
then repeated at higher temperatures (35° C - 0.5° C).
Results of the above experiments were then contrasted with
mercury sorption on A and B soil horizons developed under
coniferous, deciduous, and grass vegetations. Vaporous
mercury uptake by <150 mesh, dried, ground glass, crystalline
sodium chloride (NaCl) and activated charcoal was also
measured to contrast these three materials which vary
widely in surface area.

Experimental Results

Results of vaporous mercury sorption on the above-
mentioned humic-rich samples are shown in Table 35.

Table 35

Sorption of Mercury Vapor on Humic-Rich and
Clay-Rich Samples

Sample	*Hg° sorbed after 5 days at 30 ± 0.5° C (in ppm)*	*Hg° sorbed after 5 days at 35 ± 0.5° C (in ppm)*
Peat	24.0	1050
Pine Mull	20.0	226
Illite	4.5	not determined
Montmorillonite	1.0	116
Kaolinite	0.8	6.8
Activated Charcoal	135.0	not determined
Ground Glass	<0.1	not determined
NaCl	<0.1	not determined

Humic-rich samples were found to be capable of sorbing far more vaporous mercury than clay-rich samples lacking humus materials. Higher mercury content in the peat and pine mull appears roughly to parallel the organic contents of these samples (peat, 5000 ppm C; pine mull, 1500 ppm C).

Vaporous mercury sorption appears to be related to the surface area of the sample, as is suggested by the data for activated charcoal, ground glass, and crystalline NaCl.

The effect of different vegetative types on vaporous mercury sorption for A and B soil horizons developed under coniferous, deciduous, and grass vegetations is shown in Table 36.

Table 36

Effect of Vegetation on Vaporous Mercury Sorption

Sample	Hg° sorbed (ppm) Run #1	Run #2	Sample	Hg° sorbed (ppm) Run #1	Run #2
Pine A	910.0	900.0	Pine B	18.2	19.0
Aspen A	54.0	60.0	Aspen B	31.0	30.0
Grass A	270.0	280.0	Grass B	42.5	40.0

The organic-rich A soil horizons all sorbed more vaporous mercury than did the clay-rich, B, soil horizons. This experiment, together with the sorption experiments on clays (Table 34), suggests that distribution of vaporous mercury in soils may also be controlled by soil organics.

Variations of mercury sorbed by the A horizons may again reflect the chemical variations in the type of humus matter forming under the three different vegetations.[12]

Field Studies

In order to determine soil mercury distributions when a vaporous mercury source exists, soil horizons (Mull, A, B, C), developed over known mercury mineralization, were sampled near the Bonanza, Palmer Cr., and War Eagle mercury mines in southwestern Oregon. Samples of both residual and transported soils were taken and stored in polyethylene bags to prevent loss of vaporous mercury and contamination of other samples. Mercury and humic acid contents were determined by the previously described methods.

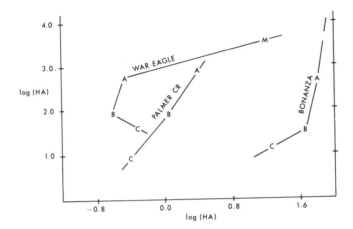

Figure 27: Mercury and Humic Acid Content of Soils
Overlying Mineralization. A general correlation appears
to exist between the mercury and humic acid content for
the soil horizons (Mull, A, B, C) developed over known
mercury mineralization.

Figure 27 shows a fair correlation between the mercury
and humic acid contents in soil horizons developed over
areas most likely emanating vaporous mercury. Since the
soil was developing over a known cinnabar deposit, some
ionic mercury may be present.

X-ray diffraction analysis of the Bonanza Mine soil
horizons indicated kaolinite was the major clay type. Each
soil horizon was analyzed chemically for SiO_2, AlO_3, MgO,
CaO, Fe_2O_3, MnO, K_2O and SrO.* From these analyses, matrix
correction factors were calculated and used to determine
the relative kaolinite distributions in the soil horizons.
Calculations of the relative kaolinite distributions in the
soil were not greatly affected by the matrix correction
factors, and in fact, such corrections proved unnecessary.
A graph of the kaolinite and mercury distribution for the
Bonanza soil is shown in Figure 28.

---

*Analyses conducted by G. T. Burrow and Violet Merrit,
USGS.

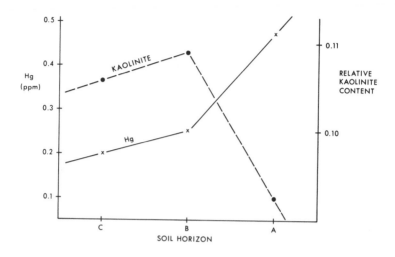

Figure 28: Mercury and Kaolinite Content in the Bonanza Soil. No apparent correlation exists between the clay and mercury contents of this soil developed over mercury mineralization.

Mercury distribution in these soils bears no obvious relationship to kaolinite content. The lack of a relationship between clay and mercury, compared to the correlation between humic acid content and mercury, suggests that humic acids, or at least humic-acid-type organics, primarily control the distribution of mercury in these soils developed over mineralized areas.

Results of vaporous mercury distribution in southwestern Oregon were then contrasted to mercury distribution in soils from Central Colorado developed over traceable faults and sulfide veins. Previous independent work had shown mercury anomalies, 5-7 times background, and apparently of vaporous origin, directly overlaying the permeable fault zones and sulfide veins.[14] Table 37 shows the relationship between mercury content, soil horizons, and geologic features.

Assuming a vaporous source organic-rich A horizons appear to be far better sorbers of elemental mercury than do the clay-rich B soil horizons. Again an excellent agreement between the data from southwestern Oregon and Central Colorado areas exists, suggesting that the vaporous mercury-humic-acid-type organic interaction is independent of climatic and geologic variations.

Table 37

Relationship Between Mercury Content, Soils Horizon,
and Geologic Features

Sample Site and Soil Horizon	Depth, inches	Hg Content ppm	Geologic Feature
1A	5	0.50	sulfide vein
B	12	0.01	sulfide vein
2A	3	0.01	background
B	12	0.00	background
3A	3	0.25	sulfide vein
B	14	0.01	sulfide vein
4A	2	0.23	sulfide vein
B	8	0.02	sulfide vein
5A	0-0.5*	0.00	fault
B	10	0.27	fault
6A	3	0.36	fault
B	11	0.05	fault

*Poorly developed to non-existent A soil horizon

Conclusions

Field and laboratory studies are consistent in suggesting
humic-acid-type soil organics control the distribution of
vaporous mercury in soils to a far greater extent than do
clays. This was evidenced in the laboratory by a much
larger sorption of vaporous mercury on humic-rich samples
than on clay-rich samples. Vegetation type appears to
exert a strong influence on vaporous mercury sorption
capacities, as evidenced by the large uptake of mercury by
the coniferous A horizons and the relatively small uptake
by the deciduous A horizons.

Soils developed over areas most likely emanating vaporous
mercury displayed a fairly consistent relationship between
their humic acid and mercury contents but no correlation
between their clay and mercury contents.

Neither the nature of the soil (residual or transported),
topography, lithology or geographic location affected the
relative distribution of vaporous mercury and its predominance
in the humic-rich parts of the soil.

References

1. Hawkes, H. E. and J. S. Webb. Geochemistry in Mineral Exploration (Harper and Row, 1962).
2. Gruner, J. W. "Organic Matter and the Origin of the Biwabic Formation of the Mesabi Range," Econ. Geol., *17*, 407 (1952).
3. Graham, E. R. "Colloidal Organic Acids as Factors in the Weathering of Anorthite," Soil Science, *52*, 291 (1941).
4. Schnitzer, M. "Reactions Between Fulvic Acid, a Soil Humic Compound and Inorganic Soil Constituents," Soil Sci. Soc. Amer. Proc., *33*, 75 (1969).
5. Trost, P. B. and R. E. Bisque. "Differentiation of Vaporous and Ionic Mercury in Soils," Proceedings, Int. Geochem. Symposium (1970), to be published.
6. Malcolm, R. L. Mobile Soil Organic Matter and Its Interactions with Clay Minerals and Sesquioxides. Unpublished Ph.D. thesis, North Carolina State University (1964).
7. Allison, L. E. "Organic Carbon," in Methods of Soil Analysis, C. A. Black, ed. (1965), pp. 1367-1378.
8. Pyrih, R. Z. and R. E. Bisque. "Determination of Trace Mercury in Soil and Rock Media," Econ. Geol., *64*, 825 (1969).
9. Pyrih, R. Z. and R. E. Bisque. "Determination of Trace Mercury in Soil and Rock Media--A Reply," Econ. Geol., *65*, 358 (1970).
10. Weast, R. C. Editor-in-Chief. Handbook of Chemistry and Physics, 49th ed. (Cleveland, Ohio: The Chemical Rubber Co., 1968), p. B218.
11. Schnitzer, M. and S. I. M. Skinner. "Organo-metallic Interactions in Soils. 5. Stability Constants of Cu^{++}, Fe^{++}, and Zn^{++} - Fulvic Acid Complexes," Soil Science, *102*, 361 (1966).
12. Waksman, S. A. Humus: Origin, Chemical Composition and Importance in Nature (Baltimore: Williams and Wilkins Co., 1938).
13. Grim, R. E. Clay Mineralogy (McGraw-Hill, 1953).
14. Stevens, D. N., D. N. Bloom, and R. E. Bisque. "Evaluation of Mercury Vapor Anomalies at Colorado Central Mines, Clear Creek County, Colorado," Colorado School of Mines Quarterly, *64*, 573 (1969).

Research Needs: Study of the Environmental
Dynamics of Mercury

Rolf Hartung

This is a brief outline of some important parameters
which need to be studied so that we may better understand
the behavior and effects of mercury in the environment.
It is hoped that the subsequent discussion will concentrate
on specific interests or needs.

It is obvious that we must study the physical behavior
of the different compounds of mercury. That is, we must
study solution properties of metallic mercury, Hg^{++}, $R-Hg^{+}$,
and $R-Hg-R'$ compounds. These properties need to be measured
in defined natural waters, so that we can relate the observed
phenomena to natural processes. In doing this, we must also
examine the tendencies of various mercury compounds to form
complex ions and to complex with naturally occurring organic
ligands. Partitioning coefficients between water and lipids
need to be derived, so that a theoretical base can be formed
in our study of absorption rates into biota. The study of
uptake would also be greatly aided by a knowledge of the
binding energies of various mercury compounds to -SH groups
and other biochemically active moieties.

In the study of environmental transport we have to contend
with air transport, water transport, storage, and interconversions in sediments and soils. The study of the behavior
of mercury compounds at the various air-water-solids interfaces
should have a great deal of bearing on our interpretation of
the behavior of mercury in the environment. Some of this
physical-chemical information has already been developed
for relatively pure systems. The more difficult, but
necessary, task is to extend this work into impure and
multiple systems as found in nature. This relatively basic
knowledge, in conjunction with information on biotransformation
and biological dynamics, is required to develop practical
working models which will serve a predictive function.

The central phenomenon, which conveys much of the toxicological impact to environmental mercury, is the methylation
process. The basic work which has been done on this
phenomenon in Sweden, in the United States, and elsewhere,
has given us a good start. But already it is becoming
apparent that there may be several distinct methylation
processes at work, which would conceivably give us several
important avenues of influence on the transformation process.

The behavior of methyl mercury and its various analogues is tightly interwoven with biological processes. It seems obvious that these compounds can be concentrated from water and then amplified in food chains and food webs. Our understanding of the mechanics of this process is only qualitative and simplistic. We will need to know absorption rates, concentrating ability, metabolism, and excretion rates in many large phyla, orders, and perhaps even families of plants and animals. To date, for instance, we know very little about the relative importance of absorption of methyl mercury in fish through gills, epidermis, or via food intake. However, such information is vital to any prediction of the relative importance of food chains, the effects of changes in water concentration of CH_3Hg^+ on body burdens in fish. The biological availability of organo-mercurials such as dimethylmercury in water needs to be studied. It is doubtful that it solely disappears into the atmosphere as often assumed.

I have briefly outlined the complexity and importance of studying the environmental dynamics of mercury. This study becomes especially important in predicting and interdicting adverse effects, waste management, and in planning possible alterations of transformation processes.

Beyond these requirements, there are important needs in determining the chronic toxicity of the important compounds of mercury for plants, invertebrates, fish, birds, and mammals, including man, so that we may develop a better appreciation for environmental and human safety requirements.

Discussion Paper

Contributions by: T. W. Clarkson, A. J. Coble, F. M. D'Itri, J. C. Gage, L. Goldwater, R. Hartung, A. Hinman, A. Jernelöv, R. E. Jervis, H. F. Kraybill, P. A. Krenkel, V. W. Lambow, D. J. Lisk, J. A. McGroarty, L. W. Muir, N. Nelson, R. Reinert, H. L. Rook, J. E. Spaulding, W. T. Sullivan, P. B. Trost.

The environmental dynamics of mercury are obviously greatly complicated by the existence of several compounds of mercury which have drastically different properties, and by the fact that interconversions between these mercury

compounds occur. The most important of these is the
methylation of mercury in natural systems.

It is important to identify the biological and other
factors which influence the methylation process. Wood
et al.[1] have described the nonenzymatic methylation of
mercury by methylated vitamin B_{12} from bacterial extracts.
There are reasons to believe that some algae can form B_{12}
and methyl B_{12}, but so far the methylation process has not
been demonstrated in algae. Experiments on the blue-green
alga *Microcystus* also failed to demonstrate methylation of
mercury. In a related vein, while most intestinal bacteria
appear to have the ability to methylate mercury, they do
not appear to do so to any appreciable extent under normal
conditions in higher vertebrates.

In addition to the nonenzymatic methylation of mercury
by methyl B_{12}, recent studies have pointed out the possibility of an enzymatic methylation involving the addition
of mercuric ions to the sulfhydryl group of cysteine or
homocysteine which then accepts a methyl group. The
resulting methylmercuric homocysteine, or the dimethylmercury derived from another pathway, may mean that the
mercury is biologically inactivated, since all valences of
mercury are filled. There appears to be a good correlation
in sedimentary bacteria between their ability to methylate
mercury and their resistance to high concentrations of
mercury in the substrate. The relative importance of the
various methylating pathways is not entirely clear. However,
alkyl mercury compounds are known to be highly effective
inhibitors of most enzymes, so that it may require some
rather unusual enzymes to be able to synthesize a mercury-
carbon bond.

While the methylated mercury is toxicologically most
important, the majority of the mercury in natural systems
will usually be found in the sediments. In a nonpolluted
deep lake, the dominating proportion might be in the water,
but the biomass would rarely, if ever, contain a high
proportion of the total mercury in an aquatic system.

The methylating process apparently can be greatly influenced by environmental conditions. The presence of
large amounts of sulfides will make mercury less available
in the sediments because of the formation of the almost
insoluble mercuric sulfide. The presence of large amounts
of chloride ions, as in sea water, will in contrast tend
to solubilize mercury as the complex $(HgCl_4)^{++}$ ion. The
methylating process has been found to proceed readily in
sediments from the North Sea and the Baltic Sea, but appears
to be related primarily to total microbiological activity.

The relative roles of monomethyl mercury and dimethyl mercury in the environment are difficult to assess. Monomethyl mercury has by far the greater stability and has a strong tendency to bind to proteins. Dimethyl mercury has a low water solubility, but a high fat solubility. At the same time, dimethyl mercury has a low boiling point (90° C), which makes escape into the atmosphere very likely, and which may provide little opportunity for fish to absorb dimethyl mercury from the environment. In rodents, Ostlund has demonstrated that dimethyl mercury has a much shorter biological half-life than monomethyl mercury and that only a small amount of the dimethyl mercury was converted into monomethyl mercury.

The overall rate of methylation of mercury in the environment is low. The amount that is likely to be solubilized from the sediments, and subsequently methylated per year under "normal" Swedish conditions, is generally below 1%. It is conceptually possible to decrease this conversion rate by decreasing microbiological activity, or by binding the mercury in a less available form, such as the sulfide.

The methylation process requires the presence of free Hg^{++} ions. The environmental conversion of metallic mercury to ionic mercury is usually not the rate-limiting step. The thermodynamic feasibility of this conversion has been estimated by

$$E = 850 + 30 \log \frac{[Hg^{++} \text{ total}]}{\alpha}$$

where α is a coefficient which estimates the binding energy of Hg^{++} ions to organic sediments.[3] Whether mercury is added to the aquatic environment as the metal or the ionic form does not affect the methylation rate, because under those conditions the methylation itself becomes the rate-limiting event. However, when mercury occurs as HgS, which has an extremely low water solubility, then the reaction $HgS \rightarrow Hg^{++} + S^{--}$ becomes the rate-limiting step in the overall methylation process. The possible role of environmental chelating agents in this process has as yet not been properly investigated.

So far it has not been possible to differentiate clearly between inorganic and organic mercury in water samples from lakes and rivers. There also is a sporadic variability for total mercury in environmental water samples. The Swedish experience has been that most water samples contain approximately 0.1 ppb mercury, but about 10% of the samples from the same waters contain 5 to 10 ppb mercury. While some of this variability may be due to analytical error, there is a strong possibility that much of the mercury is

associated with microparticulates. Thus, Westermark has
demonstrated that the mercury content of natural water
samples may be reduced by 80% after filtration and aluminum
hydroxide precipitation. In comparison, the concentration
of a clean solution of Hg^{++} cannot be substantially reduced
by this treatment. Since it is apparent that our understanding of the nature of the mercury in water is very
incomplete, it has not been possible to establish meaningful
correlations between the total mercury content of water and
the mercury content of the biota living there. For those
reasons, it has not been possible to derive consistent
concentration factors.

However, as some of the previous papers have indicated,
a partial qualitative and quantitative assessment of the
presence of mercury in food chains has been attempted, but
some of the mercury levels found in aquatic organisms are
not readily explainable. Thus, fresh water mussels tend
to contain very little mercury, but crustaceans tend to
have high levels of mercury, only part of which is organic
mercury. This appears to be especially true for estuarine
crustaceans, such as the Blue Crab. Terrestrial plants
concentrate only small amounts of mercury and thus appear
to play only a minor role in the terrestrial mercury food
chain. The role of aquatic plants may be similar, but
requires additional study.

It must be admitted that some of the present theories
on the environmental dynamics of mercury are based upon
relatively small samples, especially when compared with
the data from environmental monitoring for pesticides.
Many monitoring studies of environmental mercury have
concerned themselves exclusively with total mercury
determinations, which have provided adequate information
for the general distribution of mercury. Studies on the
rates, food-chain dynamics, and environmental toxicology
have benefitted most from the few studies which have
attempted to identify the mercury compounds in addition
to quantifying them.

References

1. Wood, J. M., F. S. Kennedy, and C. G. Rosen. "Synthesis
   of Methylmercury Compounds by Extracts of a Methanogenic
   Bacterium," Nature, 220: 173-174 (1968).
2. Ostlund, K. "Studies on the Metabolism of Methyl Mercury
   and Dimethylmercury in Mice," Acta Pharmacologica et
   Toxicologica, 27 (Suppl. 1): 13-132 (1969).
3. Jernelöv, A. "Conversion of Mercury Compounds," Chapt. 4.
   Chemical Fallout (C. C. Thomas Publ., 1969).

PART IV

BIOLOGICAL EFFECTS OF MERCURY COMPOUNDS

CONTRIBUTORS TO PART IV

William J. Adams, Department of Fisheries and Wildlife, Michigan State University, East Lansing, Michigan

Don B. Chaffin, Ph.D., Department of Industrial Engineering, The University of Michigan, Ann Arbor, Michigan

T. W. Clarkson, M.D., Department of Radiation Biology and Biophysics and Department of Pharmacology and Toxicology, University of Rochester, Rochester, New York

Bertram D. Dinman, D.D., Sc.D., Department of Environmental and Industrial Health, School of Public Health, The University of Michigan, Ann Arbor, Michigan

Leonard J. Goldwater, M.D., Professor of Community Health Sciences, Duke University Medical Center, Durham, North Carolina

Hoda A. Guirgis, Ph.D., Department of Preventive Medicine, Creighton University, Oklahoma, Nebraska

Lawrence H. Hecker, Ph.D., Institute of Environmental and Industrial Health, The University of Michigan, Ann Arbor, Michigan

I. T. T. Higgins, M.D., Department of Epidemiology, School of Public Health, The University of Michigan, Ann Arbor, Michigan

A. Hinman, M.D., New York State Department of Health, Albany, New York

R. F. Korns, M.D., New York State Department of Health, Albany, New York

Harold H. Prince, Ph.D., Department of Fisheries and Wildlife, Michigan State University, East Lansing, Michigan

Ralph G. Smith, Ph.D., Department of Environmental and Industrial Health, School of Public Health, The University of Michigan, Ann Arbor, Michigan

W. K. Stewart, MRCPE, Department of Medicine, Dundee University, Scotland

Tadao Takeuchi, M.D., Department of Pathology, Kumamoto
University School of Medicine, Kumamoto, Japan
W. Taylor, Ph.D., M.D., MRCPE, Department of Social
Medicine, Dundee University, Scotland
L. Tryphonas, D.V.M., Ph.D., Western College of Veterinary
Medicine, Saskatoon, Saskatchewan, Canada

Dose-Response Relationship Associated with
Known Mercury Absorption at Low Dose
Levels of Inorganic Mercury

Ralph G. Smith

Many years before mercury in the total environment
became a matter of universal concern, the effects of mercury
in the industrial environment were known and studied by
industrial physicians and industrial hygienists. Occupational mercurialism is a recognized disease entity, and
there are all too many well-documented cases describing
the symptoms displayed by workers engaged in the extraction of mercury from its ores or in the subsequent use of
the metal or its compounds. Although occupational exposure
to mercury may involve organic as well as inorganic compounds, the greatest number of employees have been exposed
to elemental mercury, usually occurring as a vapor.✦ In
this discussion we shall confine our attention to a consideration of the effects of exposure to inorganic mercury
only, most of which in practice derives from vapor exposures.
We shall further limit our consideration to "low-level exposures," a definition of which is clearly required.
✦ For many years the industrial air standard for inorganic
mercury and its compounds, or "Threshold Limit Value" (TLV),
as it is called in the United States, has been 0.1 milligram
or 100 micrograms per cubic meter. In relatively recent
times, this TLV has been lowered to 50 micrograms per cubic
meter, and it appears likely that this standard will prevail
in the United States and in some other countries. In general, concentrations at or around this level are considered
to be relatively "low" and do not result in the appearance
of clinical symptoms of mercurialism. In the general atmosphere of cities, however, mercury levels are very much
lower yet, with reported concentrations ranging from a few
nanograms per cubic meter to perhaps 1 microgram per cubic

meter. By comparison with these ambient air levels, the occupational air levels are relatively high, but are nonetheless much lower than the concentrations required to produce what is generally considered acute or chronic mercurialism with textbook clinical manifestations.

It is apparent that occupational exposures to mercury offer an excellent opportunity to determine dose-response relationships, for the effects on health, if any, can theoretically be related to the quantity of mercury absorbed from the air of the occupational environment, if mercury levels are properly measured. In fact, however, measuring the amount of mercury to which workers have been exposed has always been a difficult matter, and the rather voluminous literature on this subject contains relatively few examples of well-defined mercury intake with which clinical findings can be correlated. Individual reports tend to be confusing and contradictory, but a report that was prepared by an international committee which met in Stockholm in 1968[1] probably provides the best integration of available information extant, and represents an authoritative statement of the known relationships between mercury intake and the probable effects. This report deals with all forms of mercury, but reference will be made here only to the summary dealing with chronic exposure to inorganic mercury.

Chronic Exposure to Inorganic Mercury

In general, absorption of mercury is stated to take place primarily as a result of inhalation of the vapor or its inorganic salts. Skin absorption is not thought to be a major route of entry, but skin contamination or other external contamination can cause additional exposure to mercury by inhalation. Once inhaled, the report states, as much as 75% to 85% of the mercury vapor may be absorbed,[2] which may thereafter diffuse rapidly through the alveolar membrane. Some oxidation of the elemental mercury occurs in the blood, and the mercuric mercury formed is then bound to plasma proteins or to hemoglobin in the erythrocytes. Prior to this oxidation, however, the blood contains a quantity of elemental mercury which readily diffuses across membranes, giving rise to substantially higher brain concentration than would occur if all of the mercury were present as mercuric ion. Once mercury is stored in the brain it is excreted very slowly; hence, long-term exposures to mercury tend to affect the central nervous system.

A number of symptoms and signs involving the central
nervous system as a result of long-term exposure to mercury
vapor have been reported. The most frequently observed are
tremor and the symptom complex known as erethism. There is
conflicting evidence concerning the effect of long-term
exposure to low levels of mercury on the kidney, but numerous investigators have reported proteinuria and in some
cases, a nephrotic syndrome.[3,4] Disorders of the mouth
such as gingivitis, stomatitis, and excessive salivation
have also been reported, but, as in the case of kidney
damage, the evidence tends to be conflicting. It should
be noted that a number of very specific findings are observed as a result of substantially higher intake of
mercury compounds, or due to extended exposure to somewhat
higher levels than those under consideration (*ca.* 100 μg/
m^3). This has inevitably led to some confusion concerning
the effects of mercury in the occupational environment.

One of the earlier studies which was intended to establish the dose-response relationship of inorganic mercury
was that performed in the felt hat industry and reported
by Neal *et al.*[5,6] as early as 1937. On the basis that no
clinical evidence of mercurialism was found among workers
exposed to less than 100 micrograms of mercury per cubic
meter, the TLV which prevailed for the next two decades
was established in the United States. Numerous other
studies[7-11] have been reported in which the presence or
absence of disease has been related to air concentrations
in the working atmospheres, but, in most cases, the data
have been incomplete and the differentiation between inhaled mercury and that taken in unintentionally by ingestion
has been difficult to make.

Studies of Mercury in Chlorine Manufacture

In 1962, the chlorine-producing industry, which uses
considerable quantities of mercury in certain cell rooms,
manifested its concern with occupational mercurialism by
contracting with Wayne State University to perform an
epidemiological study of workers engaged in the manufacture
of chlorine. This study, supported by The Chlorine Institute,
Inc., and only recently published,[12] is one of the most
ambitious attempts thus far to clearly relate the inhaled
dose of mercury to response. It involved a large industrial
group located in many plants throughout the United States
and Canada. The following condensation of the study is

presented in the belief that it represents a major effort
to establish the dose-response relationship for elemental
mercury vapor.

It was not possible to study all the plants producing
chlorine in North America, but a representative and fair
cross-section of the industry was reflected in the more than
25 plants that cooperated in the study.   Geographically,
the plants were widely distributed in the United States and
Canada, from the Atlantic seaboard to California and from
the Gulf Coast to Quebec, so no specific climatic or geographic features should have affected the results unduly.
The essential features of the study plan were as follows:

1. A "study year" was selected, during which time
all required data would be collected. (Although ideally
it was desirable that each plant observe the same year,
in practice it was not possible; so the actual "study
year" extended over a period of approximately two years.)

2. Every employee potentially exposed to mercury and
engaged in the manufacture of chlorine would be given a
thorough medical examination once during the year.

3. At least four times during the year, blood and
urine specimens would be obtained from each employee for
the purpose of determining mercury levels.

4. Each cell room and adjacent areas to which employees spent working hours would be studied to select
a number of sampling points which would permit characterization of the degree of exposure to mercury
throughout the working day.

5. The percentage of time normally spent by each
employee at each of the specified points, or areas
represented by them, would be determined. In addition,
the length of time that each employee was required to
wear respiratory protection against exposure to mercury
was also to be noted.

6. At least six times during the year, air sampling
for mercury was to be performed at each sampling location
by a method agreed upon by cooperating industrial
hygienists.

7. On the basis of the information derived from
items 4, 5 and 6, above, time-weighted average exposures
for all employees were to be calculated and used as the
basis for estimating exposure to mercury during the year.

8. All data were to be received by the department
and subjected to examination and analysis for the purpose
or arriving at conclusions concerning the degree of
exposure and the presence or absence of effects.

9. To assist in reaching conclusions, a control population consisting of as large a group as possible of plant employees not occupationally exposed to mercury would be selected and treated in the same fashion as exposed employees.

Medical examinations were made by the regular plant physicians and/or by physicians in the area of the plant acceptable to the participating company authorities and the study director. The physical examination of workers was made at any time during the study year and was not repeated. Preferably, the examinations were completed during the first six months of the study year. Exhaustive medical and occupational histories and results of physical examinations of all individuals in the study were recorded by examining physicians on a standard form by checks and code numbers, with additional information recorded on notation sheets where necessary.

Special efforts were made to record dates and descriptions of any unusual exposure to chlorine. Any previous history of respiratory illnesses was noted; pertinent symptoms of tooth decay, frequent colds, sore mouth, sore throat, sore gums, cough, sputum, shortness of breath, heart trouble and palpitations, nausea, diarrhea and constipation, weight loss and loss of appetite, various psychosomatic complaints of headache, dizziness, fatigue, nervousness, shyness, anxiety, tremors, insomnia, etc. were recorded as absent, present and stable, present and better, present and worse, or progressive or regressive from onset. The use of alcohol and use of tobacco in different forms was also noted.

In addition to the physical examination, certain relevant blood and urine studies were undertaken. These included hematocrit, white blood cell count, urinary proteins and urinary specific gravity. These were performed on specimens obtained at the original plant at the time of physical examination. In addition, blood and urine specimens were collected four times during the year and were analyzed to determine their mercury content. Chest x-rays (inspiration and expiration) were taken and interpreted initially by local physicians, and again by radiologists at Wayne State University, who had no knowledge of the exposure status of given individuals. Electrocardiograms were also obtained and, where possible, interpreted at Wayne State University.

Measurements of Mercury in the Plants

The measurements of mercury in the plants were made primarily by means of ultraviolet meters made by several manufacturers (generally called mercury vapor meters). In recognition of the fact that such meters respond only to mercury if present as a vapor, some concern was evidenced that mercury compounds present as dust would go undetected, and accordingly, each plant was requested to sample from time to time in such a manner as to determine total mercury levels, which could be compared to vapor levels.↓ Suggested sampling procedures included absorption in iodine or potassium permanganate solutions, with subsequent determination by a dithizone procedure. It was also suggested that if a filter preceded the absorption vessel, a differentation between particulate and vapor phase mercury could be made.

Among the problems related to determining mercury vapor levels by means of meters are the strong magnetic fields existing within the cell rooms, particularly in the newer plants where amperages are high, and the difficulty of obtaining satisfactory zero readings in large cell room areas. In most plants, the effects of the magnetic fields could be nullified by instrument shielding, but in some of the newer plants it was reported that no means could be found to assure reliable instrument performance. As far as is known, most plants participating in the study were able to obtain reliable data by solving the various problems involved. In order to minimize sampling errors, calibration procedures for vapor meters were devised, and those plants not wishing to perform the calibrations themselves were invited to send meters to the study director for calibration.

A total of 1624 workers participated in the study, but only 642 were employed in mercury cell rooms and constituted the true study population with respect to exposure to mercury and its effects. An additional 600 employed in diaphragm cell plants were the study population for chlorine-only exposure, and 382 workers not exposed to mercury or chlorine constituted the control group. The mercury-exposed group came from 21 different plants located throughout the United States and Canada, and plant populations varied from 12 to 91 employees. Within the group of 642 mercury-exposed workers on whom medical data were obtained, there were 75 for whom no exposure data were forthcoming; hence, the useful study population was 567 workers.

The age distribution of both the study group and the control group is summarized in Table 38, and it is evident that the two groups were quite similar. Table 39 presents

Table 38

Age Distribution of Study Population

Age Range	Exposed Workers %	Control Workers %
19-29	22.4	22.5
30-39	36.1	24.9
40-49	27.6	32.7
50-59	12.2	16.5
60-	1.7	3.4

Table 39

Length of Employment in Mercury Cell Rooms

Years Employed	% of Employees
1	13.3
2-5	29.4
6-9	26.3
10-14	25.0
15-20	5.1
20+	0.9

(551 employees only)

a summary of employment histories, showing that more than half of the study group had worked between 6 and 14 years in the industry, a length of time which would seem to be entirely adequate to result in effects due to mercury, if exposure levels were sufficiently high.

Table 40 shows that 63%, or nearly two-thirds, of the study population smoked cigarettes, compared to approximately 56% of the controls. When the number of individuals who admitted to consuming alcoholic beverages was compared, the two groups were remarkably similar, with 51.0% of the exposed group and 50.5% of controls consuming alcohol, respectively. No attempt was made to define the quantity of alcohol consumed, nor the frequency of drinking.

Table 40

Cigarette Smoking Habits of Study Population

Packs of Cigarettes per Day	Exposed %	Controls %
0	37.2	43.7
Less than 1	7.2	12.9
1-2	55.0	42.9
2+	0.6	0.5

Finally, it should be noted that all study employees were males, and that no breakdown by race or nationality was made. Most of the members of the control population were workers comparable to cell-room workers, and relatively few office employees were included in the group. Thus, it can be stated that the control group was, in general, similar to the exposed group in most respects, even though the method of interpreting data on the basis of dose-response tended to minimize the importance of having a perfectly matched control group.

Time-Weighted Average Exposures

The many thousands of mercury-in-air measurements can be summarized in several ways, but the significant figures with which the study was primarily concerned were the time-weighted average exposures, computed as previously indicated. It should be kept in mind that these values are not the average cell-room mercury levels, but do bear an obvious relationship to such levels. In Table 41 the time-weighted average exposures have been grouped as shown for convenience; when so grouped, 88 employees, or approximately 14% of the total group, experienced at least a year of exposure to concentrations of mercury in excess of the previous threshold limit value of 0.1 mg/m^3. The mean exposure level for the 567 employees for whom data were available was 0.065 mg/m^3, with a standard deviation of ± 0.085. In the case of 12 plants, every employee had a time-weighted average exposure of 0.1 mg/m^3 or less, while in the remainder some employees were exposed to higher concentrations.

Table 41

Mercury Exposures of Study Group
Time-Weighted Averages

Exposure mg/m³	*No. of Workers*	*% Workers*
<0.01	58	10.2
0.01-0.05	276	48.7
0.06-0.10	145	25.6
0.11-0.14	61	10.7
0.15-0.23	--	--
0.24-0.27	27	4.8

The actual cell-room concentrations of mercury in air ranged from <0.001 mg/m³ to 2.64 mg/m³ (cell-bed grinding), with most values below 0.1 mg/m³. It should be kept in mind that most, if not all, plants require workers to wear respirators at certain times when high mercury levels can be anticipated, and although measurements may have been made at such times, they were not to be used in calculations of time-weighted exposure data.

Useful data regarding urinary levels of mercury were obtained from 627 employees, of whom 67 lacked the necessary air data for computing time-weighted averages (TWA's). Only 339 persons provided useful blood data, of whom 31 lacked air concentration information. All told, some 2500 urinalyses and 1400 blood analyses were performed.

The correlations between TWA's of mercury and blood and urine levels were very strong, exhibiting the highest t-values for any variables compared. For air and blood, the t-value was 18.1, and for urine 18.7, for values corrected to specific gravity 1.024. Both are significant at $P<0.001$. Figure 29 shows the mean blood levels plotted versus TWA's, and Figure 30 shows the same relationship for urine corrected to specific gravity 1.024. The very considerable variability of individual points is clearly observed, but the regression lines which have been drawn, using the method of least squares, are useful in suggesting the responses of groups of employees. Using these lines, it appears that the urine level of 0.25 mg/l suggested by Elkins[13] as a "biological threshold limit value" is confirmed, and from Figure 29 the corresponding blood level

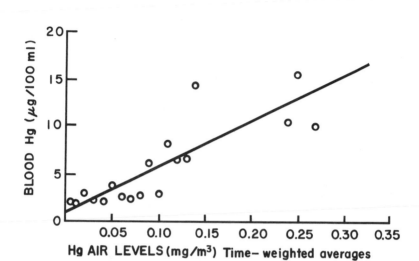

Figure 29:   Mean Lead Levels of Mercury Versus Time-Weighted
Averages of Mercury in Air

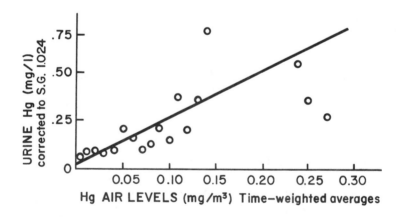

Figure 30:   Urine Levels of Mercury Versus Time-Weighted
Averages of Mercury in Air

would seem to be about 6 μg/100 ml. A literal interpretation of the regression lines indicates that the air threshold limit value of 0.1 mg/m³ corresponds to a blood level of 6 μg/100 ml, and to a urine level of 0.26 mg/1 for samples corrected to specific gravity of 1.024. All blood and urine data were also compared directly, using mean values for all individuals whose samples were analyzed by our laboratory. The resulting regression line is plotted in Figure 31, and the relationship between blood and urine

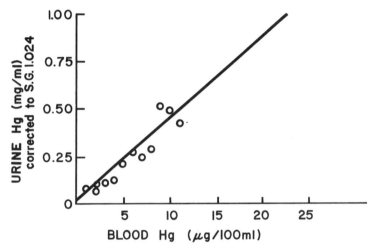

Figure 31: Relationship Between Blood and Urine Levels of Mercury

levels is identical with that deduced from the previous curves comparing TWA's and blood and urine. This rather remarkable agreement would appear to argue strongly for the validity of the air analyses and the TWA calculations, for the blood urine relationships are completely independent of any air analyses; yet the levels corresponding to threshold limit value (0.1 mg/m) exposure are found to be exactly the same as those derived by comparison to air data. In addition, the actual values agree with the data of others, notably Goldwater *et al.*[14] and Joselow *et al.;*[15] it therefore seems probable that the blood, urine, and air data are accurate as well as internally self-consistent.

Although diaphragm cell workers exposed only to chlorine failed to show well-defined evidence of adverse effects due to chlorine,[16] mercury cell workers gave considerable evidence of showing some response to mercury, based on the medical findings. (Whenever exposure to mercury is indicated, it is understood that the actual exposure in virtually every case was to mercury plus a low background level of chlorine.)

Summary of Results

The results of the study can be summarized by stating that, in all major respects, the employees examined were in good health and in no way distinguishable from the control population with respect to such basic matters as impairment of the cardiorespiratory, gastrointestinal, or hepatorenal systems. Most measurable properties, including laboratory hematological data, chest x-rays, EKG, were found to be completely normal. The clinical picture that does emerge, however, is one of a group of workers who apparently exhibit a dose-related response to mercury exposure by evidencing somewhat higher incidences of a number of neuropsychiatric symptoms (see Table 42 and Figure 32).

Table 42

Medical Findings Related to Mercury Exposure
(Based on Dose-Response Relationship)

Findings	Basis	t-Value of Correlation Coefficient	Significant at P-level
Loss of Appetite	Symptom	19.55	0.001
Weight Loss	Symptom	16.51	0.001
Object. Tremors	Sign	7.06	0.001
Insomnia	Symptom	6.98	0.001
Shyness	Symptom	4.54	0.001
Diastol. Blood Pres.	Sign	− 3.38	0.001
Frequent Colds	Symptom	3.09	0.001
Nervousness	Symptom	2.79	0.005
Diarrhea	Symptom	2.41	0.020
Alcohol Consump.	Symptom	2.33	0.020
Dizziness	Symptom	2.08	0.040

Symptoms--subjective findings, reported by patient
Signs--objective findings, measured by physician or lab

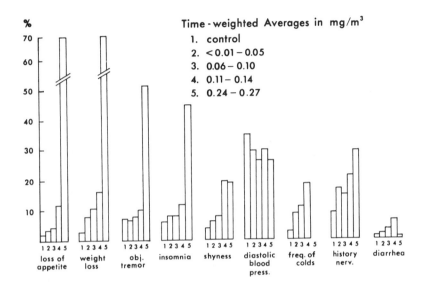

Figure 32: Percentage Incidence of Certain Signs and Symptoms Related to Exposure of Workers to Mercury

Although the findings are based largely on subjective responses, the initial awareness that the central nervous system was expected to be affected by sufficiently high concentrations of mercury makes it logical to believe the findings. It is easy to see, however, that individuals displaying the symptoms found to be more prevalent with increased mercury exposure would be hardly distinguishable from other employees exhibiting similar symptoms for a variety of reasons unrelated to exposure to mercury.

The results just summarized, together with those from many other studies considered by the international committee, were influential in suggesting that the dose-response relationship between mercury vapor and exposed workers was such that the time-weighted average exposure should be kept below 100 micrograms per cubic meter, and preferably below 50 µg/m^3, if a reasonable safety factor were to be incorporated into the limit. The American Conference of Governmental Industrial Hygienists took similar action, and recommended that its Threshold Limit Value (TLV) be lowered to this same value, a change which has now become permanent.[17] However, the international committee felt that, should the occupational exposure be limited to the inorganic salts of mercury rather than mercury vapor, a higher concentration could be tolerated, and accordingly, suggested a time-weighted average exposure maximum of 100 micrograms per cubic meter. Although this recommendation was based on sound evidence that mercuric salts do not enter the brain as efficiently as elemental mercury vapor, the ACGIH elected not to adopt a dual standard for inorganic mercury.

This brief review has been confined to a consideration of several studies which have involved human exposure to inorganic mercury. Toxicological studies involving controlled animal exposures have not been reviewed. In general, however, they tend to reinforce the evidence obtained from human studies. Unfortunately, the problems of species differences, varying lengths of life, etc. tend to make it difficult to use animal data to predict human responses, even though many similarities in observed effects are noted.

It can be implied from the occupational health standards that, at levels below 50 micrograms per cubic meter, no adverse effects on exposed workers will be found. Present-day concern with environmental mercury pollution, however, has stimulated a great deal of atmospheric sampling, both in our cities and in areas adjacent to industries which may release mercury. As previously noted, concentrations very much lower than those found within the plant are generally found. Do such concentrations pose any threat to the health of urban populations?

The problem of establishing an ambient air quality standard for mercury is inevitably complicated by the fact that the population at risk is greatly different from an industrial population. Additionally, exposure may be continuous rather than limited to a 40-hour work week. There are little or no data to support any ambient air quality standard for mercury at this time, but studies of the type described involving industrial populations would seem to suggest that ambient levels as presently known are well below any standard that might be based on the direct effects of inhalation on human health. Possibly situations will occur, however, in which localized concentrations will be excessive; perhaps from such incidents will come data to assist in determining the magnitude of a rational ambient air standard for mercury.

It is unlikely that standard-setting will be deferred
while awaiting such data, though; it is much more probable
that some arbitrary fraction of the TLV will be selected
instead. As in the case of several other trace metals,
the dietary intake will doubtlessly prove to be of over-
riding importance in determining the body burden of mercury,
and even this factor is further complicated by the possibility that much of the ingested mercury may be present
as the far more toxic compound, methyl mercury. At the
present time, in fact, it appears that the ingestion of
certain foods containing excessive quantities of methyl
mercury constitutes the single threat to human health
resulting from general environmental pollution by mercury,
and it is to be hoped that actions presently being taken
will serve to bring this problem under control.

References

1. International Committee Report. "Maximum Allowable
    Concentrations of Mercury Compounds," Arch. Environ.
    Health, *19*, 891 (1969).
2. Teisinger, J. and V. Fiserova. "Pulmonary Retention
    and Excretion of Mercury Vapors in Man," Industr. Med.
    Surg., *34*, 580 (1965).
3. Kazantzis, G., *et al.* "Albuminuria and the Nephrotic
    Syndrome Following Exposure to Mercury and Its Com-
    pounds," Quart. J. Med., *31*, 403 (1962).
4. Joselow, M. M. and L. J. Goldwater. "Absorption and
    Excretion of Mercury in Man: XII. Relationship Between
    Mercury and Proteinuria," Arch. Environ. Health, *15*
    155 (1967).
5. Neal, P. A., *et al.* "A Study of Chronic Mercurialism
    in Hatters' for Cutting Industry," U.S. Public Health
    Service, Bulletin 234 (1937).
6. Neal, P. A., *et al.* "Mercurialism and Its Control in
    the Felt-Hat Industry," U.S. Public Health Service,
    Bulletin 263 (1941).
7. Bidstrup, P. L. *et al.* "Chronic Mercury Poisoning in
    Man Repairing Direct-Current Meters," Lancet, *2*, 856
    (1951).
8. Fribert, L. "Aspects of Chronic Poisoning With
    Inorganic Mercury," Nord. Hyg. T., *32*, 240 (1951).
9. Goldwater, L. J. "Occupational Exposure to Mercury,"
    The Harben Lectures, *1964* (Royal Institute of Public
    Health: December, 1964).
10. El-Sadik, Y. M. and A. A. El-Dakhakhny. "Effects of
    Exposure of Workers to Mercury at a Sodium Hydroxide

Producing Plant," <u>Amer</u>. <u>Ind</u>. <u>Hyg</u>. <u>Assoc</u>. <u>J</u>., *31*, 705 (1970).

11. Ladd, A. C., E. Zuskin, F. Valic, J. B. Almonte, and T. V. Gonzales. "Absorption and Excretion of Mercury in Miners," <u>J</u>. <u>Occup</u>. <u>Med</u>. <u>Balt</u>. <u>Mar</u>., *8*, 127 (1966).
12. Smith, R. G., A. J. Vorwald, L. S. Patil, and T. F. Mooney, Jr. "Effects of Exposure to Mercury in the Manufacture of Chlorine," <u>Amer</u>. <u>Ind</u>. <u>Hyg</u>. <u>Assoc</u>. <u>J</u>., *31*, 687 (1970).
13. Elkins, H. B. "Excretory and Biologic Threshold Limits," <u>Amer</u>. <u>Ind</u>. <u>Hyg</u>. <u>Assoc</u>. <u>J</u>., *28*, 305 (1967).
14. Goldwater, L. J., M. B. Jacobs, and A. C. Ladd. "Absorption and Excretion of Mercury in Blood and Urine," <u>AMA</u> <u>Arch</u>. <u>Env</u>. <u>Health</u>, *5*, 537 (1962).
15. Joselow, M. M., R. Ruiz, and L. J. Goldwater. "Absorption and Excretion of Mercury in Man, XIV. Salivary Excretion of Mercury and Its Relationship to Blood and Urine Mercury," <u>AMA</u> <u>Arch</u>. <u>Env</u>. <u>Health</u>, *17*, 35 (1968).
16. Patil, L. S., R. G. Smith, A. J. Vorwald, and T. F. Mooney, Jr. "The Health of Diaphragm Cell Workers Exposed to Chlorine," <u>Amer</u>. <u>Ind</u>. <u>Hyg</u>. <u>Assoc</u>. <u>J</u>., *31*, 678 (1970).
17. Amer. Conf. of Governmental Ind. Hygienists. <u>Threshold Limit</u> <u>Values</u> <u>of</u> <u>Airborne</u> <u>Contaminants</u> (1970).

Surface Electromyography in
Chronic Inorganic Mercury Intoxication

Don B. Chaffin and Bertram D. Dinman

The Institute of Environmental and Industrial Health was contacted in August, 1970, by a small metal salvage shop regarding possible occupational mercury intoxication. The operation in question separated tungsten-carbide tool-bit scrap from the associated steel by an ingenious differential floatation method. Unfortunately for those involved, metallic mercury permitted adequate separation of the two alloys in question because of the relatively higher specific gravity of the tungsten-carbide. The process consisted of skimming the floating steel off the surface of a metallic mercury bath, then recovering the more valuable alloy from the bottom of the bath, this being accomplished by raising a

perforated basket which had been previously inserted in
the mercury bath. The associated skimming, drag-out of
the basket, and other operations required manipulation of
several hundred pounds of mercury. This contamination was
further aggravated by a heated tumbler used to separate
the metallic mercury from the recovered tungsten-carbide
alloy.

On the basis of a telephone description of this operation, it appeared practically certain that a mercury vapor
hazard existed in this plant. This was confirmed by a
rapid industrial hygiene survey of the operation. The
airborne concentration of mercury vapor (Table 43) clearly

Table 43

Airborne Mercury Concentrations

Location	Mercury in mg/m^3*
1. At mercury tub	0.215
2. At tumbler-crusher	0.239
3. At sizer	0.178
4. General work-room air	0.093
5. Outside plant, at exhaust	0.039
6. Secretary's office	0.038

*Method of analysis = Campbell-Head single extraction
dithizone method.[1] Collection method = 1% $KMnO_4$ in N H_2SO_4,
fitted bubbler at breathing 3 ml.

indicated that probable health hazard existed. Accordingly,
the four workers in the shop were examined at The University
of Michigan at the Institute of Environmental and Industrial
Health, and in the Laboratories of the Department of Industrial Engineering.

Methods of Evaluation

Medical evaluation: Extensive historical and physical
evaluation was carried out, with specific attention
directed toward psychomotor and emotional status of those
examined. A series of psychological evaluations were performed and will be reported at a later date. In addition,

blood, urine, and hair were obtained for the determination of total mercury.

Surface electromyographic evaluation: Recently some electromyographers have advocated the use of frequency analyzers to gain a more quantified representation of muscle action potentials. In essence, this technique simply treats the detected muscle action potential as a summation of many simpler wave forms, each of which has a varying frequency and amplitude. Briefly, frequency analysis breaks a complex muscle action potential into the basic components occurring in preselected frequency bands. The "outcome" of such an analysis is then a graphical and numerical plot of the amplitude of these components (usually in terms of the power developed by the components) in each of these frequency bands. This is reported as a histogram of muscle action potentials, with the frequency bands being plotted on the abscissa (horizontal axis), and the power developed by the components being plotted (for each band) on the ordinate (vertical axis). Refer also to Figure 33.

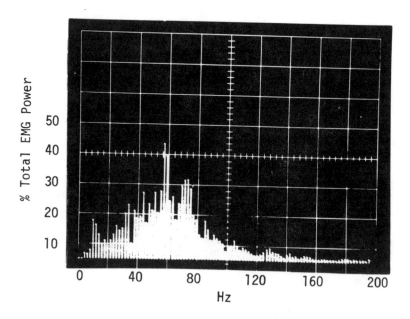

Figure 33: Histogram of Muscle Action Potentials, with Frequency Bands Plotted on the Abscissa and Power Developed by the Components Plotted on the Ordinate

A sensitive quantification of the EMG involves a transformation of the continuous EMG signal into discrete
quantities via a high speed digital computer, and then
numerically computing the power of the components existing
within various defined frequencies. For example, the
frequency bands used in research here are centered at
intervals of two Hertz, over a range from four to 200 Hertz.
Thus each spectrum analysis provides 98 power measures.

Over the past four years, over 5000 EMG power spectra
have been developed from healthy individuals isometrically
contracting various muscle groups. These have all been
based on the muscle action potentials being detected by
the use of surface electrodes--one on the skin over the
active muscle, and one on the skin over an electrically
quiet area. The outcome of these studies have been EMG
power spectral "norms." (Figure 33 displays the normal
EMG power spectra for the biceps brachii.) Normal EMG
power spectra from a monopolar surface electrode are
(1) unimodal, (2) major power between 30-80 Hz, (3) insensitive to degree of contraction between 10% and 40%
maximum voluntary strength, and (4) shifted to low frequency spectra (e.g., major power below 30 Hz) after
sustained exertions.

The four persons suspected of mercury intoxication were
tested with 10, 15, and 20 pound loads on a wrist strap.
They supported each load by holding their forearm horizontal
for eight seconds while an EMG was obtained from the con-
tracted biceps brachii.

Results of Evaluation

Clinical: The production worker (patient #1) and the
owner of this small firm (patient #2) evidenced signs and
symptoms of chronic mercurialism, while the secretary
working in the adjoining room and a salesman who usually
worked away from the shop appeared unaffected. Patients
1 and 2 both reported loss of appetite and weight, impaired
sleep and nightmares, ease of fatigue, and personality
changes. These latter were reported variously as increased
irritability with family and friends, an inability to perform tasks requiring either motor-cognitive function or
fine finger coordination. For patient 2, consciousness of
this impairment made him increasingly irritable with him-
self, as well as withdrawn, since he feared that others
could observe this psychomotor disability. Both patients
noted fine tremors of both hands at rest, which could
successfully be suppressed with intention. Curiously, it

appeared that patient 2 had more severe involvement, despite
the fact that patient 1 had a higher mercury content of
biological media (Table 44). It should be noted that a

Table 44

Mercury Concentrations in Blood, Hair, and Urine

Patient	Blood Hg (μg/100 ml)	Urine Hg (μg/l)	Hair Hg (μg/gm)
1	18.6	1486	27.4 Free end 29.3 Scalp end
2	8.7	726	15.0 Free end 4.5 Scalp end
3	---	330	16.0 Free end >3 Scalp end
4	3.2	221	4.3 Free end 2.0 Scalp end

history of increased salivation could not be clearly
detected and that gingival changes were not found. On
physical examination, a fine intention tremor was noted;
otherwise their physical examinations were not remarkable.
Examination of the secretary (patient 3) and salesman
(patient 4) were unremarkable.

The analysis of total mercury in blood, urine and hair
was performed by the method of Campbell-Head,[1] and is given
in Table 44.

Electromyographic: Spectral analysis of the electro-
myograms revealed signal abnormalities in patients 1 and 2,
while patients 3 and 4 appeared normal. The abnormalities
were noted with the 10, 15, and 20 pound weight, though
such aberrations were more definitive with the greater
weight. In contrast to the normal single peaked power
distribution at 30 to 40 Hz (Figure 33), patients 1 and 2
demonstrated a bimodal power distribution, with peaks at
about 30-40 Hz and at 60 Hz (Figure 34). Statistical
analysis of 200 normals permitted definition of a two
standard deviation limit about such a derived normal power

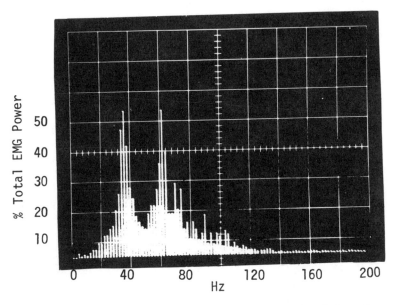

Figure 34: Histogram of Muscle Action Potentials of
   Patients 1 and 2

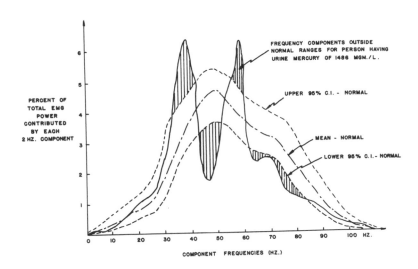

COMPARISON OF NORMAL VALUES WITH PERSON HAVING ELEVATED
MERCURY LEVELS

Figure 35: Comparison of Normal Values with Person Having
   Elevated Mercury Levels

distribution. This is illustrated in Figure 35, wherein the normal power distribution, the two standard deviation range, and the power distribution of patient 1 are compared.

Patient 1 can be seen to demonstrate increased power extending beyond the two standard deviation limits in the 30-40 Hz and 50-60 Hz portions of the spectrum, at the expense of electromuscular activity centering about the 50 Hz area.

Discussion of Results

The significance of the observed changes at this time is unknown. However, that such objective changes occurred in patient 2 is of particular interest, in view of the report of Smith, *et al.*[2] In that study of 642 chloralkali (mercury) cell-room workers, correlations between atmospheric and blood mercury and the appearance of highly subjective, nonspecific symptoms indicated that health aberrations appeared when blood mercury concentrations were in the range of 6-8 µg per 100 ml of blood. Patient 2 had a blood concentration in this range, and also had such subjective symptoms as noted in the population believed by Smith to represent minimal mercury intoxication. Although Smith could identify such groups of minimally intoxicated workers by study of symptom frequency within a population, the nonspecific nature (shyness, nervousness, loss of weight and appetite, frequent colds, diarrhea) of these changes makes it extremely difficult to identify an individual with minimal poisoning who manifests only subjective symptomatic change. Thus, the objective nature of the electromyographic approach might make it possible to identify individuals with minimal mercury body burdens as in the case of patient 2.

Application of this method to such populations requires further investigation. The patients reported here had been chronically exposed to mercury over a period of approximately 1 1/2 years, without remission of exposure; they did not have the benefit of medical or industrial hygiene controls. Since continued inadequately controlled mercury exposure is required to produce the loadings these two patients experienced, such a prolonged period of uptake and loading may not be too common. Also, chronic continuous exposure may be required to produce the changes seen here.

Other factors are known to affect the electromyographic record, *e.g.*, drugs and medications, concomitant pathological states, physical fitness, recent physical work. The usefulness of this technique may well be dependent upon our ability to standardize testing conditions. Nevertheless, the highly abnormal EMG power density distributions do not resemble any others seen among 200 normal individual previously tested. Accordingly, application of this method to the study of cases of mercury intoxication--as well as other toxicants, *e.g.*, lead, arsenic, halogenated aliphatics, acetylcholinesterase inhibitors, etc.--would seem appropriate.

References

1. Campbell, E. E. and B. M. Head. Amer. Indust. Hyg. Assoc. Quart., *16*, 275 (1955).
2. Smith, R. G., A. J. Vorwald, L. S. Patil, and T. F. Mooney, Jr. Amer. Indust. Hyg. Assoc. J., *31*, 687 (1970).

Biotransformation of Organo-Mercurials in Mammals*

T. W. Clarkson

Introduction

Organo-mercurial compounds have been defined as those compounds in which the mercury atom is covalently linked to at least one carbon atom.[1] In general, two pathways of biotransformation of organo-mercurials may be considered (Figure 36). One pathway is the cleavage of the carbon-mercury bond resulting in the release of inorganic mercury. The other pathway starts with a chemical change in the organic moiety to give a modified organo-mercuric compound. This compound may then undergo further chemical reaction, perhaps eventually leading to the release of inorganic mercury. | Most of the studies of biotransformation of organo-mercurials have described the first pathway. The paper by Daniel *et al.*[2] is one of the few studies describing metabolic changes by the second pathway.

Weiner, Levy, and Mudge[3] reported that the carbon-mercury bond in organo-mercurials used as diuretic agents may be

*This work was supported in part by GM1-5190-04 and in part under Contract No. W-7401-Eng-49 from the U.S. Atomic Energy Commission and has been assigned Report No. UR 1486.

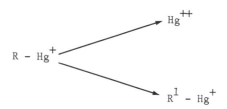

Figure 36:   Alternative Pathways in the Biotransformation
of Organo-Mercurial Compounds. R-Hg$^+$ Represents the
Unchanged Mercurial Ion, Hg^{++} Inorganic Mercury, and
R^1-Hg$^+$ an Organo-Mercurial Metabolite of the Parent
Compound

rapidly split *in vitro*, in the presence of a thiol compound
in solution buffered at pH 4.0. The phenyl and alkyl
mercury compounds were stable under these conditions. A
slow *in vitro* breakdown of methylmercuric cysteinate, in
the presence of excess cysteine at pH 7.0, has been reported to occur at a rate of approximately 0.4% per day.
No significant breakdown took place in the absence of
cysteine.

Several investigators have studied the rate of cleavage
of the carbon-mercury bond in experimental animals.[2,4-9]
The rate of *in vivo* conversion to inorganic mercury cannot
be accurately estimated until a complete pharmacokinetic
model is developed. However, it is known that inorganic
mercury is well accumulated by kidney tissue.[10,11] Thus,
an approximate idea of the relative rates of biotransformation may be obtained by comparing the fraction of
inorganic mercury in kidneys following single doses of
different organo-mercurial compounds.

The short chain alkyl mercurials undergo conversion to
inorganic mercury much more slowly than the other main
classes of organo-mercurials listed in Table 45. The
mercurial diuretics and the aryl mercurials are converted
so quickly that virtually all the mercury in the kidneys
is in the inorganic form within 24 hours of a single dose
of the mercurial. In contrast, methyl mercury compounds
yield less than 50% inorganic in kidney even 8 days after
injection. Ethyl mercury compounds are also slowly
metabolized but at a faster rate than the methyl compounds.

Table 45

The Fraction of Total Mercury Present in Rat Kidneys as
Inorganic Mercury Following Single Injections of
Organo-Mercurial Compounds

*Organo-Mercurial Ion	Time (Days)	Inorganic Hg in Kidneys % Total
CH_3-Hg^+	8	39
$CH_3-CH_2-Hg^+$	4	57
$R-CH_2-\underset{OY}{CH}-CH_2-Hg^+$	1	93
$C_6H_5-Hg^+$	1	87
$CH_3O \cdot C_2H_4 \cdot Hg^+$	1	100
$HOOC \cdot C_6H_4 \cdot Hg^+$	2 hours	100

*The anion is not specified, as it has only a secondary
effect on rates of biotransformation.

**The general formula for organo-mercurials acting as
diuretics.[12]

The Role of Inorganic Mercury in Determining
The Toxic Effects of Organo-Mercurial Compounds

The acute LD_{50} of mercuric chloride, parenterally
administered, is approximately ten times lower than LD_{50}'s
of organo-mercurial compounds.[13] Thus, it is possible that
inorganic mercury released from organo-mercurial compounds
may be responsible for the acute toxicities, if not the
chronic effects, of these compounds. For example, the conversion of 10% of an LD_{50} dose of a phenyl or short-chain
alkyl mercurial would release into the body an amount of
inorganic mercury equivalent to the LD_{50} of mercuric
chloride.

The idea that organo-mercurial diuretics elicit their
therapeutic action via release of inorganic mercury dates
back several decades.[14] The so-called "mercuric ion"
hypothesis has recently been reaffirmed by Weiner, Levy
and Mudge.[3] Arguments supporting the mercuric ion hypothesis may be summarized as follows: Inorganic mercury,
administered to dogs as mercuric cysteine, elicits diuresis
at a lower dose, expressed as mg of Hg/kg body weight, than

the doses required of organo-mercurial diuretics. Organo-mercurial diuretics release inorganic mercury *in vitro* at pH 4.0 in the presence of thiol compounds. Organo-mercurial compounds that are stable under these conditions do not possess diuretic properties. The diuretic potency of the organo-mercurials is greatly enhanced when the experimental animal and human subject is in an acidotic state--a finding consistent with the *in vitro* lability under acid conditions. Diuresis elicited by administration of inorganic mercury is relatively independent of the acid-base balance of the animal.[15]

The "mercuric ion" hypothesis received further support when it was demonstrated that the mercurial diuretic chlormerodrin deposited inorganic mercury in kidney tissues of the rat, rabbit, and chicken,[7] and of the dog.[16] Organo-mercurial diuretics are virtually ineffective in producing diuresis in rats. The changes in urinary excretion elicited by the diuretics in the rat suggest a toxic rather than pharmacologic action in these species.[7,16] Nevertheless, the effects seen in renal function in the rat are similar to those induced by mercuric salts, and the levels of inorganic mercury in rat kidney associated with these effects are similar.[16] These arguments, although persuasive, are not conclusive. Vostal and Clarkson[17] initiated a more detailed quantitative study on dogs to further investigate the "mercuric ion" hypothesis. The findings confirmed that diuretic doses of organo-mercurial diuretics, such as chlormerodrin and mersalyl, release inorganic mercury which accumulates in the kidney tissue of dogs.

However, several facts came to light that were unfavorable to the "mercuric ion" hypothesis. First, the levels of mercuric ion in kidney tissue following minimally effective diuretic doses of mercuric cysteine were higher than levels of mercuric ion released from diuretic doses of chlormerodrin and mersalyl. Second, nondiuretic mercurials produced higher kidney levels of inorganic mercury than were observed following diuretically effective doses of chlormerodrin and mersalyl. Third, changes in the acid base balance of the dogs did not elicit the expected changes in breakdown of the diuretics as predicted by the *in vitro* tests of Weiner *et al.*[3] For example, diuretics administered to alkalotic dogs failed to elicit diuresis, but nevertheless deposited inorganic mercury in renal tissue in amounts at least as great as under acidotic conditions when diuresis ensued. These findings indicated that, despite many years of investigation in several laboratories, the "mercuric ion" hypothesis is still in doubt.

Single doses of methyl mercury salts produce brain damage in experimental animals following a latent period lasting several days and weeks.[13,18-20] The possibility has been raised that the toxic effects on the central nervous system may be caused by inorganic mercury split off from the methyl mercury radical.[9] A slow cumulative build of inorganic mercury in the brain might account for the characteristic latent period. However, the weight of evidence is against this hypothesis. The data of Table 46 indicate that the fraction of total mercury present in

Table 46

Percentage Inorganic Mercury in Brain after
1 and 10 mg Hg/kg Given as Methylmercuric Chloride

Days after Injection	Inorganic Mercury (% Total Hg in Brain)	
	Low Dose	High Dose
1	3.5	0.7
3	3.9	3.7
6	---	1.1
8	1.1	---
9	---	0.4
16	3.0	---
24	0.8	---
28	---	2.2

brain as inorganic mercury was never more than 4% with no significant change with time after both dosage levels.[21]

*The Role of Biotransformation in Distribution
and Deposition of Mercury*

Inorganic mercury is accumulated and stored in cortical tissue of the kidneys. One day following a single injection of mercuric chloride, approximately 50% of the dose was found in the kidneys.[10] Several weeks later, over 90% of the mercury remaining in the body was found in the kidneys.

The distribution of mercury in the body following single doses of organo-mercurial compounds exhibits two characteristic patterns. The first pattern, seen shortly after injection, depends upon the type of organo-mercurial injected. The second pattern is typical of inorganic mercury. The organo-mercurial diuretic chlormerodin gives kidney levels higher than seen with inorganic mercury, but urinary excretion is very rapid, and the intact mercurial rapidly disappears from the body. Mercury remaining in the body 24 to 48 hours after injection is present entirely as inorganic mercury, giving a pattern of distribution characteristic of this form of mercury. The rate of change from the first to the second pattern of distribution depends upon the rate of biotransformation of the organo-mercurial and the relative rates of excretion of the intact molecules of the organo-mercurial versus the excretion rate for inorganic mercury. The change is most rapid for the organo-mercurial diuretics because they are rapidly metabolized and rapidly excreted. The methyl mercury salts undergo the change in patterns of distribution more slowly than all other compounds of mercury tested to date.[21] The pattern of distribution of mercury following a single dose of methylmercuric chloride is characterized by a more uniform distribution in various tissues as compared to other mercury compounds, and by high red blood cell to plasma distribution ratios. This pattern persists in rats for many weeks. As long as seven weeks after a single injection of methylmercuric chloride, significant fractions of the intact mercurial were found in the livers and kidneys of rats. One would have to wait, then, a great deal longer to see a distribution pattern characteristic of inorganic mercury.

The toxicological significance of the change in tissue distribution and deposition of mercury as a result of biotransformation cannot be fully assessed at this time. In the case of the mercurial diuretics, biotransformation will result in residual levels of inorganic mercury in the kidneys. This may account for clinical findings that repeated frequent doses of organo-mercurial diuretic may give rise to mercurialism. Repeated doses of the other rapidly metabolizable mercurials may lead to renal accumulation of inorganic mercury (Figure 37). Fitzhugh *et al.*[22] have reported that chronic oral intake of phenyl mercury compounds produces kidney damage in rats.

The Role of Biotransformation in the Excretion of Mercury

The mercurial diuretics are excreted much more rapidly than inorganic mercury.[3] Therefore, biotransformation of

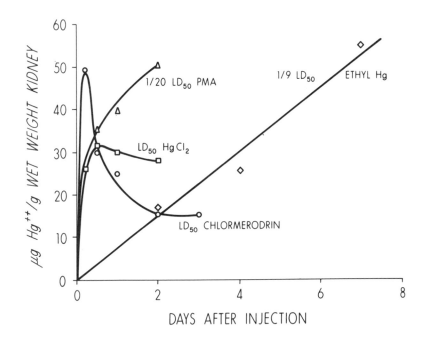

Figure 37: The Levels of Inorganic Mercury in Kidney Tissue
of Experimental Animals Given a Single Dose of a Mercury
Compound. The Dose is Expressed in Units of LD_{50} for
that Compound. The line Labeled Ethyl-Hg is from Data
by Miller *et al*. (1961). The Curve Labeled PMA
(Phenylmercuric Acetate) is from Data by Miller *et al*.
(1960), and the Curves Labeled $HgCl_2$ and Chlormerodrin
are from Data by Clarkson (1969).

these compounds to inorganic mercury will result in increased
retention of mercury in the body, as demonstrated in the case
of chlormerodrin.[7] The phenyl and methoxyethyl mercurials
appear to be excreted at approximately the same rate as
inorganic mercury, so that biotransformation should not
greatly affect excretion.[4,6,11]
    In principle, one would expect that biotransformation
would play its most important role in the case of the alkyl
mercurials, since these compounds are excreted much more
slowly than inorganic mercury.[11] Norseth and Clarkson[21,23]
have demonstrated the importance of biotransformation in
the excretion of mercury from rats dosed with methylmercuric
chloride. The fecal pathway is the most important route of
excretion, accounting for over 80% of the total excretion

of mercury in the first ten days after a single dose. Inorganic mercury accounted for at least 50% of the total mercury in feces during this period--a finding in agreement with the original observation of Gage.[6]

Rats given methylmercuric chloride excrete large amounts of mercury in the bile. Most of this mercury, in the form of methyl mercury complexes, is reabsorbed in the small intestine back into the blood stream. However, a small amount of inorganic mercury is also excreted in the bile. This form of mercury is very slowly absorbed across the intestine so that most of the biliary inorganic mercury appears in the feces.

The importance of a slow rate of biotransformation of methyl mercury in the liver is demonstrated by the data in Table 47.

Table 47

Total and Inorganic Mercury in Plasma and Liver
in Control and Bile Duct-Ligated Rats
3 Days after a Single Dose (1 mg Hg/kg)
of Methylmercuric Chloride

Tissue	Treatment	No. of Experiments	Total Mercury $\mu g/g$ (ppm)	Inorganic Mercury $\mu g/g$ (ppm)
Plasma*	Control	4	0.022 ± 0.001	0.006 ± 0.0007
	Ligated	4	0.052 ± 0.003	0.025 ± 0.0014
Liver	Control	7	0.91 ± 0.06	0.10 ± 0.015
	Ligated	5	1.56 ± 0.12	0.33 ± 0.027

*The mercury concentrations in plasma are in $\mu g/ml$ (approx. ppm).

Bile duct ligation produced not only an increase in the total mercury in liver, as may be expected, but a greater relative increase in the amount of inorganic mercury. The increase in the total mercury levels in plasma from 0.022 to 0.055 $\mu g/ml$ can be accounted for as due entirely to the increase in levels of inorganic mercury from 0.006 to 0.025 $\mu g/ml$. Thus when the bile duct is ligated, the biotransformation process in the liver no longer leads to excretion of mercury. But inorganic mercury accumulates in the organ and diffuses into plasma where it may distribute to other tissues.

References

1. MAC Committee. "Maximum Allowable Concentrations of Mercury Compounds: Report of an International Committee," Arch. Environ. Health, *19*, 891 (1969).
2. Daniel, J. W., J. C. Gage, and P. A. Lefevre. "The Metabolism of Methoxyethylmercury Salts," Biochem. J., *121*, 411 (1970).
3. Weiner, J. M., R. I. Levy, and G. H. Mudge. "Studies on Mercurial Diuresis," J. Pharmacol. Exp. Ther., *138*, 96 (1962).
4. Miller, V. L., P. A. Klavano, and E. Csonka. "Absorption, Distribution and Excretion of Phenylmercuric Acetate," Toxic. and Appl. Pharmac., *2*, 344 (1960).
5. Miller, V. L., P. A. Klavano, A. C. Jerstad, and E. Csonka. "Absorption, Distribution, and Excretion of Ethylmercuric Chloride," Toxic. and Appl. Pharm., *3*, 459 (1961).
6. Gage, J. C. "Distribution and Excretion of Methyl and Phenyl Mercury Salts," Brit. J. Indus. Med., *21*, 197 (1964).
7. Clarkson, T. W., A. Rothstein, and R. Sutherland. "The Mechanism of Action of Mercurial Diuretics in Rats," Brit. J. Pharmacol., *24*, 1 (1965).
8. Clarkson, T. W. and M. R. Greenwood. "The Mechanism of Action of Mercurial Diuretics in Rats; the Renal Metabolism of P-Chloromercuribenzoate and its Effects on Urinary Excretion," Brit. J. Pharmacol., *26*, 50 (1966).
9. Norseth, T. and T. W. Clarkson. "Biotransformation of Methylmercury Salts in the Rat Studied by Specific Determination of Inorganic Mercury," Biochem. Pharmacol., *19*, 2775 (1970).
10. Rothstein, A. and A. H. Hayes. "The Metabolism of Mercury in the Rat Studied by Isotope Techniques," J. Pharmacol. Exp. Ther., *130*, 166 (1960).
11. Swensson, A. and U. Ulfvarson. "Distribution and Excretion of Mercury Compounds in Rats over a Long Period Injection," Acta Pharmacol. Toxic., *26*, 273 (1968).
12. Kessler, R. H., R. Lozano, and R. F. Pitts. "Studies on the Structure Diuretic Activity Relationships in Organic Compounds of Mercury," J. Clin. Invest., *36*, 656 (1957).

13. Swensson, A. and U. Ulfvarson. "Toxicology of Organic Mercury Compounds Used as Fungicides," Occup. Health Rev., *15*, 5 (1963).
14. Sollman, T. A Manual of Pharmacology (London: W. B. Saunders Co., 1957), p. 1324.
15. Mudge, G. H. and I. M. Weiner. "The Mechanism of Action of Mercurial and Zanthine Diuretics," Ann. N. Y. Acad. Sci., *71*, 344 (1958).
16. Clarkson, T. W. "Isotope Exchange Methods in Studies of the Biotransformation of Organo-Mercurial Compounds in Experimental Animals," in Chemical Fallout, M. Miller and G. G. Berg, Eds. (Springfield, Illinois: Charles C. Thomas, 1969), pp. 244-293.
17. Vostal, J. and T. W. Clarkson. "The Release of Inorganic Mercury from Diuretic and Non-Diuretic Organomercurials in Dogs," Fed. Proc. (1970).
18. Hunter, D., R. R. Bomford, and D. S. Russel. "Poisoning by Methylmercury Compounds," Quart. J. Med., *33*, 193 (1940).
19. Yoshino, Y., T. Mozai, and K. Nakao. "Distribution of Mercury in the Brain and its Subcellular Units in Experimental Organic Mercury Poisonings," J. Neurochem., *13*, 397 (1966).
20. Yoshino, Y., T. Mozai, and K. Nakao. "Biochemical Changes in the Brain in Rats Poisoned with an Alkylmercury Compound, with Special Reference to the Inhibition of Protein Synthesis in Brain Cortex Slices," J. Neurochem., *13*, 1223 (1966).
21. Norseth, T. and T. W. Clarkson. "Studies on the Biotransformation of [203]Hg-Labeled Methyl Mercury Chloride in Rats," Archiv. Environ. Health, *21*, 717 (1970).
22. Fitzhugh, O. G., A. A. Nelson, E. P. Lang, and F. M. Kunze. "Chronic Oral Toxicities of Mercuric-Phenyl and Mercuric Salts," Arch. Ind. Hyg. and Occup. Med., *2*, 433 (1950).
23. Norseth, T. and T. W. Clarkson. "Intestinal Transport of [203]Hg-Labeled Methyl Mercury Chloride," Archiv. Environ. Health, *22*, 568 (1971).

The Binding of Inorganic and Organic Mercury Compounds (^{203}Hg) to Constituents of Normal Human Blood

Hoda A. Guirgis, W. K. Stewart, and W. Taylor

Blood is of physiological importance both as a "carrier" and as a "distributing" agent for various substances within the body, including metals. In this present investigation, the uptake of ^{203}Hg labelled mercuric chloride (Hg Cl$_2$), phenylmercuric acetate (PMA) and methylmercuric nitrate (MMN) by normal human blood was studied *in vitro*. Table 48 shows that the relative uptake of HgCl$_2$, PMA and MMN by

Table 48

The Uptake of Mercuric Compounds (^{203}Hg) by Erythrocytes and Plasma of Normal Human Blood

Mercuric Compound	Range: R.B.C./Plasma	Mean: R.B.C./Plasma	Standard Deviation
HgCl$_2$	1:3.3 to 1:7.8	1:5.7	1.3
PMA	1:0.7 to 1:1.3	1:0.96	0.2
MMN	2.3:1 to 3.9:1	3.0:1	0.6

erythrocytes and plasma varied from one compound to another. The amount of HgCl$_2$ taken up by the plasma ranged from 3.3 to 7.8 times that taken by erythrocytes, PMA was essentially equally distributed, and the amount of MMN taken by erythrocytes ranged from 2.3 to 3.9 times that taken by plasma.

It thus appears that the affinity of PMA and MMN to erythrocytes is greater than that of HgCl$_2$, the latter being mainly bound to the serum proteins. These observations indicate that the chemical structure of the individual compound influences both the site and extent of its interaction with blood cells and proteins.

The uptake of organic mercury compounds by the erythrocytes may result from the tendency of these compounds to be bound to the lipid components of the erythrocyte envelope.+

Table 49 shows the electrophoretic separation of HgCl$_2$, PMA, and MMN-serum mixtures. This indicates that the

Table 49

Binding of Labelled Mercuric Chloride ($HgCl_2$),
Phenylmercuric Acetate (PMA) and
Methylmercuric Nitrate (MMN) to Normal Serum

Procedure	Compound	% Activity in Each Fraction				
		Albumin	α_1	α_2	β	γ
^{203}Hg + Serum:	$HgCl_2$	89.9	3.9	3.3	1.0	0.4
electrophoresis	PMA	64.5	7.5	1.7	5.9	20.2
after 15 minues	MMN	51.7	10.5	8.4	7.6	21.9
Control:	$HgCl_2$	1.5	3.4	5.5	82.3	7.1
electrophoresis	PMA	0.9	1.5	1.3	1.1	95.1
	MMN	7.0	7.6	6.9	7.2	71.3
^{203}Hg + serum:	$HgCl_2$	2.4	19.2	67.8	4.6	5.7
24-hour incuba-	PMA	66.6	4.2	3.4	3.5	21.3
tion and 24-hour	MMN	46.9	10.2	6.9	8.0	28.2
dialysis at 4°C,						
then electrophoresis						

organic forms of mercury compounds are bound preferentially
to the albumin and γ-globulin fractions. The presence of
some radioactivity in the γ-globulin fractions, in addition
to that associated with the albumin, may be due to (1) the
tendency of this fraction specifically to bind the organic
types of mercury compounds, or (2) the presence of unbound
mercuric compounds that have not moved from the electrophoretic starting point. By contrast, in the case of
mercuric chloride there was a shift in the binding fraction
from the albumin to the γ-globulins when it was incubated
and dialyzed. The presence of more than one binding site
for the $HgCl_2$ may be due to the high degree of ionization
of the inorganic mercury compounds. This may account for
their rapid combination with readily accessible binding
sites present in the albumin fraction, while the sites in
the γ-globulin are only available following incubation.
These results confirm the views of Linderstrom-Lang and
Schellman[1] who believe that the bound molecules "slide
between groups on the protein."

Table 50

The Uptake of ^{197}Hg by Plasma and
Erythrocytes *in vivo*

Sample	*dpm in 1.0 ml. whole blood*	*dpm in 1.0 ml. plasma*	*dpm in 1.0 ml. erythrocytes*	*Ratio of Plasma: erythrocytes*
before injection	81	81	83	--
25 minutes after injection	58070	93678	27294	3:1
20 hours after injection	5164	4008	6036	1:1.5

Table 50 shows the uptake of mercury by human blood *in vivo* among a group of patients injected with a therapeutic dose of radioactive mercury (^{197}Hg)-labelled chlormerodrin. The blood mercury content was 3.3 µg/100 ml before the injection of chlormerodrin (^{197}Hg), 69.0 µg/100 ml after 25 minutes, and 5.2 µg/100 ml after 20 hours. The loading of ^{197}Hg by plasma and erythrocytes, shown in Table 50, demonstrates marked decreases 20 hours after the injection. One might hypothesize that enzymic factors operate *in vivo* to release the mercury from its binding sites in the blood, thereby enhancing the transport of mercury compounds to storage tissues or excreting organs.

Figure 38 shows that, after electrophoretic separation, the maximum radioactivity was detected in the albumin and γ-globulin fractions. This supports the previous results *in vitro* that the albumin and the γ-globulin fractions have great tendency to bind mercury.

We then studied the effect of mercuric chloride and phenylmercuric acetate for enzyme systems in blood. The blood enzymes chosen for study were (a) glutathione reductase, (b) phosphoglucose isomerase, (c) glucose-6-phosphate dehydrogenase, and (d) caeruloplasmin.

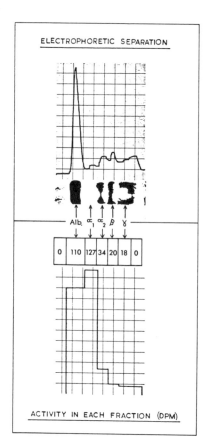

Figure 38: Radioactivity in Each Blood Fraction after Electrophoretic Separation

Mersalyl sodium was also injected in patients, and the enzymatic activities were compared with the preinjection levels.

Our *in vitro* work was designed so that the sample of normal human blood was divided into two portions, one of which was mixed with the mercuric compound and the other was used whole. The two portions were tested for the enzymatic activities.

(a) Glutathione reductase: Table 51

The glutathione reductase of sera from 11 healthy volunteers had a mean activity of 17 M.I.U. (Mean International Units). When activity was tested in serum mixed with $HgCl_2$ or PMA, in concentrations equivalent to 1.0 and 10 μg Hg per 100 ml respectively, there was 100% inhibition.

Table 51

The Effect of Mercuric Chloride (HgCl) and
Phenylmercuric Acetate (PMA) on Four Human Blood Enzymes

Enzyme	No. of Experiments	Basic Activity M.I.U.	With $HgCl_2$		With PMA	
			Activity M.I.U.	Inhibition %	Activity M.I.U.	Inhibition %
Glutathione reductase	11	17	zero	100	zero	100
Phosphoglucose isomerase	8	65	34	48	7	89
Glucose-6-phosphate dehydrogenase	5	1739	1635	6	1647	5.3
Caerulaplasmin*	6	191	183	4	173	9

*The activity is expressed as o.d. units.

(b) Phosphoglucose isomerase: Table 51

After the addition of mercuric chloride to serum, the percentage inhibition of phosphoglucose isomerase ranged from 24.1% to 75.6% with a mean of 48.3%. Using PMA, the inhibition was 63% to 100% with a mean of 89%. With both compounds, there were significant differences between the test and the control solutions at the 5% level.

(c) Glucose-6-phosphate dehydrogenase: Table 51

No difference was demonstrated between the activity of glucose-6-phosphate dehydrogenase of red blood cell hemolysate measured before and after the addition of $HgCl_2$ and PMA.

(d) Caeruloplasmin: Table 51
    $HgCl_2$ and PMA had no significant effect on serum
caeruloplasmin activity.

These results are in agreement with the findings of
Txuboi *et al.*[2] However, the findings that mercuric compounds had no significant effect on the glucose-6-phosphate
dehydrogenase and caeruloplasmin activities are contrary to
that of Curzon[3] and of King.[4] It is possible that the
inhibition observed by the previous authors was due to
their use of higher concentrations of mercury compounds.
By contrast, in this study only concentrations likely to
be present in human blood under ordinary conditions of
occupational exposure were used.

In the course of one *in vivo* study, therapeutic doses
of 10% mersalyl were injected into patients. Blood samples
were withdrawn before dosing, then 30 minutes and 24 hours
after the injection. Table 52 shows that the degree of

Table 52

Enzymic Activity Before and After Injection of Mersalyl

Enzyme	No. of Patients	Activity Before Injection M.I.U.	Activity M.I.U.	Inhibition %	Activity M.I.U.	Inhibition %
Glutathione reductase	2	16	5	72	13	19
Phosphoglucose isomerase	3	91	37	57	41	55
Glucose-6-phosphate dehydrogenase	2	1489	1473	1	1382	7
Caeruloplasmin*	2	265	250	6	245	8

*The activity is expressed as o.d. units.

inhibition of glutathione reductase was 72% at 30 minutes
after the injection and 19% after 24 hours.

In the case of serum phosphoglucose isomerase activity
(Table 52) there was significant inhibition of the enzymes

in each of the three cases. The mean inhibition after 30 minutes was 37%. After 24 hours, the mean inhibition was 55%.

No detectable inhibition of the enzyme activity was observed in the case of glucose-6-phosphate dehydrogenase or caeruloplasmin (Table 52).

It was of particular interest to compare the inhibition of glutathione reductase with that of phosphoglucose isomerase after the injection of mersalyl *in vivo* (Figure 39). The findings were: (1) There was a marked decrease

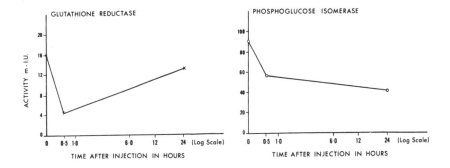

Figure 39: Percentage Activity of Glutathione Reductase and Phosphoglucose Isomerase 30 Minutes and 24 Hours After Musalyl Injection

in the activity of glutathione reductase 30 minutes after injection, possibly due to an interaction with the SH groups of this enzyme system. It is possible that the interaction is reversible, since the activity was restored to 80% of its initial level after 24 hours. On the other hand, there also exists the theoretical possibility that further synthesis in the body may provide more enzymic material. (2) The phosphoglucose isomerase was inhibited after 30 minutes, as was the glutathione reductase. However, there was a further decrease in the activity after 24 hours. The reaction would, therefore, appear to be irreversible. This finding may well account for the low serum values observed in the activity of the phosphoglucose isomerase in the blood of seed-dressers exposed to organo-mercurial fungicides, as we have previously reported.

Summary

Blood is of physiological importance as a "carrier" and "distributing" agent for various substances including metals within the body.

In the present investigations, the uptake of labelled mercuric compounds (^{203}Hg), mercuric chloride (HgCl$_2$), phenylmercuric acetate (PMA) and methylmercuric nitrate (MMN) by normal human blood was studied *in vitro*. The relative uptake by the erythrocytes as contrasted with the serum proteins was measured. The binding of the mercury compounds to the serum proteins was confirmed, using both dialysis and gel-filtration techniques. Electrophoretic separation of the mercuric compound and serum mixture was utilized to identify the protein fraction which binds each of the mercuric compounds *in vitro*.

In vivo inhibition of glutathione reductase, phosphoglucose isomerase, glucose-6-phosphate dehydrogenase and caeruloplasmin were unaffected by mercuric chloride, phenylmercuric acetate and mersalyl.

References

1. Linderstrom-Lang, K. and J. A. Schellman. "The Structure of Insulin as Compared to that of Strang's A-Chain," Biochim. Biophys. Acta, *15*, 156-157 (1954).
2. Txuboi, K. K., J. Estrada, and P. B. Hudson. "Enzymes of the Human Erythrocyte. VI. Phosphoglucose Isomerase, Purification and Properties," J. Biol. Chem., *231*, 19-29 (1958).
3. Curzon, G. "The Effect of some Ions and Chelating Agents on the Oxidase Activity of Ceruloplasmin," Biochem. J., *77*, 66-73 (1960).
4. King, J. Practical Clinical Enzymology (London: Van Nostrand Co., 1965), p. 70.

Biological Reactions and Pathological Changes in
Human Beings and Animals Caused by
Organic Mercury Contamination

Tadao Takeuchi

Organic mercury contamination may result from (1) mercury residue produced during manufacturing processes in
chemical plants (methyl mercury), (2) agricultural chemicals
used widely on the farm (methyl, ethyl, and phenyl mercury),
(3) erratic use of disinfectants and fungicides for medical
supplies (ethyl mercury) and clothes (phenyl mercury), and
(4) other unknown factors.

Among these factors, (1) and (2) are presently increasing,
especially that contamination due to the discharge of mercury
into the water from chemical manufacturing plants. Some of
these mercury compounds may enter the aquatic food chain.
They are then absorbed by river and seabottom vegetation or
plankton, which are in turn eaten by small fish and shellfish, which are then eaten by large fish. Thus the mercury
becomes concentrated in ever-greater amounts, at which point
it may reach human beings and domestic animals. Poisoning
may then take place, and an outbreak of illness may occur.
These eventualities have transpired with "Minamata disease,"
named for the place in Japan where the first mysterious
poisoning occurred. The second outbreak of this poisoning
occurred in Niigata, Japan. Much new knowledge was obtained
from the investigation of Minamata disease. I will try here
to summarize some of the biological effects of organic
mercury contamination.

Pollution of Water by Methyl Mercury

The mercury residue from manufacturing operations in
chemical plants has been thought in many instances to be
inorganic mercury. However, it was found by Irukayama *et
al.*[1] and Kitamura *et al.*[2] that methyl mercury is produced
in the process of manufacturing acetaldehyde from acetylene.
In the chemical plants studied, acetaldehyde was synthesized
by the hydrogenation of acetylene. In the reaction, mercuric oxide dissolved in sulfuric acid had been used as the
catalyst. In the process, methylmercuric chloride (MMC)
could be formed; this was the case in the mercury sludge
of the reaction tube of the acetaldehyde plant. It also
was experimentally shown in the laboratory that MMC was
formed in a mixture of acetaldehyde, mercuric oxide in

sulfuric acid, ferro- and ferrisulfates, manganese dioxide and sodium chloride under conditions similar to those occurring at the manufacturing plants. Furthermore, MMC can also be formed in a mixture of acetaldehyde, inorganic mercury and sodium chloride.

Methyl mercury was experimentally formed during the process of manufacturing vinyl chloride, which is produced from the reaction of acetylene with hydrogen chloride gas by using mercury chloride as a catalyst.[2] MMC was also found in a vinyl chloride plant in Minamata by Irukayama et al.[1]

In addition, methyl mercury compounds may also be synthesized from other operations using inorganic mercury and alcohol compounds.[2,3,4] Furthermore, Swedish investigators found that methyl mercury may be synthesized from inorganic mercury by some naturally occurring bacteria.[5]

In Minamata, it was thought that methyl mercury was produced mainly by the acetaldehyde manufacturing plant, and partly by the vinyl chloride manufacturing operation in the same factory. Effluent containing mercury from the acetaldehyde plant was discharged into the small bay of Minamata through iron scraps in an attempt to eliminate metal ions according to the ion exchange principle; however, this did not lead to the elimination of the organic mercury compound. This discharge continued from the years before 1953, when Minamata disease occurred, to September, 1958. Thereafter, the effluent was dumped into the mouth of the Minamata River outside the small bay of Minamata, until waste treatment equipment was completed in January, 1960. The effluent from the vinyl chloride manufacturing operation was also poured into the Minamata Bay until September, 1959.

In Niigata also, methyl mercury was presumably formed by the acetaldehyde plant of another firm, and it was poured into the Agano River until 1964, when the outbreak of disease occurred.

Outbreak of Minamata Disease Resulting from Mercury Contamination

From 1953 to 1956, when the production of acetaldehyde and vinyl compounds was rapidly increasing, the outbreak of a neurological disease occurred in Minamata. The same disease occurred in Niigata between 1964 and 1965, when the production of acetaldehyde increased (Figure 40).

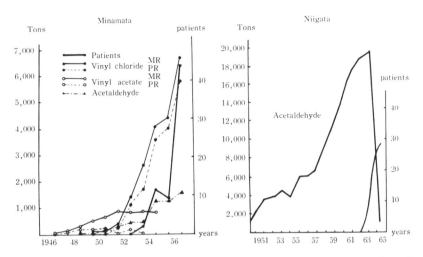

Figure 40: Production of Vinyl Compounds and Acetaldehyde, Compared with the Occurrence of Minamata Disease in the Early Stage

(a) Occurrence of the Disease in Humans

In Minamata, between 1953 and 1961, 88 cases of Minamata disease were recorded. Thereafter, 33 additional cases were discovered as a result of detailed clinical investigation. The total of 121 cases consisted of 68 cases in adults, 30 in children and 23 of so-called fetal Minamata disease (Figure 41). Classified by sex, 72 males and 49 females were affected. Out of these 121 cases, there were 46 deaths. About half of the adults, one-third of the children, and about one-eighth of the fetal patients died. The mortality seemed to be higher in adults than children, and lowest in the fetal cases. Of the adult deaths, 11 (one-sixth of total adult cases) were acute and subacute deaths; that is, the patients died less than a year after clinical onset of the disease (Table 53).

In Niigata, 30 cases, including 5 deaths, were reported in 1965.[7,8] Thereafter, 17 cases, including one death and one fetal case, were reported from 1966 to 1970.

In both places, the disease broke out mainly among fishermen and their families, and also among other people who fished frequently or liked to eat fish and shellfish.[9] Characteristically, the patients in Minamata as well as in Niigata had eaten a great amount of fish and shellfish that had contained a considerable amount of mercury, from 1 ppm to 50 ppm in some organs on a wet weight basis. In fetal

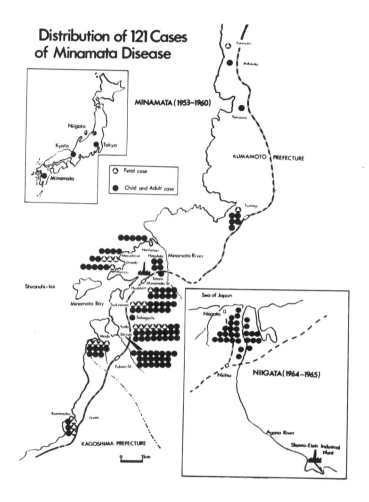

Figure 41: Distribution of 121 Cases of Minamata Disease
in Minamata and in Niigata

cases, all of the mothers had eaten a large amount of seafoods and river fish. This provided evidence that alkyl
mercury penetrates the placental barrier in humans.[10-13]

Table 53

Annual Distribution of the Patients of Postnatal
and Prenatal Minamata Disease

Year	Postnatal Adults Patients	(Death)	Postnatal Children Patients	(Death)	Prenatal Patients	(Death)	Total Patients	(Death)
1953			1				1	
1954	7	(3)	5	(2)			12	(5)
1955	8	(2)	2	(1)	5		15	(3)
1956	24	(7)	21	(3)	8		53	(10)
1957	2	(1)		(1)	6		8	(2)
1958	4	(4)		(1)	2		6	(5)
1959	19	(5)	1	(2)	2		22	(7)
1960	4	(2)					4	(2)
1961						(1)		(1)
1962		(1)				(1)		(2)
1963								
1964		(1)						(1)
1965		(3)						(3)
1966~70		(4)				(1)		(5)
Total	68	(33)	30	(10)	23	(3)	121	(46)

(b) Incidence Among Animals

In 1953, about one year before the outbreak of the disease in human beings, cats in the contaminated areas died after developing nervous symptoms such as ataxic gait, abnormal movement and convulsion. According to Nagano *et al.*,[14] 48 of 123 cats died from this illness. Kitamura *et al.*[15] reported that forty families affected with Minamata disease had 61 cats, of which 50 (82%) died between 1953 and 1956. Of 60 cats belonging to 68 unaffected families in the same area, 24 (40%) died during the same period.

On the basis of these results, cats which had the opportunity to eat fish were most likely to be affected with this disease. Therefore, cats were most frequently used in our experimental investigations.

Other domestic animals also manifested the disease.[16,17] Dogs, pigs and sea birds that ate seafood were frequently affected. However, domestic fowls in the same area were less sensitive to the causative agent in seafood. Herbivores such as rabbits, horses, and cows in the same area were not affected.[15]

Crabs, fish, and shellfish also were affected and died of mercury contamination.[13,18] In 1959, when the causative agent of the disease was found to be an organic mercury,[6,19,20] the mud of Minamata Bay contained an extremely large amount of mercury. The maximum concentration (133 ppm to 2010 ppm) was found near the drainage channels from the chemical plants. A sharp drop in the concentration was observed near the mouth of the small bay (12.2 ppm to 22.2 ppm) and there were only slight deposits outside the bay (0.25 ppm to 3 ppm). The bottom mud of the Shiranui Sea outside the bay also contained mercury from 0.06 ppm to 0.55 ppm.

Shellfish such as *Hormomya mutabilis* (Gould), which were used for experimental induction of the disease in animals, contained mercury from 11.4 ppm to 39.0 ppm wet weight in the bay, and from 2.4 ppm to 20.4 ppm outside the bay. It was noted that mercury contained in the sea water became concentrated in shellfish because the mercury content in the mud was much lower than the content in the shellfish.

Clinical Symptoms and Biological Reactions of
Minamata Disease

(a) Humans

Clinical symptoms of this disease were reported by Katsuki *et al.*,[21] Nagano *et al.*,[14] Tokuomi,[22,23] McAlpine and Araki,[9] Kurland *et al.*,[24] and Harada;[10] Tokuomi *et al.*

made detailed observations of adult cases, while Harada *et
al.* studied infant cases exclusively--including fetal. Of
the various nervous symptoms they described, Takeuchi *et
al.*[6,20] pointed out that, from a pathological point of
view, the three main symptoms were cerebellar ataxia, con-
triction of visual fields, and dysarthria. These had been
described by Pentschew[25] as the Hunter-Russell Syndrome.
At present, it may be reasonable to add to those major
symptoms others resulting from lesions of the cerebral
cortex and peripheral nerves, particularly the sensory
peripheral nerves of extremities.

The onset of illness was acute or subacute, and usually
unattended by fever. In all the adults observed in detail
(34 cases),[23] numbness developed in the extremities (100%)
and frequently around the mouth, often accompanied or followed by slurred speech (88.2%) unsteady gait (82.4%), and
increasing disability. Most of the patients complained of
deafness (85.3%), and concentric constriction of visual
fields (100%). Cerebellar ataxia and dysarthria were
always present (100%). Tremor was frequently observed
(75.8%), distal hypaesthesia and disturbances of super-
ficial and deep sensations were always noticed (100%), and
choreiform (14.7%), athetotic movements (8.8%), and ballism
(14.7%) were sometimes noted in severe cases. The deep
reflexes were exaggerated in some cases (38.2%) and de-
pressed in a few cases (8.8%). An extensor plantar response
was noted twice. Muscular rigidity was infrequently found
(20.6%), and increased salivation and sweating were seldom
noted (23.5%). Epileptiform attacks occurred in one adult,
though more frequently these were seen in infants. Slight
mental disturbance was noted frequently (70.5%), and sometimes a more severe mental disorder was observed.

Among the children observed in detail (18 cases),[10]
mental disturbance, ataxia, and impairment of the gait were
manifested in every case (100%). Speech disturbance was
noted in 17 cases (94%), and deafness (67%), dysphagia
(89%), and exaggerated reflex (72%) were found frequently.
Pathological reflex (50%), involuntary movement of the
limbs (39%), and forced laughing (28%) were sometimes observed. Increased salivation occurred frequently (55.6%),
and convulsions were noticed occasionally.

In infants with fetal disease, disturbances in mental
and motoric development were noted in all cases, being
accompanied with impairment in gait, disturbance of speech,
and impairment in chewing or swallowing (100%). However,
difficulty in hearing was present only in 4.5%, and blindness was absent. Visual fields and acuity as well as

hearing acuity could not be examined in infants. Over-
activity of the tendon reflex (81.7%), primitive reflexes
(72.7%), pathological reflexes (54.5%), involuntary movement (72.7%), and increased salivation (77.2%) were often
observed. Convulsions also occurred more often than in
the cases of the older children.

Table 54 illustrates the differences in clinical

Table 54

Frequency of Occurrence of Various Symptoms and
Signs in Minamata Disease (%)

Symptoms	*Fetal*	*Children*	*Adults*
Mental disturbance	100	100	71
Ataxia	100	100	94
Impairment of the gait	100	100	82
Disturbance in speech	100	94	88
Hearing impairment	4.5?	67	85
Constriction of visual fields		100?	100
Disturbance in chewing and swallowing	100	89	94
Brisk and increased tendon reflex	82	72	34
Pathological reflex	54	50	12
Involuntary movement	73	40	27∿76
Primitive reflex	73	0	0
Impairment of superficial sensation	?	?	100
Salivation	72	56	24
Forced laughing	27	29	

symptoms among the adults, the children and the infants
with fetal cases. These differences might result from
differences in the pathological lesions stemming from
different biological reactions for methyl mercury in the
adult, child, and fetus.[13]

In Minamata disease observed in Niigata, the same nervous symptoms were observed by Tsubaki *et al.*,[7,8] who
pointed out joint pain (in 72% of the cases) as the only
symptom not observed in Minamata. Also, the other symptoms
were relatively less severe than in Minamata. There were

no other general symptoms characteristic of Minamata disease, although slight or moderate anemia was observed in some cases in the early stage.

The course of the disease fluctuated, and its results were variable. The most severely affected died, while others remained incapacitated in varying degrees. Improvement in the hospital was occasionally followed by relapse on returning home. After a long period of time, some symptoms improved, but the main symptoms are still present after approximately 15 years.

Laboratory examination: Mercury excretion in urine varied according to the lapse of time after onset of the disease. The cases examined within five months after the onset revealed a markedly high excretion, amounting to 40-116.3 µg per day, in contrast to values of less than 16 µg per day in controls. In those cases observed more than one year after the onset of disease, excretion of mercury was generally below 30 µg per day. A 2- to 4-fold increase of mercury in urine occurred with administration of EDTA-Ca or BAL which was not so effective for improvement of the symptoms as penicillamine. Mercury in the hair increased exceedingly after the onset of the disease, ranging from 30 ppm to 570 ppm.

The cerebrospinal fluid was normal. There were no specific changes in liver function tests and electrolytes in urine. Some adult patients, as well as infants, manifested abnormal EEG's during the course of the illness.

(b) Symptoms in Animals

Cats were most frequently affected spontaneously. Unsteady and slow movement, ataxic gait, and paroxysmal convulsions (Figure 42) were the usual three main symptoms in these animals.[13,17,26] Epileptiform convulsions occurred subsequently. Although this symptom was very rarely seen in human adults, it was always observed in the fetal and infantile Minamata disease of cats. Gait was frequently ataxic, particularly manifested by false steps while going down stairs. The rightening reflex on falling was disturbed in early stages of this disease. Dashing and circling around, standing on their heads, fits, tremors and other abnormal movements were occasionally seen. Blindness occurred occasionally. Cats had frequent attacks of paroxysmal convulsions with dilation of pupils and foamy salivation prior to death.

Crows (Figure 43) and sea birds in the Minamata bay area also fell ill, presenting such symptoms as unsteadiness, frequent falling and abnormal movement. Spastic paralysis was also identified in a crow.[17]

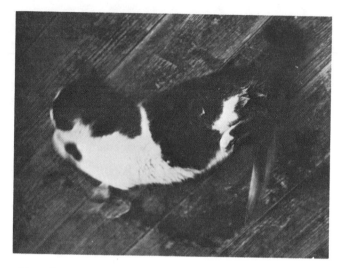

Figure 42: Paroxysmal Convulsion of Cat Affected with Minamata Disease

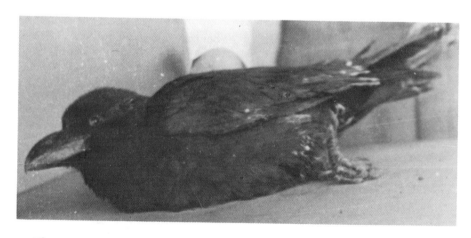

Figure 43: Crow Affected with Minamata Disease

Affected fish could easily be caught by hand. They died after emaciation with abnormal movements (Figure 44). Cataracts, which were never found in land animals, were very often observed in fish in the Minamata bay.[27]

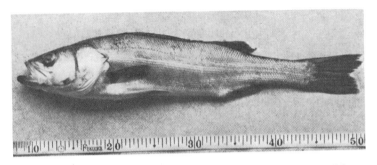

Figure 44: Emaciated Fish Affected with Minamata Disease

Rats fed contaminated fish and shellfish also suffered from the same disease.[27,28] Rats first showed a decrease in body weight, but there was neither loss of hair nor diarrhea. After 20 to 40 days of feeding, nervous symptoms appeared in the limbs, particularly in the hind legs. The movement of their limbs became slow, and they assumed a paretic posture. Strong flexion of limbs was usually observed (Figure 45) when the animals were held by the tail, while wide extension of limbs occurred then in control rats. Ataxic gait and clumsy climbing up a wire-net wall was noted. Occasionally, running in circles, tremor, and other abnormal movements appeared. Mice showed almost the same symptoms, and they occasionally could not hold millet seeds for feeding with their paws.[29]

Pathology of Minamata Disease

(a) Pathologic Changes in Humans

Autopsies were performed on 28 cases of Minamata disease. Twelve of these cases had died within 19 to 120 days after clinical onset of the disease (acute and subacute type); the remaining 16 cases had died between 1.4 and 13.7 years later (chronic type).[6,13,30-32] Two additional cases revealed a characteristic type of congenital infantile cerebral palsy, and were recognized at post-mortem examinations as instances of fetal Minamata disease.[11,12] Pathological findings of these cases were mainly identified in the nervous system.

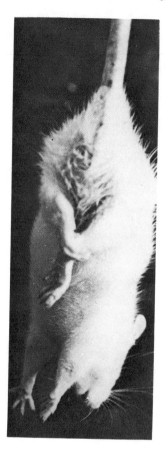

Figure 45: Rat Experimentally
Affected by Feeding with
Powder of Shellfish from
Minamata Bay

Macroscopic examination: In acute cases, the brain was
swollen and the pia arachnoid was slightly edematous and
turbid. In subacute and chronic cases, the leptomeninges
were slightly thickened and turbid or normal; atrophy of
the brain and compensatory increase in fluid volume was
noticed (*hydrops ex vacuo*). In chronic cases, there was
minimal symmetrical convolutional atrophy of the hemispheres, relatively more marked over both occipital lobes,
especially in both calcarine regions (Figure 46). In the
cerebellum, there was gross atrophy of the folia in both
lateral lobes and also in the vermis. On sections, considerable convolutional atrophy was generally observed.
It was particularly marked in the medial aspects of both
occipital lobes, mainly about the anterior ends of both
calcarine fissures. The normal cortical striation of

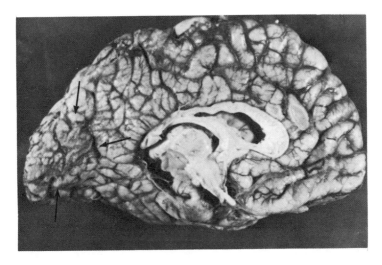

Figure 46: Atrophic Brain of Chronic Case (a Female Child
    Aged 8 Years). Intense Atrophy of Calcarine Cortex
    Noted.

Gennari was destroyed. Occasionally small foci of atrophy
were also found in the cortex of other convolutions such as
the pre- or postcentral and lateral convolutions.

In chronic cases, the ventricles were slightly dilated,
particularly in the occipital horns, while the sulci were
also slightly widened. In the prolonged chronic cases, the
white matter was also atrophied. The most conspicuously
severe cases revealed widespread destruction of cerebral
convolutions, in which the grey matter was colliquated and
absorbed, appearing as a sponge network; the cerebellum
was also extensively atrophied and its grey matter was
thin. In most cases, no severe macroscopic changes were
observed in the brain and spinal cord.

Microscopic examinations: The most conspicuous changes
were noted in the cerebellum and the calcarine cortex.

In the cerebellum, the disintegration following diffuse
loss of granular cells was most severe, while the Purkinje
cells were, in general, spared (so-called granular cell
type of cerebellar atrophy). In severe cases, both cell
types entirely disappeared, being accompanied with proliferation of Bergmann's glial cells in the Purkinje cell layer.
In these cases, the first disappearance of granular cells
occurred diffusely under the Purkinje cell layer and then
spread out over all the granular cell layer. The slight
loss of granular cells under the Purkinje cell layer, as

well as the slight "thinning out" or decrease of neurons in the calcarine cortex, were often observed in the latent patients who had not been diagnosed as having Minamata disease during their lifetime (Figure 47). The molecular

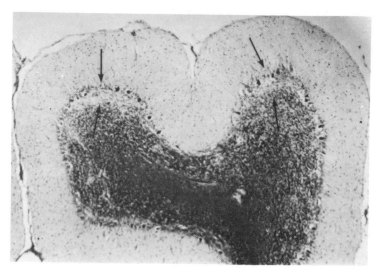

Figure 47: Slight Loss of Granule Cells under the Purkinje Cell Layer and Slight Disappearance of Purkinje Cells in Cerebellum of Latent Minamata Disease

layer became narrow, and sometimes assumed the pseudolaminar appearance of gitter cells containing the myelin debris. The changes were most advanced in the depths of the sulci, particularly in the central regions (Figure 48). The cortex at the surface of the cerebellum was relatively normal, except for loss of the granular cells, which was usually rather slight. The slight loss of the granular cells under the Purkinje cell layer produced the "apical scar" appearing later after a prolonged clinical course. The white matter was atrophied, with accompanied diffuse demyelination being found only in the prolonged cases. In the dentate nuclei, degenerative atrophy of the nerve cells, without loss, was sometimes observed in chronic cases.

In all cases the cortex of the calcarine region (visual area) was most grossly disturbed in both the hemispheres. Disintegration and loss of neurons therein were generally striking (Figure 49) and most marked in the depths of the hemispheres, namely in the anterior regions of both visual

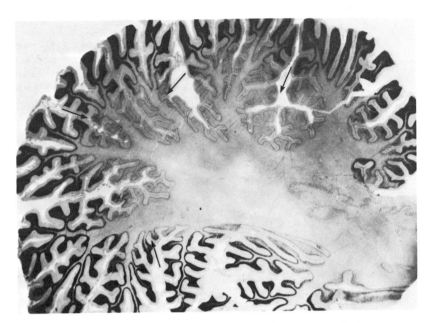

Figure 48: A Typical Disappearance of Granule Cells of
Central Type

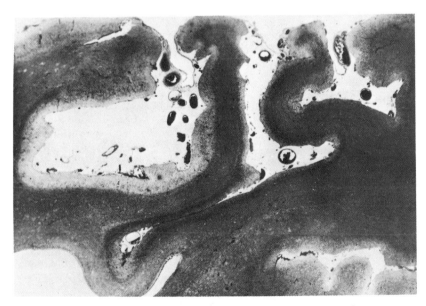

Figure 49: Intense Disturbance Following Loss of Neurons
in the Calcarine Cortex (in Chronic Case)

centers and also in the depths of sulci. These changes
caused concentric constriction of visual fields. In the
severe cases, the neurons in these portions almost always
disappeared entirely, forming a spongy matrix. In the
relatively less severe cases, the neurons were gradually
thinned out (Figure 50), and were accompanied by a slight
but diffuse proliferation of the glial cells.

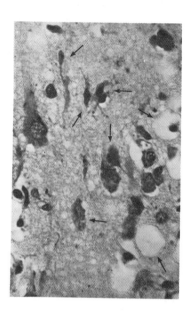

Figure 50: Disintegration
of Neurons During a
Process of Gradual
Disappearance of Nerve
Cells

   The loss of neurons varied considerably in different
fields of the other cerebral cortices. Conspicuous atrophy
of the other cortices, with loss of neurons, was seen
occasionally. The "thinning out" of neurons was observed
in general in various convolutions. In a very severe case,
loss of almost all cortical neurons was observed in the
occipital, parietal, temporal (except for insula and
hypocampi), and frontal lobes. In the prolonged cases,
the white matter was reduced and accompanied by degenerative
changes.
   In acute and subacute cases, acute swelling, hydropic
vacuolar degeneration, chromolysis, severe destruction and
necrosis of neurons were noted, with neuronophagia being
observed often. Small hemorrhages and perivascular edema
was generally seen in acute and subacute cases. As a rule,
cell infiltrations in the walls of blood vessels were not

observed, but a small number of round cells and phagocytes
containing brown pigment were occasionally observed in
subacute and chronic cases.

In cerebral nuclei, slight disintegration occurred occasionally. No marked changes were observed in brain stems.
No conspicuous changes were seen, except for occasional
slight hemorrhages, edema, and degeneration of neurons
without loss in acute and subacute cases. Symmetrical
demyelination of the pyramidal tracts was observed occasionally in chronic infantile cases, and was presumably
related to the severe disturbance in the precentral
cortices. After a prolonged clinical course, slight sys-
temic degeneration with demyelination sometimes appeared
in the posterior tracts of the spinal cord. This change
presumably resulted from disturbances of the sensory
peripheral nerves.

In the peripheral nerve, it was previously reported that
no gross changes were observed, except on rare occasions
when localized demyelination, mild perivascular cuffing
with macrophages containing pigmentary granules, and scar
formation were seen. The cranial nerve rootlets, including
the optic, acoustic, and other nerves were almost free of
lesions, with the exception of slight changes in some
cases.[33]

However, after detailed reinvestigation, the peripheral
sensory nerves were found to be considerably disturbed.
The destruction of nerve fibers with demyelination was
seen. These changes still remained after more than ten
years.[34] In the biopsy of the sural nerve containing only
sensory fibers,[35] disappearance of nerve fibers with
collagen proliferation, irregular size and irregular
arrangement of nerve fibers, irregular proliferation of
Schwann's cells, and macrophages containing pigments were
observed by light microscopy. The incidence of fibers
below 3 μ in diameter, which presumably were incompletely
regenerated, increased; by contrast, normal fibers had two
distributional peaks of 5 μ and 11 μ in diameter (Figure
51).

Upon examination by electron microscopy, the sural nerve
had scars with increasing amounts of collagen. There were
variable changes in nerve fibers which revealed irregular
and incomplete regeneration. Extremely small axons, irregular in size, were surrounded by incomplete myelin and
lamellar processes of the cytoplasm of Schwann's cells.
The latter were increased in number (Figure 52).

No conspicuous changes were demonstrated in the optic
nerves and retinas of eight cases examined by light

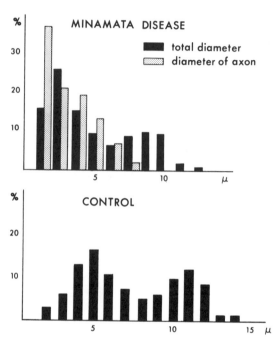

Figure 51: Decrease of Larger Fibers and Increase of
Smaller Fibers Following Degeneration and Regeneration
of Human Sural Nerve Observed in Chronic Minamata
Disease.

microscopy, in spite of the clinical observation of visual
disturbances.

Pathological features of other organs: In acute and
subacute cases, hypoplasia and aplasia in the bone marrow,
hypoplasia of lymph nodes, fatty degeneration of parenchymatous cells in the liver and kidney were found.
Erosion and catarrhal inflammation of mucous membranes of
the digestive tract, particularly in the duodenum, were
also found in some cases. Irregular spermatogenesis of
the testis occurred in some cases, but no changes were
seen in ovaries.

The remaining organs appeared normal, except for
generalized atrophic changes of the viscera in subacute
and chronic cases. Bone marrow activity remained reduced,
probably resulting from poor nutrition in chronic cases.

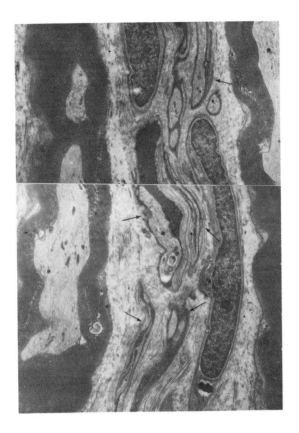

Figure 52: Irregularly Regenerated, Smaller Fibers with
Schwann's Cells Containing Dense Granules and Collagen
Proliferation

Except for a few cases, death was usually caused by an
accompanying illness such as aspiration pneumonia or acute
pneumonia. The pathological findings did not suggest that
the nervous disorders in the cortical regions of cerebrum
and cerebellum were sufficient by themselves to cause
death.

(b) Differences in Minamata Disease Among Adults, Infants,
and Fetal Cases
   From the pathological observations of human autopsy
cases and experimental results, it is presumed that the
essential changes in Minamata disease are expressions of

a toxic neuroencephalopathy, in which the nerve cells in the cerebral and cerebellar cortex are selectively involved, irrespective of age and sex. The toxic agent, methyl mercury, gives rise to the cortical disturbance, which may occur throughout the whole cortex in cerebrum and cerebellum, but is preferentially localized in the calcarine region and in the granular layer of the cerebellum. The distribution of the lesions is believed to be related to the intensity and amount of the toxic agent absorbed, and to the growth stage of the brain and individual condition of the patient.[13]

Fetal Minamata disease, in which the fetuses examined had become involved *in utero* in the sixth and eighth month of pregnancy (as manifested by maternal episodes), has two characteristic pathological features. One of these coincides with the neuropathological findings seen in nonfetal infantile Minamata disease. The other is related to the age (growth of the brain) at the time of fetal exposure, when the mother had eaten contaminated fish and shellfish. The latter change is represented by the hypoplastic and dysplastic changes in the central nervous systems, which are never seen in the nonfetal cases exposed after birth. Resting matrix cells at the ventricular wall, appearance of nerve cells in the cerebral medulla, columnar grouping of nerve cells in the cerebral cortex, abnormal cytoarchitecture of nerve cells in cerebral and cerebellar cortices, hypoplasia and dysplasia of nerve cells with poor myelination of nerve fibers, specific hypoplasia of the cerebellar cortex, and hypoplasia of the corpus callosum were observed. The disturbance of development in the cytoarchitecture of the brain suggests that the disease results from the poisoning during the fetal period (Table 55).[13]

Particularly in the fetus and infants, the neurons throughout the whole cortex of the brain tend to be involved by this toxin. The cortical lesions of the brain are distributed more widely and are more severe in the fetal form of the disease than in the infantile form. In the adult brain, there is a tendency for lesions to become more localized, particularly in the calcarine cortex and in the granular layer of the cerebellum. The small type of neuron is more readily involved than the large type of neuron such as Betz's cells, Purkinje cells, neurons of the nuclei, and other pyramidal nerve cells. Therefore, the neurons in the second to upper third or fourth layer in the cerebral cytoarchitecture tend to be attacked more frequently in this disease. The granular cells of the cerebellum also are frequently involved, being preferentially disintegrated in deep central regions of the hemispheres and vermis as well.

Table 55

Comparison of Pathology of Minamata Disease among
Fetal, Non-fetal, and Adult Cases

Pathological features	*Fetal infantile*	*Non-fetal infantile*	*Adult*
1. Cortical disturbance of cerebrum	+++	+++	+++
2. Cerebellar disturbance of granule cell type	+++	+++	+++
3. Central type of granule cell atrophy	+	++	++
4. Intense reduction of brain	+++	+++~++	+
5. Wide distribution of lesions	+++	+++	+
6. Preferential localization of lesions	±	++	+++
7. Degree of the granule cell disturbance	+	+++	+++
8. Hypoplastic changes of cytoarchitecture (a, b, c, d, e)*	+++	−	−
9. Malformation of neurons	+++	−	−

*a), b), c), d), and e) are included. a) Remaining matrix cells, b) Evidence of nerve cells in cerebral medulla, c) Abnormal cytoarchitecture (columnar block, etc.), d) Hypoplastic narrowing of granular layer in cerebellum, 3) Hypoplastic corpus callosum.

Both underdevelopment and regressive changes of the brain in fetal infantile Minamata disease produce a specific microcephalia in which the weight of the brain is reduced by two-thirds or one-half when compared with that of normal brains for the same age (Table 56).[13] On the other hand, the weight of the brain in the nonfetal infantile cases may also be decreased by two-thirds or one-half as the result of severe atrophic changes. Therefore, the differentiation between fetal and nonfetal Minamata disease must be based on the microscopic findings and the presence of the specific hypoplastic changes mentioned above.

In spite of severe underdevelopment, there were no malformations in the extremities or other parts of the

Table 56

Brain Weight in Minamata Disease and Comparison with Normal Brain Weights

| Average of brain weight in normal Japanese | | | Minamata disease | | | | Rate of atrophy |
Age	Sex	Brain weight (W) g	Age	Sex	Clinical course	Brain weight (W') g	($\frac{W'}{W}$ x 100)
1-2	F	1053	2.6	F	2.6 yrs.	650*	38
3-5	F	1175	4	F	1.6 yrs.	700	40
			5		26 days	950	19
6-9	F	1250	6.3	F	6.3 yrs.	630*	50
			8		2.9 yrs.	890	29
	M	1303	7	M	4.0 yrs.	600	54
20-29	F	1318	28	F	2.9 yrs.	1250	5
			29		53 days	1150	13
30-39	M	1450	34	M	19 days	1200	17
			34		96 days	1150	21

40-49	M	1426	47	M	45 days	1300	9
			49		86 days	1320	7
50-59	F	1250	50	F	90 days	1200	4
			58		60 days	1050	16
	M	1417	52	M	100 days	1430	0
			56		48 days	1290	9
			57		1.4 yrs.	1050	26
			59		93 days	1250	12
60-more	M	1400	60	M	2.0 yrs.	1170	16
			61		76 days	1410	0
			66		10.2 yrs.	1300	7
			78		9.9 yrs.	1000	29
			79		4.3 yrs.	1230	12

*Fetal Minamata Disease.

body, except for abnormal dentition, in the two autopsy cases or in the other 21 patients. In general disturbances of nerve cells in early fetal life may give rise to mal-formations of the extremities and body. Therefore, the hypoplastic and dysplastic changes in the brain in fetal Minamata disease suggest that the causative agent did not disturb the primitive immature nerve cells in the early period of gestation. The nerve cells were probably affected after considerable differentiation had occurred, during the intermediate or later period of fetal life.

Actually, in Case #1 the patient presumably had been affected in the eighth month of fetal life, when the mother complained of numbness of the fingers and the father suf-fered from typical Minamata disease. The patient in Case #2 had been involved in the sixth month of fetal life when the brother fell ill with Minamata disease, despite the fact that the mother showed no symptoms. Takeuchi's work[13] has shown that the signs of this disease appear about one month after the first effective exposure to the causative agent. Therefore, it can be suggested that these patients were exposed as fetuses about one month before the clinical onset of disease in parents or siblings. The pathological findings observed in two cases of "congenital cerebral palsy" represented the offered conclusive evidence of the fetal type of Minamata disease.

The pathological findings on human beings can reasonably explain why clinical signs varied in adults, infants, and fetal cases.

(c) Pathological Changes in Animals

In cats affected with Minamata disease, loss of granular cells in the cerebellum was usually found (Figure 53),[17,28,36] particularly of the central type; there were the same various changes in neurons of cerebral cortex as in the human brain. As in humans, small hemorrhages, edema, and slight gliosis were found and were accompanied by perivascular cell infiltration more frequently than in humans.

Crows and sea birds which were affected revealed various changes in the nervous system, e.g., regressive changes following neuronophagia, loss of neurons with gliosis in the brain, and loss of granular cells in the cerebellum.[17] The ill fish were always emaciated and revealed lesions of nervous tissues, with loss of granular cells in the small brain. No conspicuous changes occurred in the retina of animals. Cataracts were occasionally observed, but only in fish.[27]

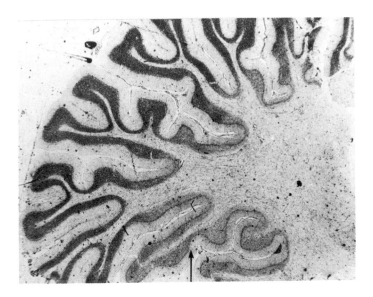

Figure 53: Loss of Granule Cells of Central Type in Cat
Affected with Minamata Disease

In rats affected with the experimentally induced
disease, loss of granular cells in the cerebellum and
disturbance of neurons in the cerebrum occurred.[19],[28]

Mercury Content in Organs of Human Beings and Animals Affected

(a) Mercury Content in Human Beings
The mercury content of human organs in autopsy cases
was investigated by the dithizone method. A large amount
of mercury was found in the liver, kidney, and brain in
acute and subacute cases;[6],[13] the ratio of mercury content
in the brain to that in the liver and kidney was higher,
showing a characteristic pattern of alkyl-mercury poisoning
(Table 57). Kurland *et al.*[24] pointed out that the ratio
of the percentage of mercury content in the brain to that
in the liver or kidney amounts to more than 20:1 in organic
mercury poisoning, and is less than 5:1 in inorganic mercury poisoning. During a three-month period it decreased
gradually. However, considerable amounts still were
demonstrated between 3 months and 1.5 years. Thereafter,
the second decrease occurred between 1.5 years and 2.5
years. After about three years, the mercury content

Table 57

Mercury Content in Organs of Human Autopsy Cases of Minamata Disease

Number of Autopsy	Sex	Age	Clinical course (days)	Liver (ppm)	Kidney (ppm)	Brain (ppm)	Brain/Liver x 100 (%)	Brain/Kidney x 100 (%)
1 3159	M	35	19	70.5	144.0	9.6	13.6	6.7
2 2774	F	5	26	38.2	47.5	15.4	40.3	32.4
3 3350	M	48	45	38.8	68.2	24.8	63.9	36.7
4 2791	M	56	48	34.6	99.0	7.8	22.5	7.9
5 2776	F	29	53	39.5	40.5	9.0	22.7	22.1
6 3201	F	58	60	42.1	106.0	21.3	50.6	20.1
7 3349	M	62	70	34.7	64.2	7.8	22.5	12.1
8 2775	M	49	86	/	/	9.5	/	/
9 3209	F	50	90	36.2	21.2	4.9	13.4	22.9
10 3388	M	59	90	32.6	49.8	6.4	19.5	12.8
11 3355	M	34	96	30.0	22.6	4.6	15.3	20.4
12 3290	M	52	100	22.0	42.0	22.6	11.8	6.2
13 3497	M	57	480	21.3	36.5	2.8	20.2	14.0
14 3018	F	4.5	553	26.0	37.4	5.3		
15 3216	F	8	993	6.4	12.8	1.3		
16 3139	F	28	1000	2.1	3.1	0.1		
17 3298	M	7	1467	5.4	5.9	2.2		
18 3567	F	2.6	*	0.3	9.4	0.4		
19 3764	F	6.4	*(years)	5.7	11.3	0.7		
20 3732	M	60	2.0	8.3	19.6	1.0		
21 4292	M	79	4.3	2.0	17.6	2.0		
22 4473	M	78	9.9	35.0	12.6	3.0		
23 4312	M	66	10.2	2.3	21.6	0		
24 4951	M	63	11.3	0.97	10.70	2.64		
25 5360	F	68	11.7	0.14	/	0.14		
26 5539	M	14	*	0.16	5.47	0.04		
Control (15 cases)				0-2	0-3	0-0.5		

*Fetal Minamata disease

decreased considerably, but it did not revert completely
to normal (Figure 54).[13]

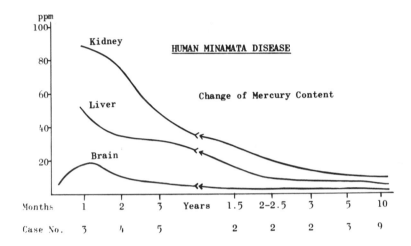

Figure 54: Change of Mercury Content in Organs during
Human Minamata Disease

Alkyl mercurials, for example, methyl mercury, were
deposited more abundantly in the parenchymatous organs
such as kidney and liver than in the brain. However, in
spite of smaller amounts of mercury in the brain, its toxic
effect on the nerve cells appeared to be most striking and
severe, while even large amounts of mercury left the
parenchymatous cells of liver, kidneys and other organs
mysteriously unaffected with the disease. Obviously, it
appears reasonable to assume that there are variations in
sensitivity to methyl mercury among different cells of the
body. It is very well established that the central nervous
system is the most sensitive organ to alkyl mercury exposure.
However, according to our examinations, bone marrow and
testes also are critical organs, as described below.

Mercury in the organs was also demonstrated histo-
chemically.[37-39] In the brain, mercury was deposited in
nerve cells as well as in glial cells, seemingly in the
lysosomes, particularly when investigated in the subacute
and chronic cases. It was abundantly demonstrated in liver
cells and Kupffer cells, as well as in the epithelium of
the convoluted tubules of the kidney.

(b) Mercury Content Among Animals

A large amount of mercury was found in the kidney, liver, and brain of cats affected with Minamata disease, and also among cats fed fish and shellfish contaminated in the Minamata area (Table 58).[6]

Table 58

Mercury Content (ppm wet weight)* in Organs of Cats
Affected with Minamata Disease and of
Control Cats in 1959

Cat No.	Minamata disease			Control		
	Liver	Kidney	Brain	Liver	Kidney	Brain
1	54.0	30.0		0.6	0.7	
2	37.0	17.2		3.7	0.5	
3	58.5			3.0		
4	101.1			1.2	0.8	0.1
5	54.5	12.2	8.1	1.3	0.1	0.1
6	68.0		10.4	1.6	0.3	0.1
7	66.0			1.6	0.6	0.1
8	105.6			0.7	0.3	0.1
9	145.5		18.1	1.3	0.2	0
10	53.5		8.1	0.6	0.3	0
11	78.3	12.8		1.7		
12	57.5	36.1		2.7		
13	63.0		18.6	6.6	0.1	0
14	47.6	15.6	10.0			
15	52.5	15.9	9.1			

*Mercury content was estimated by the dithizone method.

In an experiment with rats (Irukayama),[40] methyl mercury gradually increased in the liver, kidney, brain, and hair during oral administration of 0.8–1.6 mg/kg/day for 28 days. The methyl mercury began to accumulate in the early phase of administration in the liver and kidney, increasing gradually, while the deposition in the brain occurred slowly and to a lesser extent because of the blood-brain barrier. After cessation of administration, mercury gradually decreased in the liver and kidneys, but decreased more slowly in the brain. By contrast, mercury appeared very slowly in hair

after the administration, and increased in a step-wise
fashion, until it reached its maximum on the 25th day after
administration ceased.

After the oral administration of methyl mercury compounds, mercury was absorbed and deposited in every organ.
It was deposited abundantly in the liver, kidneys, and
hair, moderately in the stomach, intestine, muscles, heart,
bone marrow, spleen, pancreas, adrenals, lungs, testes,
and brain, and slightly in the trachea, etc.

*Study of Various Mercury Compounds Administered in
Order to Produce Similar Symptoms and
Pathological Findings as Minamata Disease*

The clinical and pathological features of Minamata
disease in animals were experimentally compared with those
of organic mercury poisoning (Table 59), using various
species of animals (especially cats and rats) in which
typical Minamata disease was produced by feeding contaminated fish and shellfish as well as methyl mercury.

Organo-mercuric compounds may disturb the nervous
system, in contrast to inorganic mercury, which tends to
injure parenchymatous visceral organs. However, different
kinds of organic mercury seem to give rise to changes of a
different pattern and degree of nervous system involvement.
From our investigations,[13,36,41,42] intoxication by alkyl
mercury compounds like R-Hg- (R: methyl), R'-Hg- (R':
ethyl), and R-Hg-S- (S: sulfide) compounds usually result
in severe injury to the nervous system, especially to the
brain cortex. These show a characteristic pattern of
cerebral and cerebellar pathomorphological changes with
corresponding signs. Compounds like R-Hg-R, R'-Hg-R',
R-Hg-S-R and R'-Hg-S-R' can also produce similar changes.
The sulfide compounds are less toxic than the other
compounds.

The complicated alkyl mercury compounds (R-Hg-X-)
binding cystein, gluthatione, thiourea, etc. are less
toxic than the simple alkyl mercury substances. They do
not always produce the same changes in the brain.

According to Sebe *et al.*[43] brain damage produced by
alkyl mercurials increased when the alkyl group contained
fewer carbon atoms. Methyl and ethyl mercury were more
toxic to the nervous system than propyl and butyl mercury.

The pathological changes resulting from the chloride,
phosphate, iodide, sulfide, and hydroxide of the same alkyl
mercury seem to be essentially the same, except for individual difference in animals, and differences due to the

Table 59

Organo-Mercury Compounds Used in the Experiments

Research year	Names (Mercury compounds)		Chemical formula
Takeuchi et al. 1958	Diethyl mercury		$C_2H_5-Hg-C_2H_5$
1959	Ethylmercuric chloride	a	$C_2H_5-Hg-Cl$
1959	Bis-ethylmercuric	a	$C_2H_5-Hg-S-Hg-C_2H_5$
1959	Diethylmercuric phosphate	a	$(C_2H_5Hg)_2=HPO_4$
1959	S-ethylmercurithiourea hydrobromide	a	$C_2H_5-Hg-D-V-(NH)$ $-NH_2-HBr$
1959	Mercuric ethylmercaptide	a	$C_2H_5-S-Hg-S-C_2H_5$
1959	Phenylmercuric acetate	a	$C_6H_5-Hg-S-C_2H_5$
1962	Methyl methylmercuric sulfide	c	$CH_3-Hg-S-CH_3$
1962	Bis-methylmercuric sulfide	b	$CH_3-Hg-S-Hg-CH_3$
1962	Methylmercuric chloride	b	$CH_3-Hg-Cl$
Tokuomi et al. 1959	Diethylmercuric phosphate		$(C_2H_5-Hg)_2=HPO_4$
1962	Bis-methylmercuric sulfide	b	$CH_3-Hg-S-Hg-CH_3$
1962	Methylmercuric iodide	b	CH_3-Hg-I
1962	Methylmercuric chloride	b	$CH_3-Hg-Cl$
1962	Ethylmercuric iodide	b	C_2H_5-Hg-I
1962	Methyl methylmercuric sulfide	c	$CH_3-Hg-S-CH_3$
Irukayama et al. 1960	Marsonin		$C_2H_5-Hg-S-C_6H_4$ $-CO_2Na$
1962	Dimethyl mercury	b	$CH_3-Hg-CH_3$
1962	Methylmercuric chloride	b	$CH_3-Hg-Cl$
1962	Methylmercuric iodide	b	CH_3-Hg-I
1962	Bis-methylmercuric sulfide	b	$CH_3-Hg-S-Hg-CH_3$
1962	S-methylmercuric cystein	b	$CH_3-Hg-SCH_2-CH$ $-(NH_2)-COOH$
1962	S-methylmercuric gluthatione	b	$CH_3-Hg-S-CH_2CH$ $-CO-NH-CH-COOH$ $NH-CO-(CH_2)_2CH(NH_2)$ $-COOH$
1963	Methylmercuric hydroxide	b	$CH_3-Hg-OH$
1963	Methyl methylmercuric sulfide	b	$CH_3-Hg-S-CH_3$

a = Synthesized by Prof. Kaku
b = Synthesized in Irukayama's Lab.
c = Uchida's substance

dose of mercury given. However, it was stated by Takeuchi *et al.*,[13] on the basis of pathological studies, that alkyl mercury sulfides most frequently cause characteristic changes similar to those of Minamata disease. On the other hand, Irukayama[40] maintained that there are no differences among poisonings with these substances, on the basis of his toxicological studies.

Poisoning with mercaptide, i.e., with the R-S-Hg-formula, is essentially different from those seen after R-Hg-S-poisoning. The former did not produce changes similar to Minamata disease in our experiments.

Aryl mercury compounds (phenyl-Hg-) are less injurious to the nervous system than alkyl mercury compounds. The nervous system is free from cerebral and cerebellar lesions. Occasionally, however, lesions in the brain may appear with these poisons, according to the electron microscopic observations by Koya.[43]

Quantity of Alkylmercuric Compounds Necessary to Produce Poisoning Similar to Minamata Disease

Since our experiments clarified the role of alkyl mercury compounds (such as methyl or ethyl mercury compounds) in the development of clinical and pathological features similar to Minamata disease, there remains no doubt that Minamata disease is due to poisoning with methyl mercury. This agent has also been extracted as methylmercuric sulfide (CH_3HgSCH_3) from shellfish in Minamata Bay by Uchida,[44,45] and as methylmercuric chloride by Irukayama *et al.*[1,40,46] from slag in the chemical plant.

It is very important for prophylatic treatment that the amount of mercury the human body and animals can tolerate be known. According to our studies,[13,47] oral methylmercuric sulfide can produce Minamata disease in cats after about one month at a dose of 1.5-2.0 mg/kg body weight per day (totalling 20.6-25.7 mg/kg for two or three weeks in one cat). Rats show the disease after 2-3 weeks at a daily dose of 5-10 mg/kg body weight daily (totalling 100-200 mg per kg body weight). According to Irukayama *et al.*,[40] methyl-mercuric chloride can produce the disease in cats at a dose of 0.8-1.6 mg/kg body weight daily (totalling 8.0-56.0 mg/kg body weight). The dosages for other methyl mercury compounds are similar (Table 60).

These amounts of organo-mercurials listed agree remarkably well with the total amounts of mercury contained in shellfish sufficient to produce the experimental Minamata disease.

Table 60

Amounts of Organo-Mercury Compounds Necessary to
Produce Poisonings Similar to Minamata Disease

		Organomercury			Cat/kg	Rat/100g
Takeuchi *et al.* (1958–1962)	Shellfish	Hormomya mutabilis		g	200 ∿ 600	120 ∿ 250
		Hg-amount	Total	mg	20 ∿ 60	12 ∿ 25
			Daily	mg	1 ∿ 3	0.5 ∿ 1
		$CH_3-Hg-S-CH_3$	Total	mg	20.6 ∿ 25.7	10 ∿ 20
			Daily	mg	1.5 ∿ 1.8	0.5 ∿ 1
		$CH_3-Hg-S-Hg-CH_3$	Total	mg	20.6 ∿ 34.1	10 ∿ 20
			Daily	mg	1.2 ∿ 2.0	0.5 ∿ 1
		$(C_2H_5Hg)_2=S$	Total	mg	43.1 ∿ 56.0	15 ∿ 25
			Daily	mg	2.6 ∿ 3.2	1 ∿ 1.5
		Hg-amount in fish (20ppm)		mg	50	9.4
Irukayama *et al.* (1962–1963)		$CH_3-Hg-Cl$	Total	mg	8.0 ∿ 56.0	5.5 ∿ 13.5
			Daily	mg	0.8 ∿ 1.6	1.0 ∿ 2.0
		CH_3-Hg-I	Total	mg	14.0 ∿ 25.2	
			Daily	mg	0.6 ∿ 1.4	

The amount of methyl mercury compounds necessary to
produce Minamata disease in human beings is unknown.
Extrapolating from the cat experiments, a person with a
body weight of 50 kg would have to ingest 0.7–1.0 g of
organic mercury over a certain period to become ill. However, as fishermen and their families used to eat about
200 g of fish containing about 20 ppm wet weight mercury,
they ingested about 120 mg of alkyl mercury per person
during a month. This amount is less than the experimental
dose. Therefore, the sensitivity of human beings to alkyl
mercury is presumably higher than cats, which in turn is
higher than rats. Imai[45] of the Tokyo University Medical
School reported a case in which a 13-year-old boy showed a
nervous illness with the typical Hunter-Russell's syndrome.
Because of an intense hypoproteinemia, he was treated for
one month with 8000 ml of stock human serum, containing
0.01% ethylmercuric thiosalicylic acid (totalling 0.8 g of

organic mercury) as a disinfectant. The resulting mercury
loading seemed to be between 0.1 and 1.0 gram. If one-tenth
of this dose could be dangerous to human beings, 2 mg per
kg body weight (i.e. 2 ppm) may be tolerated in human beings.
As the fetus seems to be about four times more sensitive
than the postnatal cases, according to Irukayama, 0.5 mg/kg
body weight (0.5 ppm) should be a tolerated dose.

Biological Reaction of Tissue Cells to Alkyl Mercury

Alkyl mercury compounds, e.g., methyl mercury, are lipid-
soluble and may penetrate the blood-brain barrier as well
as the placental barrier. It can be transported (about 90%
with erythrocytes) in blood to all of the organs.[48,49]
However, injury of tissue cells by alkyl mercury does not
occur in any organ, except for the nervous system. Why
only the nervous tissue should be injured is unknown. As
SH-containing enzymes are present in various organs, the
mechanism of poisoning can be explained only by blocks of
these important enzymes. Some metabolic event must occur
only in neurons in order for methyl mercury to produce the
injury discussed previously. According to the histochemical
investigation by Koya,[41] mitochondrial enzymes of nerve
cells were not disturbed in the early stage of administration of methyl mercury. Phosphorylase activity of granular
cells disappeared rapidly. Free ribosomes in granular cells
also disappeared rapidly after the administration of methylmercuric sulfide.[50,51] The chromatin of nuclei of granular
cells tended to be destroyed in the early stage after the
administration. As incorporation of cytidine-^{3}H into the
granular cells of the cerebellum was rapid, metabolism of
RNA seems to be remarkable in normal granular cells. Incorporation of cytidine-^{3}H into RNA-synthesis was disturbed
by methyl mercury (Otsuka).[52]
These results indicate what happens to the intracellular
metabolism of granular cells in the cerebellum after the
administration of the methyl mercury. However, it is still
unknown which metabolic process of the neurons may be
disturbed by methyl mercury.
Umeda *et al.*[53] demonstrated that methyl mercury inhibits
cell division of cultured Hela cells. In this case, the
inhibition mechanism was very similar to the effect of
colcemide.
Ascites hepatoma AH 13 cell growth was inhibited by
methylmercuric chloride, particularly by concentrations
over 10^{-7}M (Figure 55). In this study there were increases

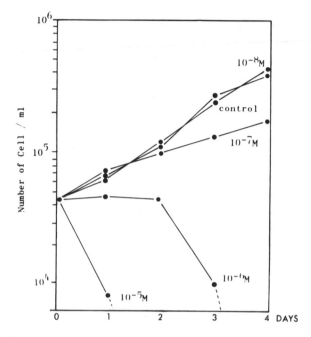

Figure 55: Effect of Methylmercuric Chloride on Cell
   Growth of AH 13 *in vitro*

is abnormal mitosis, irregular cells, and polynuclear cells.
DNA-synthesis in nuclei of AH 13 cells was also disturbed
(Otsuka),[52] and incorporation of thymidine-^{3}H into nuclei
of AH 13 cells was inhibited by more than 10^{-6}M concentrations of methylmercuric chloride (Table 61). The incorporation of cytidine-^{3}H in nucleoli and cytoplasms of AH
13 cells was also disturbed (Table 62).
     Spermatogenesis in experimental rats was inhibited by
the administration of methylmercuric chloride (Sakai and
Takeuchi);[54] incorporation of thymidine-^{3}H into
spermatogonia was decreased conspicuously (Table 63).

Congenital Effects of Methyl Mercury

     On the basis of the results seen in human Minamata
disease, methyl mercury is a fetotoxic substance. This
position is taken since fetal Minamata disease, which was
expressed by the clinical sign of a congenital cerebral
palsy, was caused by the effect of the toxin after the
formation of the placenta in pregnancy. There were no

Table 61

Frequency Distribution of Silver Grains by ^{3}H-Thymidine
Incorporation over Nuclei of AH 13 Cells after
Administration of Methylmercuric Chloride
(MMC) for 24 Hours*

Grains	Control	$10^{-7}M$ MMC	$5X10^{-7}M$ MMC	$10^{-6}M$ MMC
0	58	63	130	180
1- 20	14	13	8	10
21- 41	12	12	5	2
41- 60	10	11	5	3
61- 80	16	11	6	1
81-100	20	15	8	2
101-120	25	15	9	1
121-140	23	22	10	1
141-160	12	28	8	0
161-180	13	17	7	0
181-200	3	3	5	0
201-220	2	0	1	0
grains/ labeled cell	106	115	108	43

*data taken 6 hrs after ^{3}H-thymidine administration

Table 62

Frequency Distribution of Silver Grains by ^{3}H-cytidine
Incorporation in Nucleoli and Cytoplasms of AH 13 Cells
After Administration of Methylmercuric Chloride
(MMC) for 24 Hours*

Grains	Control	$10^{-7}M$ MMC	$5\ 10^{-7}M$ MMC	$10^{-6}M$ MMC
0	24	56	76	82
1- 40	50	82	86	93
41- 80	38	32	22	15
81-120	38	19	11	8
121-160	21	8	5	2
161-200	16	2	0	0
201-240	10	0	0	0
241-280	3	0	0	0
grains/ labeled cell	90.0	48.2	39.0	32.5

*data taken 2 hrs after ^{3}H-cytidine administration

Table 63

Distribution of Silver Grains by ^{3}H-thymidine Incorporation
over Nuclei of Rat Spermatogonia after the Administration
of Methylmercuric Chloride (125 mg for 16 days)*

Distribution	Control	CH_3HgCl Expt. No. 9	CH_3HgCl Expt. No. 10
Number of non-labeled tubes	31	30	43
Number of labeleled tubes	69	70	57
Number of labeled cells	652	309	200
Number of grains			
1-2	97	84	35
3-4	254	104	93
5-6	202	78	48
7-8	49	28	13
9-10	28	11	8
11-12	6	4	3
13-	16	0	0
grains/labeled cell	4.78	4.22	4.34

*data taken 4 hrs after a ^{3}H-thymidine injection

true malformations in prenatal Minamata disease. Embryotoxic
effects which may give rise to malformations of the newborn
were not observed in the Minamata area. The frequency of
miscarriages was not found to have increased in this area.

However, the experimental administration of contaminated
fish and shellfish, or of methyl and ethyl mercury compounds,
frequently produced miscarriages among rats and cats.[55,56]
In these experiments, no malformations of the extremities
or bodies were observed. Fetal Minamata disease could be
induced by the experimental administration of the agent to
animals, but no embryotoxic effects were found. The fact
that spermatogenesis was inhibited by Minamata disease in
human beings and by the experimental administration of the
toxin may result in decrease of fertility, although there
are no data to confirm this possibility.

When methylmercuric chloride is fed to domestic fowl,
it appears in the eggs, mainly in the white. When inorganic
mercury is administered, it is mainly deposited in the

yolk.[57] Eggs contaminated with the organic mercury were
less successfully hatched. The contaminated developing
embryos died in 85% of the cases during incubation, while
only 15% of control embryos died. The hatching time was
also prolonged to 22 to 23 days. However, the newborn
looked relatively normal, except for a decrease in body
weight. No malformations were found. Only slight disturbances in gait were noted in some cases. Pathological
changes of the neurons in the brain were occasionally
observed.[58]

The question of genetic effects of alkyl mercury still
remains unanswered.

Summary

On the basis of investigations on Minamata disease
induced by organic mercury contamination, the biological
reactions and pathological changes were discussed. It was
found that alkyl mercury, particularly methyl mercury compounds, which may contaminate the environment, are absorbed
in organisms, accumulated in various organs and tissues,
and can give rise directly or indirectly to various disturbances of human beings and animals.

References

1. Irukayama, K., S. Tajima, and M. Fujiki. "Studies on
   the Origin of the Causative Agent of Minamata Disease
   (VIII). On the Formation of Methyl Mercury Compounds in
   an Acetaldehyde Plant - Methyl Mercury Compounds Formed
   from the Reaction of Acetaldehyde and Inorganic Mercury
   Compounds," Jap. J. Hygiene, *22*, 392-400 (1967) Japanese
   edition.
2. Kitamura, S., K. Hayakawa, K. Sumino, and K. Sebe.
   "Accessory Reaction in Acetylene Hydrolytic Reaction
   (I) Formation of Methyl Mercury," Folia Pharmacol.
   Japon., *63*, 228-243 (1967) Japanese edition.
3. Kitamura, S., K. Sebe, K. Hayakawa, and K. Sumino.
   "Formation of Alkylmercury Compounds from Acetylene,"
   Folia Pharmacol. Japon., *64*, 531-543 (1968) Japanese
   edition.
4. Sebe, E., and Y. Itsuno. "Organic Mercury Compounds
   and Minamata Disease," Nisshin-Igaku, *49*, 607-631 (1962)
   Japanese edition.
5. Jensen, S. and A. Jernelöv. "Biological Methylation of
   Mercury in Aquatic Organisms," Nature, *223*, 753-754
   (1969).

6. Takeuchi, T., N. Morikawa, H. Matsumoto, and Y. Shiraishi. "A Pathological Study of Minamata Disease in Japan," Acta Neuropath. (London), 2, 40-57 (1962).
7. Tsubaki, T. and K. Kondo. "Outbreak of Organic Mercury Poisoning in Niigata City. Second Minamata Disease?" Rodo - Eisei, 6, 627-631 (1965) Japanese edition.
8. Tsubaki, T. "Organic Mercury Poisoning Around the River Agano. A Study in Niigata University," Clin. Neurology, 8, 511-520 (1968) Japanese edition.
9a. McAlpine, D. and S. Araki. "An Unusual Neurological Disorder Caused by Contaminated Fish," Lancet 1958 II, 629-631 (1958).
9b. McAlpine, D. and S. Araki. "Late Effects of an Unusual Neurological Disorder Caused by Contaminated Fish," A. U. A. Arch. Neurol., 1, 522-530 (1959).
10. Harada, Y. "Infantile Minamata Disease," and "Congenital Minamata Disease," in Minamata Disease (Shuhan Co., 1968) pp. 73-117.
11. Matsumoto, H., G. Koya, and T. Takeuchi. "Fetal Minamata Disease. A Neuropathological Study of Two Cases of Intrauterine Intoxication by a Methyl Mercury Compound," J. Neuropath. Exper. Neurol., 24, 563-574 (1965).
12. Takeuchi, T., H. Matsumoto, and G. Koya. "A Pathological Study on the Fetal Minamata Disease, Diagnosed Clinically So-Called Infantile Cerebral Palsy," Advances in Neurol. Sci., 8, 867-883 (1964) Japanese edition.
13. Takeuchi, T. "Pathology of Minamata Disease," and "Experiments with Organic Mercury, Particularly with Methyl Mercury Compounds; Similarities Between Experimental Poisoning and Minamata Disease," in Minamata Disease (Shuhan Co., 1968), pp. 141-252.
14a. Nagano, S. et al. "Pediatrical Observation of Encephalopathy from Unknown Cause in Minamata District of Kyushu, Japan," J. Kumamoto Med. Soc., 31 (Suppl. 1), 10-22 (1957) Japanese edition.
14b. Nagano, S. et al. "Studies on Encephalopathy from Unknown Cause in Minamata District (II). General Checkup of Children in That Area and on the Statistical Survey Together with Specific Examination," J. Kumamoto Med. Soc., 31 (Suppl. 2), 243-250 (1957) Japanese edition.
15. Kitamura, S. et al. "Epidemiological Studies on Encephalopathy from Unknown Cause in Minamata District of Kyushu, Japan," J. Kumamoto Med. Soc., 31 (Suppl. 1), 1-9 (1957) Japanese edition.

16. Takeuchi, T., H. Matsumoto, T. Fujii, and H. Ito. "Pathological Studies of Cats Affected Spontaneously by Minamata Disease," J. Kumamoto Med. Soc., *31* (Suppl. 2), 268-275 (1957) Japanese edition.

17. Takeuchi, T., N. Morikawa, H. Matsumoto, and E. Higashi. "On Minamata Disease of Crows and Other Birds," J. Kumamoto Med. Soc., *31* (Suppl. 2), 276-281 (1957) Japanese edition.

18. Kitamura, S. "Mercury Poisoning from the Fish," J. Jap. Med. Ass., *57*, 488-498 (1967) Japanese edition.

19. Takeuchi, T. "Causative Pathogenesis of Minamata Disease," Medicine (Tokyo), *18*, 323-334 (1961) Japanese edition.

20. Takeuchi, T. *et al.* "Pathological Observation of Minamata Disease, Especially on the Cause of this Disease," J. Kumamoto Med. Soc., *34* (Suppl. 3), 521-530 (1960) Japanese edition.

21. Katsuki, S., H. Tokuomi, *et al.* "Clinical Observation on Encephalopathy from Unknown Cause in Minamata District of Kyushu, Japan," J. Kumamoto Med. Soc., *31* (Suppl. 1), 23-36 (1957) Japanese edition.

22. Tokuomi, H. "Minamata Disease (Symposium). Clinical Observation and Pathologic Physiology," Psychiat. Neurol. Jap., *62*, 1816-1850 (1960) Japanese edition.

23. Tokuomi, H. "Clinical Investigation of Minamata Disease," in Minamata Disease (Shuhan Co., 1968), pp. 38-72.

24. Kurland, L. T., N. F. Stanley and H. Siedler. "Minamata Disease. The Outbreak of a Neurologic Disorder in Minamata, Japan, and Its Relationship to the Ingestion of Seafood Contaminated by Mercuric Compounds," Neurology (Minneap.), *1*, 370-395 (1959).

25. Pentschew, A. "Quecksilbervergiftung," Handbuch d. Spez. Path. Anat. u. Histol. XIII/2, Teil B, 2007-2023 (1958).

26. Ito, H. "Experimental Formation of Minamata Disease in Cats Fed by Fish and Shellfish, Captured in Minamata Bay," J. Kumamoto Med. Soc., *31* (Suppl. 2), 282-289 (1957) Japanese edition.

27. Takeuchi, T., Y. Shiraishi, Y. Hirata, and M. Sasaki. "Pathological Studies of the Fish Captured in the Minamata Bay," J. Kumamoto Med. Soc., *34* (Suppl. 3), 542-547 (1960) Japanese edition.

28. Shiraishi, Y. *et al.* "On the Pathological Findings of Cats and Mice Fed on Shellfish, Captured in Minamata Bay," J. Kumamoto Med. Soc., *33* (Suppl. 3), 642-652 (1959) Japanese edition.

29. Takeuchi, T., N. Morikawa, and T. Fujii. "Experimental Production of Minamata Disease in Mice Fed by Fish and Shellfish, Captured in Minamata Bay," J. Kumamoto Med. Soc., *31* (Suppl. 2), 290-298 (1957) Japanese edition.

30. Takeuchi, T. *et al.* "Pathological Studies of the Encephalopathia from Unknown Cause in Minamata District of Kyushu, Japan," J. Kumamoto Med. Soc., *31* (Suppl. 1), 37-47 (1957) Japanese edition.

31. Takeuchi, T. *et al.* "Two Autopsy Cases of the 'Minamata Disease' in Subacute Course," J. Kumamoto Med. Soc., *33* (Suppl. 3), 609-613 (1959) Japanese edition.

32. Takeuchi, T. *et al.* "Histopathological Study on the Four Autopsy Cases of the 'Minamata Disease' in Chronic Course," J. Kumamoto Med. Soc., *33* (Suppl. 3), 614-641 (1959) Japanese edition.

33. Matsumoto, H., G. Koya, and T. Takeuchi. "Pathological Finding of Peripheral Nerves in Minamata Disease," Advances in Neurol. Sci., *8*, 70-71 (1964) Japanese edition.

34. Takeuchi, T., H. Matsumoto, K. Eto, H. Kojima, and H. Miyayama. "Minamata Disease Following Ten Years and Its Pathological Changes," Nihon Iji Shinpo, *2402* 22-27 (1970) Japanese edition.

35. Eto, K. and T. Takeuchi. "Pathological Changes of Peripheral Nerves in Human Minamata Disease; An Electron Microscopic Observation," Advances in Neurol. Sci., *15*, 606-618 (1971) Japanese edition.

36. Takeuchi, T. and N. Morikawa. "Minamata Disease (Symposium). Pathological Studies on Minamata Disease," Psychiat. Neurol. Jap., 1850-1886 (1960) Japanese edition.

37a. Matsumoto, H., Y. Otsuka, Y. Ieiri, and T. Takeuchi. "A Pathological Study of Long Affected Minamata Disease, Especially on the Secondary Degenerative Changes in the Brain," Advances in Neurol. Sci., *10*, 729-736 (1966) Japanese edition.

37b. Matsumoto, H., T. Kameda, and T. Takeuchi. "Pathological Studies on Organic Mercury Poisoning. Supplement to Histochemical Demonstration of Mercury in the Brain of Minamata Disease," Advances in Neurol. Sci., *13*, 270-278 (1969) Japanese edition.

38. Oyake, Y., M. Tanaka, H. Kubo, and M. Chichibu. "Neuropathological Studies on Organic Mercury Intoxication, with Special Reference to Distribution of Mercury Granules," Advances in Neurol. Sci., *10*, 744-750 (1966) Japanese edition.

39. Shiraishi, Y. "An Experimental Study of Minamata Disease, Especially on the Histochemical Demonstration of Mercury in the Tissues," J. Kumamoto Med. Soc., *37*, 361-392 (1963) Japanese edition.

40. Irukayama, K., T. Kondo, F. Kai, M. Fujiki, and M. Hashiguchi. "The Chemical Properties of the Organic Mercury Compound in the Fish and Shellfish from Minamata Bay and the Discussion on the Causative Agent of Minamata Disease," Jap. J. Hygiene, *19*, 246-260 (1964) Japanese edition.

41. Koya, G. "Experimental Study of Minamata Disease, Especially on Intoxication of Methyl Mercury Sulfide Compounds in Cats," J. Kumamoto Med. Soc., *38*, 100-139 (1964) Japanese edition.

42. Morikawa, N. "Pathological Studies on Organic Mercury Poisoning (I). Experimental Organic Mercury Poisoning in Cats and Its Relation to the Causative Agent of Minamata Disease," Kumamoto Med. J., *14*, 71-86 (1961).

43. Sebe, E. and Y. Itsuno. "Organic Mercury Compounds and Minamata Disease," Nisshin-Igaku, *49*, 607-631 (1962) Japanese edition.

44. Uchida, M., K. Hirakawa, and T. Inoue. "Biochemical Studies on Minamata Disease (IV). Isolation and Chemical Identification of the Mercury Compound in the Toxic Shellfish with Special Reference to the Causal Agent of the Disease," Kumamoto Med. J., *14*, 181-187 (1961).

45. Uchida, M. "Biochemical Study of Minamata Disease," Biochemistry, *35*, 430-439 (1963) Japanese edition.

46. Irukayama, K., S. Ushikusa, S. Tajima, H. Nakamura, S. Kuwahara, A. Omori, and T. Tsutae. "Studies on the Origin of the Causative Agent of Minamata Disease (IX). Transition of the Pollution of Minamata Bay and Its Neighbourhood," Jap. J. Hygiene, *22*, 416-423 (1967) Japanese edition.

47. Takeuchi, T. *et al.* "Experimental Study on Etiology of Minamata Disease, Especially on Pathological Investigation of Methylmercuric Sulfide Poisoning in Rats and Cats," J. Kumamoto Med. Soc., *36*, 713-735 (1962) Japanese edition.

48. Berlin, M. "Risk of Methyl Mercury Cumulation in Man With Reference to Consumption of Fish Contaminated with Methyl Mercury," J. Jap. Med. Ass., *61*, 1047-1050 (1969).

49. Ukita, T. "Mercury Compounds Deposited in Hairs and Erythrocytes," J. Jap. Med. Ass., *61*, 1039-1046 (1969) Japanese edition.

50. Miyakawa, T. and M. Deshimaru. "Electron Microscopical Study of Experimentally Induced Poisoning Due to Organic Mercury Compound - Mechanism of Development of a Morbid Change," Acta Neuropath. (Berl.), *14*, 126-136 (1969).
51. Miyakawa, T. *et al.* "Experimental Organic Mercury Poisoning - Pathological Changes in Peripheral Nerves," Acta Neuropath. (Berl.), *15*, 45-55 (1970).
52. Otsuka, Y. *et al.* Personal communication (1970).
53. Umeda, M., K. Saito, K. Hirose, and M. Saito. "Cytotoxic Effect of Inorganic, Phenyl, and Alkyl Mercuric Compounds on Hela Cells," Jap. J. Exp. Med., *39*, 47-58 (1969).
54. Sakai, K. and T. Takeuchi. Personal communication (1970).
55. Matsumoto, H., G. Koya, and T. Takeuchi. "Pathological Studies of Fetal Minamata Disease (II). Effect of Organic Mercury on the Fetus in Rat Pregnancy," Transact. Soc. Path. Jap., *54*, 187-188 (1965).
56. Morikawa, N. "II. Experimental Production of Congenital Cerebellar Atrophy by Bisethyl Mercuric Sulfide in Cats," Kumamoto Med. J., *14*, 87-93 (1961).
57. Kuahara, S. "Toxity of Mercurials, Especially Methyl Mercury Compound in Chick Embryo," J. Kumamoto Med. Soc., *44*, 81-103 (1970) Japanese edition.
58. Kojima, H. Personal communication (1970).

Other Reference Material

Hunter, D., R. R. Bomford, and D. S. Russel. "Poisoning by Methyl Mercury Compounds," Quart. J. Med., *9*, 193-219 (1940).
Hunter, D., and D. S. Russell. "Focal Cerebral and Cerebellar Atrophy in a Human Subject Due to Organic Mercury Compounds," J. Neurol. Neurosurg. Psychiat., *17*, 235-241 (1954).
Irukayama, K., M. Fujiki, F. Kai, and T. Kondo. "Industrial Wastes Containing Mercury Compounds from Minamata Factory," Jap. J. Hygiene, *16*, 476-481 (1962) Japanese edition.
Irukayama, K., M. Fujiki, S. Tajima, S. Omori, H. Nakamura, and S. Kuwahara. "Mercury Pollution in Minamata District Before and After the Suspension of the Production of Acetaldehyde in Minamata Factory," J. Kumamoto Med. Soc., *43*, 946-957 (1969) Japanese edition.

Itsuno, Y. "Toxicologic Studies on Organic Mercury Compounds," in Minamata Disease (Shuhan Co., 1968), pp. 267-288.

Kosaka, T. and Y. Takizawa. "Investigation into Cause of Outbreak of Organic Mercury Poisoning in District Along River Agano (II). Poisonous Methyl Mercury Compound in Fishes From River Agano," J. Niigata Med. Soc., *81*, 41-48 (1967) Japanese edition.

Lofroth, G. "Hazard of Mercury Compounds Poured into Nature," (Translated into Japanese by Uyi), Science, *39*, 592-666 (1969) Japanese edition.

Matsumoto, H. "Neuropathological Study of Minamata Disease," J. Kumamoto Med. Soc., *35*, 1133-1169 (1961) Japanese edition.

Matsumoto, H. *et al.* "A Histopathological Study of the Brain of Cats Poisoned with Methyl Mercuric Compounds," J. Kumamoto Med. Soc., *40*, 1016-1022 (1966) Japanese edition.

Nomura, S. "Epidemiology of Minamata Disease," in Minamata Disease (Shuhan Co., 1968), pp. 5-35.

Shiraishi, Y. "Histochemical Demonstration of Mercury in Tissues From Individuals Poisoned with Organic and Inorganic Mercury Compounds," Proc. Jap. Histochem. Ass., *2*, 168-171 (1961).

Takeuchi, T., T. Kambara, N. Morikawa, and H. Matsumoto. "Pathological Studies on Minamata Disease, Especially on Histopathological Findings of Nerve Cells in Human Brain," J. Kumamoto Med. Soc., *31*, (Suppl. 2), 262-267 (1959) Japanese edition.

Takeuchi, T., *et al.* "Pathological Studies on Encephalopathia From Unknown Cause in Minamata District of Kumamoto Prefecture (So-Called Minamata Disease) in Japan," Acta Path. Jap., *7* (Suppl.) 607-611 (1957).

Takeuchi, T., *et al.* "Pathological Observation of Minamata Disease," Acta Path. Jap., *9* (Suppl.) 769-783 (1959).

Takeuchi, T. "Etiology of Minamata Disease - Causative Pathogenesis of this Disease (Symposium)," Jap. J. Hygiene, *16*, 72-73 (1961) Japanese edition.

Takeuchi, T. and H. Matsumoto. "Pathological Study of Bone Marrow in Minamata Disease," Acta Haem. Jap., *24*, 253 (1961) Japanese edition.

Takeuchi, T., *et al.* "Experimental Formation of Cerebellar Disturbance by Alkyl Mercuric Poisoning," J. Kumamoto Med. Soc., *40*, 1003-1015 (1966) Japanese edition.

Takeuchi, T., T. Kameda, and Y. Yano. "On Latent Minamata Disease," Saikai Iho, *252*, 1-4 (1969) Japanese edition.

The Dose-Response Relationship Resulting From
Exposure to Alkyl Mercury Compounds

Bertram D. Dinman and Lawrence H. Hecker

Introduction

With a changing body burden of a foreign substance,
the manifestations of intoxication follow pharmacologically
predictable progressions. The severe signs and symptoms
resulting from high dose levels or large body loadings are
clearly definable; however, alterations of normal bodily
functions become progressively more obscure and nonspecific
as the dose decreases. Thus, any attempt to define an
association between low dose levels and minimal symptoms,
or to define the "no effect" dose level, becomes a difficult
exercise in judgment. To mitigate this difficulty it is
the usual practice to "build in" a safety factor, so that
the highest dose level unassociated with deleterious effect
is divided by a factor of 10 or 100. The choice of which
factor is to be applied is a function--among numerous other
considerations--of the severity of the effect produced by a
toxic substance, as well as feasibility. Further, our
ability to make judgments becomes clouded as we perceive
more subtle changes whose significance to human health and
well-being is unclear; such poorly understood changes all
too frequently represent a response to a low dose level,
e.g., chromosomal breaks, enzymatic alteration, etc.
Accordingly, the exercise which we have performed in
attempting to define body burdens associated with minimal
symptoms is subject to the foregoing reservations and
shortcomings.

Our review of the more readily available literature
has considered only human experience, since attempts to
extrapolate from animal data are frought with readily
apparent hazards stemming from interspecies metabolic differences and other inconsistencies. Further, though there
is a large body of data dealing with inorganic mercury
exposure, the differences between the metabolic dynamics
of alkyl mercury compounds and inorganic mercury compounds
renders questionable the use, for this study, of knowledge
derived from experiences with inorganic mercury. In addition, since urinary excretion patterns of mercury are
essentially unrelated to whole blood levels in alkyl
mercury loadings,[1] we have not attempted to use data presenting only urinary mercury concentrations to elucidate
the dose-response relationship.

As to the relationships (*v.i.*) between hair concentration and recent levels of mercury in whole blood, our review of available data cited here suggests that the range of associations follows a somewhat more consistent pattern. Accordingly, we have used population data presenting both blood and hair-borne concentrations in an attempt to define the dose-response relationship. Finally, we shall consider the high dose loadings of mercury associated with severe symptoms only to define the full range of the spectrum of human response.

Data concerning mono-alkyl mercury body loadings stem largely from occupational exposure to various compounds (usually in dusts and vapors) or from dietary intake. Work exposures largely assume pulmonary intake as well as percutaneous absorption; while the physical properties of vapors suggest ready uptake, the uptake characteristics of dusts both upon skin or the lung epithelia are less clear. Similarly, the ratio between intake and blood concentrations of alkyl mercury compounds absorbed via the gastrointestinal tract is not completely defined. Accordingly, such considerations must be understood as variables whose importance in our evaluation is not fully known.

Normal Range of Mercury Loading

The range of mercury concentrations expected in various populations might be predicted to vary as a function of diet characteristics and local variations in mercury content of soils--and hence also a function of waters, degree and nature of industrialization, and other poorly defined factors.

The reports utilized here are drawn from populations whose daily dose of mercury (approximately 10 µg per day or less) represents normal background levels; their diets are believed not to involve contaminated fish. Data which report blood concentrations are shown in Table 64, as to source of population, mercury intake, route of entry, concentrations in biological media, etc. Because in several cases concentrations are given in the blood corpuscles, we have utilized the formula suggested by Birke, *et al.*

Concentration in rbc = 185 x concentration in whole blood

in order to calculate whole blood mercury content.

In addition to 107 normal individuals whose blood mercury levels were reported, we had 796 other normals with hair values only. It should be noted that a number of investigations dealing with healthy persons report both

Table 64

Mercury in Blood and Hair: Populations Not Known to be Exposed to
Unusual Mercury Contamination

Reference No.	Analytical Method	Dose	n	Whole Blood μg/100 ml	Blood Corpuscles μg/100 ml	Blood Plasma μg/100 ml	Hair μg/g	Corpuscles: Plasma Ratio	Hair: Blood Ratio
				Direct Blood Values Available					Hair Data Only Available
2	NAA	10μg/d	4	0.57	0.76	0.30	1.35	2.7	254
17	Dithizone	10 μ/d	83	0.55[a]	1.01	0.23		4.4	
18	NAA?	?	3	2.8	5.1	0.97	2.3	5.3	81
16	NAA	~10 g/d	5	0.57[a]	1.05	0.30			
		n	5	0.72[b]	1.34	0.24			
1	NAA+ Mod-PMV	?	7	0.6–1.2		0.5–7.4			
4	Dithizone	?	16	0.72[b]			2.29		
				1.15[b]			1.5		
3	NAA	?	776	0.50[b]					
				0.75[c]			1.5		
Totals			899						

Means, utilizing whole blood values calculated from hair concentrations
On Basis of Hair:Blood = 300:1 X̄ = 0.52 g/100 ml blood
On Basis of Hair:Blood = 200:1 X̄ = 0.74 g/100 ml blood

a = calculated from corpuscular concentration
b = calculated from hair:blood ratio of 300:1 in terms of units in this table
c = calculated from hair:blood ratio of 200:1 in terms of units in this table

blood and hair values. These reports permit the calculation of whole blood levels, on the basis of hair to blood ratios. Such ratios appear to be consistently of the order of 200:1 to 300:1 within a range of ratios of 81 to 330:1. These ratios are absolute values which take into account differences in units of measurements for blood and hair.

We might thus extend our normal population by utilizing the data of Jervis, *et al.*[3] and Kitamura[4] with another 792 persons whose hair content for mercury was determined. In this population, the mean hair concentration was 1.5 and 2.29 µg/gm of hair respectively. Thus, using the ratio of hair to blood of 300:1, the whole blood concentration in the total population of 899 individuals should be approximately 0.52 µg/100 ml whole blood; using the 200:1 ratio, the normal value would approximate 0.74 µg/100 ml of whole blood.

It should be noted that qualitative variations exist in national diets and in analytical methods, as well as in the assumptions utilized to arrive at these concentrations, so that the values given represent approximations. Nevertheless, it would seem reasonable to suggest that the normal mercury level is probably between 0.5 µg and 1.0 µg/ 100 ml of whole blood.

Range of Blood Mercury Among Populations Known to Have Absorbed Mono-alkyl Mercury Compounds and Showing Signs and Symptoms of Alkyl Mercury Intoxication

The reports of the Minamata investigations,[2,5,6] the Alamogordo episodes,[3] and the Lundgren and Swensson report[7] provide us with the most pertinent data concerning whole blood mercury concentrations in fatal or severe cases of alkyl mercury poisoning (see Table 65). Though there are numerous other medical reports with varying degrees of completeness, these do not provide blood mercury data.

The data reported by Birke, *et al.*[2] utilizing the Niigata cases of Hoshino and co-workers[6] show a mean of 130 µg/100 ml of whole blood among those clearly affected by alkyl mercury intoxication due to ingestion of contaminated fish. Utilizing data reported by Kitamura,[4] among eight patients with fully-developed intoxication, hair samples taken in close temporal approximations to the onset of disease averaged 369 µg/gm of hair. Depending upon whether one uses a 300:1 or 200:1 hair to blood ratio, we would estimate approximate whole blood concentrations of between 123 µg and 184 µg/100 ml of whole blood. The hair of five individuals severely stricken in Alamagordo (Jervis, *et*

Table 65

Mercury in Whole Blood and Hair: Populations Known to Have Alkyl Mercury Poisoning

Ref. erence No.	Analytical Method	Dose	n	Whole Blood µg/100 ml	Blood Corpuscles µg/100 ml	Blood Plasma µg/100 ml	Hair µg/g	Corpuscles: Plasma Ratio	Hair: Blood Ratio	Comments
2,6	NAA	1650 g/d		130	240b		500		385	Minamata cases
4	Dithizone	5-6 ppm	8	96b			370			Minamata cases
3	NAA	LD50?		221b			877			Alamagordo cases
7	Dithizone	Occupa-tional	1	400						Occupational alkyl exposure

a = calculated on basis RBC Hg concentration = 1.85 x concentration in whole blood
b = calculated on basis of Birke-Hoshino Hair/Blood ratio = 385

al.[3]) would suggest blood concentration estimates of between 290 µg/100 ml (using a 300:1 ratio) and 440 µg/100 ml blood (using a 200:1 hair to blood ratio). In yet another fatal case of occupational alkyl mercury poisoning reported by Lundgren and Swensson,[7] the whole blood concentration of mercury was estimated to be 400 µg/100 ml blood.

Range of Whole Blood Concentrations Among Populations Known to Have Absorbed Mono-alkyl Mercury Compounds and Believed to be Healthy

Because of the fact that the Minamata and Niigata experience stemmed from ingestion of mercury-contaminated fish, much of the data to be discussed here is based upon pouplations exposed to fish believed to be qualitatively similarly contaminated. However, either because the fish in question were less heavily dosed or because they were less frequently ingested, such persons did not suffer mercury intoxication. The discussion to follow will consider accordingly subjects ingesting such contaminated fish.

Table 66 indicates that among 100 Scandinavian fish eaters there was a range of whole blood mercury concentrations from 3.14 to 12.5 µg/100 ml whole blood, without symptoms being detected. Ui's report,[8] which considered 27 French and Italian fishermen, indicated that all their mercury levels were less than 3 µg/100 ml regardless of whether one used the 200:1 or 300:1 hair to blood ratio. In contrast, an Indian fish-eating population of 37 in Canada[3] showed hair levels of mercury that were consistent with the Scandinavian population's blood levels, *i.e.*, 6.5 µg (300:1 hair to blood ratio) or 9.8 µg/100 ml whole blood (using a 200:1 hair to blood ratio). In all, this population of 164 persons whose blood mercury concentrations were approximately 12 µg/100 ml whole blood or less were all reported to be free of symptoms.

There are, unfortunately, few data points between these levels and the 60 to 100 µg/100 ml whole blood concentrations. Kitamura[4] noted that 19 individuals from Minamata who ate less fish than those poisoned had average mercury concentrations of 38 g/g of hair. This suggests a whole blood level of between 12.7 µg and 19.0 µg/100 ml of blood.

Other points in this 12 to 100 µg/100 ml blood range are based upon industrial exposure or direct alkyl mercury ingestion. Lundgren, Swensson and Ulfvarson reported nine workers with exposure to alkyl mercurials whose blood concentrations covered a range of 7.0 to 18.0 µg/100 ml

Table 66

Mercury in Blood and Hair: Populations Known to have Absorbed Methyl Mercury and Believed Healthy

Reference No.	Analytical Method	Dose	n	Whole Blood µg/100 ml	Blood Corpuscles µg/100 ml	Blood Plasma µg/100 ml	Hair µg/g	Corpuscles: Plasma Ratio	Hair: Blood Ratio	Comments
9	Dithizone	0.3-2.6 ppm	4	1.29-1.94b			3.88			French fish-eaters
9	Dithizone	0.5-5.0 ppm	23	1.72-2.58b			5.15			Italian fish-eaters
19	Dithizone	44µg/d	51	3.14b	5.8	0.75	7.9	7.7	252	Swedish fish-eaters
20	NAA	~50µg/d	21	3.22a	5.96	0.72		8.3		Swedish fish-eaters
3	NAA	?	37	6.55-9.83b			19.65			Canadian Indian fish-eaters
1	NAA+ Mod.-PVM	?	9	7-18		0.3-1.0				Occupational exposure
17	NAA?	1-5 ppm	20	10.0a	19.6	2.9	17.3	7.0	164	Finnish fish-eaters

2	NAA	15–815 µg/d	8	12.5	20.3	3.2	37.4	8	330	Swedish fish-eaters
4	Dithizone	?	19	12.7–19.0[b]			38.0			Minamata normals – ate less fish
3	NAA	Panogen ingested	1	40–60[b]			120			

Total cases = 193

a = calculated from blood corpuscle value
b = calculated on hair/blood ratio of 200:1 and 300:1

Other points in this 12 to 100 µg/100 ml blood range
are based upon industrial exposure or direct alkyl mercury
ingestion. Lundgren, Swensson and Ulfvarson[1] reported
nine workers with exposure to alkyl mercurials whose
blood concentrations covered a range of 7.0 to 18.0 µg/100
ml whole blood. According to these investigators, the
workers were asymptomatic. Finally, Jervis, *et al.*[3] reported one case of an individual believed to have ingested
an alkyl mercury compound whose hair concentration was
120 µg/g. Using our conversion rates, this suggests a
blood concentration of between 40 and 60 µg/100 ml whole
blood; Jervis notes that this person showed no signs of
alkyl mercury intoxication.

In summary, it would appear that alkyl mercury levels
of up to 100 µg/100 ml of blood are clearly not associated
with readily detectable deleterious effects, that levels
between 10 and 20 µg/100 ml may also not produce disease,
and that perhaps levels as high as 40 to 60 µg/100 ml
whole blood might be similarly so considered. However,
one is in no position to act on the basis of these conclusions without further consideration of the problems of
detection of low dose level effects.

Problems in the Detection of Minimal Alkyl Mercury Intoxication

A listing of the progression of signs and symptoms of
alkyl mercury intoxication immediately suggests the problem
of diagnosing <u>early</u> <u>reversible</u> alkyl mercury poisoning
(Table 67).

As one reviews the literature which deals with populations at risk of developing alkyl mercury poisoning, one
frequently finds the comment that persons "... had no
visible symptoms ..." or "... were apparently healthy ..."
or "... no health effects were noted...."   Considering
the commonplace, nonspecific nature of the minimal symptoms
(Table 67), it should be apparent that only the most painstaking clinical and epidemiologic investigation might define
such slight health effects, given a sufficiently large
population at risk. The stage wherein paraesthesia of the
extremities occurs still appears to be reversible,[9,10] yet
definition of this subjective occurrence is difficult. By
the time "finger ataxia" occurs, the patient is in a gray
area as regards recovery; however, it is possible that this
symptom is susceptible to objective demonstration by use
of newer electromyographical methods.

Table 67

Progression of Alkyl Mercury Intoxication

Prognostic Zone	*Reversible*	*Possibly Reversible*	*Ir-reversible*	*Fatal*
	Fatigue	Blurred vision	Finger ataxia[20]	Involuntary mobilization
	Headache	Tingling of fingers	Loss of motor con-	Blindness
	Inability to con-		trol: hands,	Emotional
	centrate	Numbness of fingers[9]	locomotion, speech	and mental deteriora-
	Memory			tion
	impaired	Finger ataxia[10]	Sensory defects:	Loss of
			auditory,	conscious-
		Emotional irritability	visual field	ness

The point to be emphasized is that if we are to develop safety parameters, it will be necessary for populations under study to be investigated systematically and intensively so as to establish more definitively the presence or absence of the earliest stages of alkyl mercury intoxication. A model for such a study is offered by the report of Smith and co-workers.[11]

This recommendation does not imply criticism of previous investigations. It is designed to warn our political and social institutions that if society's safety is to be ob-tained, careful, intensive studies must be supported, in a fashion consistent with the considerable investment of time and resources required to define minimal changes in a rea-sonably large population. It would seem that such approaches would be needed to fill the gap of information concerning effects between the 20 μg/100 ml and 60 to 100 μg/100 ml whole blood mercury level.

When one considers the effects of alkyl mercury loading, the other caveat relates to the even more subtle biological changes that may occur. I refer to the possibility of genetic effect through the action of methyl mercury upon chromosomal material. Methyl mercury compounds caused c-micotic effects about 1000 times more potent than colchicine in plant roots. There was associated chromosomal breakage, polyploidy, and aneuploidy at levels as low as 0.040 μg/g.[13] Treatment at rather high dose levels (0.25-5 mg methylmercuric chloride/liter) have produced exceptional offspring among Drosophila Melanogaster.[14] Skerfving, according to Jernelöv,[15] has reported that studies among human populations exposed to low doses of alkyl mercurials have suggested an increased incidence of chromosomal breaks as compared to a group of normals.

Further, the experience of the Minamata group has clearly indicated the ease with which mercury accumulates within the fetus. There has also been confirmation in animals that alkyl mercury loadings insufficient to cause toxicity among adults result in significant effects upon the fetus.[16]

Accordingly, if we attempt to define a "no effect" dose level for the whole spectrum of the total population, the relative sensitivity of the fetus as well as similar possibilities concerning the sensitivity of chromosal material to alkyl mercury effects will need to be kept in mind.

References

1. Lundgren, K.D., A. Swensson, and U. Ulfvarson. "Studies in Humans on the Distribution of Mercury in the Blood and the Excretion in Urine After Exposure to Different Mercury Compounds," Scand. J. Clin. Lab. Invest., *20*, 164-166 (1957).

2. Birke, G., A. G. Johnels, L. O. Plantin, B. Sjöstrand, and T. Westermark. Svenksa Läkartidningen, *64*(37), 3628 (1967).

3. Jervis, R. E., D. Debrun, W. LePage, and B. Tiefenbah. "Mercury Residues in Canadian Foods, Fish, Wlidlife," Summary of Progress, National Health Grant, Project No. 650-7-510 for period Sept., 1969, to May, 1970.

4. Kitamura, S. "Determination of Mercury Content in Bodies of Inhabitants, Cats, Fishes, and Shells in Minamata District and the Mud in Minamata Bog," Chapter VII in Minamata Disease (Kumamoto University, Japan: Study Group of Minamata Disease, 1968).

5. Kutsuna, S. Minamata Disease. (Kumamoto University, Japan: Study Group of Minamata Disease, 1968).

6. Tanzawa, K., T. Terao, T. Ukita, A. Ohuchi, and O. Hoshino. "Quantitative Determination of Mercury in

Hair by Activation Analysis," Eisei Kagaku, *12*, 94-99 (1966).

7. Lundgren, K. D. and A. Swensson. "Occupational Poisoning by Alkyl-Mercury Compounds," J. Ind. Hyg. Toxicol., *31*, 190-200 (1949).

8. Ui, J. Mercury Pollution of Sea and Fresh Water, Its Accumulation Into Water Biomass. A report. (Tokyo, Japan: University of Tokyo, Department of City Planning, 1969).

9. Ahlmark, A. "Poisoning by Methyl Mercury Compounds," Brit. J. Ind. Med., *5*, 117-119 (1948).

10. Höök, O., K. D. Lundgren, and A. Swensson. "On Alkyl Mercury Poisoning with Description of Two Cases," Acta Med. Scand., *150*, 131-137 (1954).

11. Smith, R. G., A. J. Vorwald, L. S. Patil, and T. F. Mooney, Jr. "A Study of the Effects of Exposure to Mercury in the Manufacture of Chlorine," Amer. Indust. Hyg. Assoc. J., *31*, 687-700 (1970).

12. Ramel, C. "Genetic Effects of Organic Mercury Compounds," Hereditas, *57*(3), 445-447 (1967).

13. Ramel, C. "Genetic Effects of Mercury Compounds I," Hereditas, *61*(2), 208-230 (1969).

14. Ramel, C. and J. Magnusson. "Genetic Effects of Mercury Compounds II," Hereditas, *61*(2), 231-254 (1969).

15. Jernelöv, Arne. Personal communication (1969).

16. Tejning, S. Report No. 6802 20. (Lund, Sweden: Department of Occupational Medicine, University Hospital, 1968).

17. Tejning, S. Report No. 670206. (Lund, Sweden: Department of Occupational Medicine, University Hospital, 1967).

18. Sumair, P., A. L. Backman, P. Karli, *et al.* "Health Investigators of Fish Consumers in Finland," Report at Scandanavian Symposium on the Mercury Problem, October, 1968.

19. Tejning, S. Report No. 670831. (Lund, Sweden: Department of Occupational Medicine, University Hospital, 1967).

20. Tejning, S. Report No. 680629. (Lund, Sweden: Department of Occupational Medicine, University Hospital, 1968).

The Relationship Between Mercury Concentration in Hair
and the Onset of Minamata Disease

Tadeo Takeuchi

The causative agent of Minamata disease was not found
until six years after the first outbreak of the disease in
1953. Therefore, the relationship between the mercury
concentration in hair and the onset of Minamata disease
was not investigated at that time.
However, in Niigata,[1] a close relationship between the
concentration of mercury in hair and the onset of the
disease was finally recognized. The inhabitants whose
hair contained higher concentrations of mercury were found
to be distributed around the Agano River. The distribution
of inhabitants with higher mercury concentrations in their
hair are depicted in Figure 56. The triangles represent

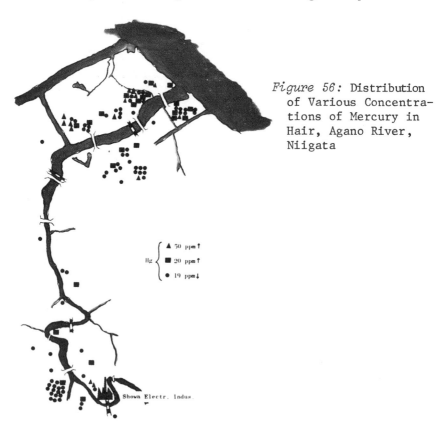

Figure 56: Distribution
of Various Concentra-
tions of Mercury in
Hair, Agano River,
Niigata

the highest concentrations (over 50 ppm), the squares show
concentrations between 20 and 49 ppm, and the circles
represent those individuals found to contain less than 20
ppm in their hair.

The disease occurred among the inhabitants of the
Niigata area who had the highest concentrations of mercury
in their hair. Figure 57 shows the occurrence of Minamata

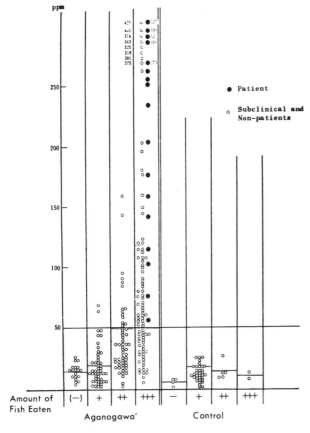

Figure 57: Occurrence of Minamata Disease among
     Inhabitants with Varying Mercury Concentrations in
     Hair (Tsubaki, 1968).

disease among inhabitants whose hair contained 52 to 570
ppm mercury. It is interesting to note that some of the
people who had the higher concentrations of mercury in
their hair were not affected by the disease.

In Minamata, on the other hand, some patients who had clinical signs of Minamata disease had only 10-20 ppm mercury in their hair. These lower concentrations can be explained by the fact that the actual mercury analyses were performed considerably after the onset of the disease.

The concentration of mercury in fetal hair had a somewhat different relationship to disease occurrence than was the case for children and adults. According to Harada,[2] the mercury concentrations in fetal hair were often less than the amount present in the mother's hair, even though those mothers did not show the clinical symptoms of Minamata disease. It was found that the fetal hair sometimes could contain only one-quarter to one-third the mercury concentration of the respective mother's hair, and yet the fetus be stricken with Minamata disease. Postnatally, infants with Minamata disease had higher mercury concentrations in their hair than unaffected infants. It is possible that these factors indicate a greater inherent sensitivity of the fetus to organic mercury loadings in comparison to children and adults.

References

1. Tsubaki, T. *et al.* Saigai Igaku, *11*, 1383-1390 (1968) *Japanese*
2. Harada, Y. "Infantile Minamata Disease - Congenital Minamata Disease," in Minamata Disease (Shuhan Co., 1968), pp. 73-117.

Organic Mercury Poisoning in Alamogordo,
New Mexico

A. Hinman

On December 4, 1969, an eight-year-old girl in Alamogordo, New Mexico, developed an illness characterized by ataxia, decreased vision, and depression of consciousness which progressed to coma over a period of three weeks. Two weeks after she became ill, her thirteen-year-old brother developed a similar illness, which also progressed to come in two to three weeks. At the end of December, their twenty-year-old sister became ill with similar symptoms and became semicomatose. All were hospitalized in El Paso, Texas, and were given supportive therapy. Investigation revealed that the patients' father had obtained waste seed grain in August, 1969, which had been treated with methylmercuric dicyandiamide. He subsequently fed this grain to the 18 hogs he was raising. In October, 1969, 14 of the hogs owned by the family became ill with blindness and a gait disturbance. Twelve of the 14 died; the survivors remained blind. The father had butchered one hog in September, 1969, at which time it appeared perfectly well. The meat from this hog was eaten on a daily basis by seven of the nine family members from September through December, 1969. Mercury determinations were performed, using the atomic absorption technique, on serum samples from the three patients, of the treated grain, and on the pork the family had been eating. Results are shown in Table 68.

Table 68

Mercury Determinations from Alamogordo
Poisoning Cases

Source	*Mercury level*
Serum - 8-year-old girl	1.92 ppm
Serum - 13-year-old boy	2.91 ppm
Serum - 20-year-old girl	2.78 ppm
Seed grain	32.8 ppm
Pork	27.5 ppm

The patients were all treated with British anti-lewisite (BAL) and, although an increase in urinary mercury excretion was demonstrated, there was no clinical improvement associated with the therapy. Subsequently all three were treated with n-acetyl-d,l,-penicillamine. No clinical improvement was noted following administration of this drug. About three to four months after onset of illness, all three patients began to show slow gradual improvement in their conditions. However, all three remain severely impaired.

Survival and Reproduction of Ring-necked Pheasants
Consuming Two Mercurial Fungicides*

William J. Adams and Harold H. Prince

Introduction

The widespread use of mercurial fungicides on cereal
grains and other agricultural crops has been a common
practice since the 1940's. Recently, the use of alkyl
mercury fungicides has been restricted and the use of aryl
mercury compounds has been encouraged. The effects of
mercury compounds on pheasants[1,2,3] and chickens[4,5] had
not been considered serious until recently, when some of
these compounds were linked to cases of mercury poisoning
in Swedish wildlife, including pheasants.[6,7] The purpose
of this study is to determine the effects of two common
mercurial fungicides, methylmercuric dicyandiamide and a
common substitute, phenylmercuric acetate, on survival and
reproduction of hen pheasants.

Thanks are due to the Michigan Agricultural Experiment
Station for providing financial support, to the Wisconsin
Department of Conservation for supplying birds for this
experiment, to the Michigan Department of Natural Resources
for providing facilities, to D. L. Haynes, Michigan State
University, for statistical advice, and to NOR-AM Agricultural Products, Inc., Woodstock, Illinois, for providing
the mercury fungicides.

Materials and Methods: Treatments

Two mercurial fungicides (NOR-AM Agricultural Products,
Inc.) were used, Panogen 15, containing 2.2% methylmercuric
dicandiamide, and Panomatic, containing 3.4% phenylmercuric
acetate (Table 69). Adult pheasant hens were fed *ad libitum*
Purina game breeder pellets treated with varied levels of
the two mercurial fungicides. The birds (males and females)
were divided into two groups, those fed treated food every
day and those fed treated food every third day. There was
an array of twelve concentrations of each compound for the
daily treatment, and five concentrations of each compound
for the hens fed every third day. There was one hen per
concentration in all treatments.

---

*Michigan Agricultural Experiment Station Paper No.
5346.

Table 69

The Experimental Design--One Hen Per Concentration

| | Mercury Compounds (mg/kg) | |
Treatment	Methylmercuric dicyandiamide	Phenylmercury acetate
Daily	0.0	0.0
	2.6	3.6
	5.1	7.1
	7.7	10.7
	10.2	14.3
	12.8	17.9
	15.4	21.5
	17.9	25.1
	20.5	28.7
	23.0	32.2
	25.6	35.8
	30.7	43.0
Every 3rd Day	0.0	0.0
	5.1	7.1
	10.2	14.3
	20.5	28.7
	30.7	43.0

The mercury compounds were sprayed with an aspirator on food pellets in a rotating jar. The food was treated in one kilogram quantities under a forced air hood.

Materials and Methods: Management

The birds were placed in outdoor pens and given three weeks to acclimate prior to receiving mercury treated food. Each female occupied a 3 x 4 meter pen containing natural vegetation. A male was placed with each hen for a 24-hour period every fourth or fifth day for insemination. New food was given each day with the previous day's food being removed and weighed to obtain a measure of consumption.

Eggs were collected daily and stored at 10°C for no longer than seven days. They were incubated at 37.5°C, 67% humidity, and rotated eight times daily. The eggs were candled and transferred to individual hatching trays on the

21st day of incubation. All chicks were weighed, banded, and placed in brooder houses. The contents of all eggs that were candled and removed or did not hatch were classified by the scheme developed by Hamburger and Hamilton[8] and Labisky and Opsahl.[9]

Statistical Analysis

Standard statistical procedures (chi square and regression analysis) were used,[10] and all values were tested at 0.05 level. Variation about the mean is denoted by the standard error.

Results: Survival of Adult Females

All birds given untreated food survived the 74-day trial. One of 11 hens fed phenyl mercury daily died. Hens given methyl mercury began to die on the 25th day, with 9 of 11 fed daily and 1 of 4 fed every third day dying. Two of 4 males died that consumed methyl mercury-treated food each day. Using a logarithmic transformation of the data, there was a linear decrease of survival time as the concentration of methyl mercury on the food increased (Figure 58). The cumulative amount of methyl mercury consumed

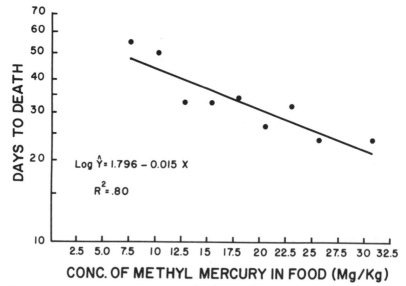

Figure 58: The Effects of Varied Concentrations of Methylmercuric Dicyandiamide Fed Daily on Survival Time of Nine Pheasant Hens

prior to death was 24.7 mg ± 0.8 mg (Figure 59). The total
amount of methyl mercury consumed by the two hens surviving
the daily treatment was 11.2 mg and 22.5 mg, suggesting
they had not yet consumed a lethal quantity. Although the
hen that consumed 22.5 mg of methyl mercury had not died,
symptoms of acute mercury poisoning were visible when the
experiment terminated.

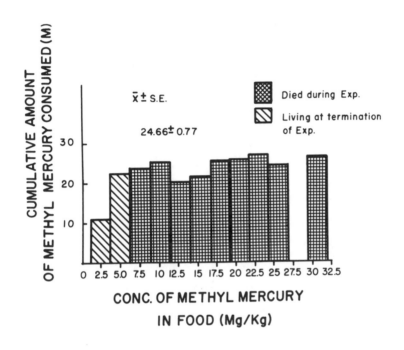

Figure 59: The Total Weight of Methylmercuric Dicyandiamide
Consumed by 11 Pheasant Hens Given Treated Food Each Day

The first visible indications of poisoning occurred after
the hens had consumed a total of 13 to 17 mg of methyl mercury. This was usually about 2 weeks prior to death; there
was also cessation in egg production at this time. Obvious
changes in behavior of the hens typically included ruffed
head feather, tameness, refusal to attempt flight, and
slight incoordination in walking. This progressed into
acute ataxia until the birds were unable to fly and walking
became difficult. Food consumption diminished from about
58 g per day prior to the 15 mg culminative total consumption

of methyl mercury, until nothing was eaten during the last two or three days prior to death (Figure 60). In the most advanced stages of poisoning the birds were unable to walk, muscle twitching of wings and legs occurred, and the birds were often found lying on their chests in a comatose state.

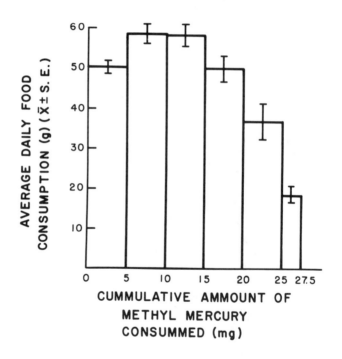

Figure 60: Average Daily Food Consumption of Hen Pheasants Influenced by the Cumulative Amount of Methylmercuric Dicyandiamide Eaten.

Results: Reproduction

The hens given untreated food produced eggs during the entire 74-day trial. Fertility of the treatment and control groups was constant throughout the experiment and averaged 96.1% and 90.4% respectively. Egg production of the hens

given methyl mercury declined during the second week of
the experiment with hens on the higher conconcentrations
going out of production first. There was a linear decrease
in the number of production days after logarithmic transformation, as the concentration of methyl mercury on the
food increased on the daily and three-day treatments
(Figure 61). No decline in the number of egg production
days was observed for either of the phenyl mercury treatments.

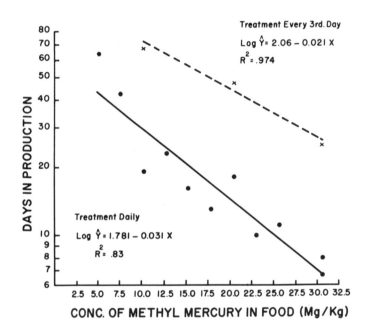

Figure 61: The Relationship of the Number of Days in
Production to the Concentration of Methylmercuric
Dicyandiamide on the Food Consumed Daily and Every
Third Day

The total number of eggs laid during the period of
greatment by hens fed methyl mercury daily followed the
same pattern of decline as the number of days in production
(Figure 62). This is not surprising, since pheasants will
lay an egg per 1.25 days.[11] Hens fed higher concentrations

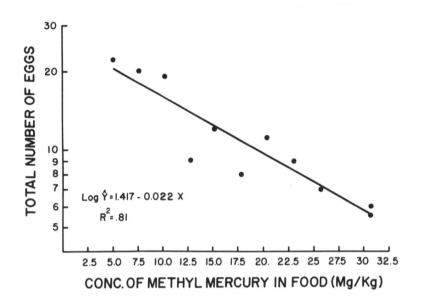

Figure 62:   The Relationship of the Number of Eggs Produced
to the Concentration of Methylmercuric Dicyandiamide
on the Food Consumed Each Day

of methyl mercury laid fewer eggs and went out of production
sooner than those on lower concentrations. There was a
decrease from a high of 40 eggs to a low of 10 eggs for the
hens fed methyl mercury every third day.

The total amount of methyl mercury consumed prior to
the last egg laid by those hens on a daily treatment was
15.8 mg ± 0.9 mg, and 15.1 mg ± 1.3 mg by the hens fed
treated food every third day.   Egg production stopped
after the consumption of approximately 16 mg of methyl
mercury, even though this occurred over a period of 10-58
days.

There seems to be no reduction in egg production due to
any of the phenyl mercury treatments within the limits of
this experiment.

Both methyl and phenyl mercury compounds affected
hatchability (Figure 63). Hatchability of the eggs laid
by hens fed methyl mercury daily increased significantly
above the control value of 74% to 93% until about 3.5 mg
of methyl mercury had been eaten.   Then hatchability

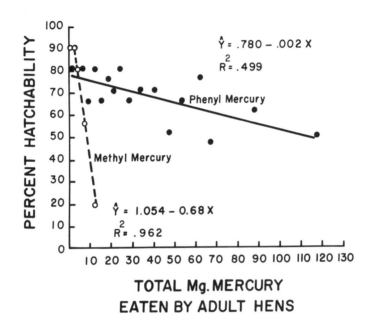

Figure 63: Hatchability of Eggs Related to Total Amount of Methylmercuric and Phenylmercuric Compounds Consumed by Hen Pheasants

decreased at a rate of 6.8 ± 0.5% for each additional mg of methyl mercury eaten (Figure 64). Hatchability decreased at a rate of 0.20 ± 0.06% for each mg of phenyl mercury consumed on a daily basis.

Embryonic mortality in the control and treatment groups was greatest during the first and last parts of the incubation period (Figure 65). There was a shift in the distribution of embryonic mortality from hens fed methyl and phenyl mercury compounds. A significant decrease of mortality in the 20-24 day developmental period occurred for both treatment groups, with consistently higher percentages of mortality in the first 3 developmental periods. The amount of embryonic mortality occurring

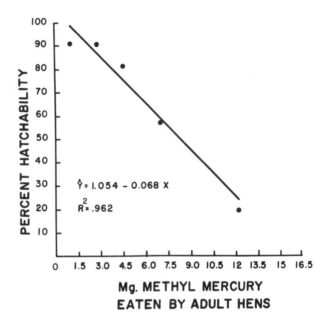

Figure 64: Hatchability of Eggs Related to Total Amount of Methylmercuric Dicyandiamide Consumed by Hen Pheasants

during the first 14 days of the developmental period was 70%, 62%, and 48% for the methyl mercury, phenyl mercury, and control groups, respectively.

Discussion

Methylmercuric dicyandiamide affected survival and reproduction in pheasants. There was a range of 31 days between the time the first and last hen went out of egg production, and a range of 34 days between the first and last death on high and low concentrations, respectively. The average amount of methyl mercury consumed at termination of egg production and at death was 15.8 mg ± 0.9 mg and

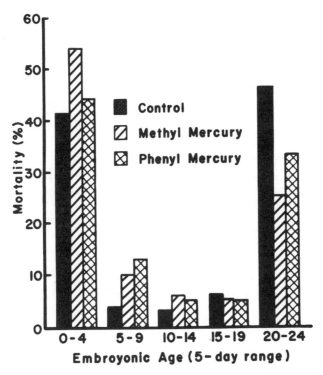

Figure 65: Distribution of Embryonic Mortality of Eggs from Hens in the Control, Methylmercuric Dicyandiamide, and Phenylmercuric Acetate Treatment Groups

24.7 mg ± 0.8 mg, respectively. The low variation about the mean over the range of concentrations suggests that methyl mercury accumulates in the body in an additive manner which is a function of concentration and time.

The hatchability of eggs from hens fed methylmercuric dicyandiamide declined at a rate of 6.8% per mg consumed. Borg *et al.*[6] reported a decline in hatchability to 55% after feeding pheasant hens 15–20 mg/kg methylmercuric dicyandiamide for 9 days. Based on an average daily consumption of 54 grams of food, their birds would have consumed 8.5 mg, which according to our regression equation would give 51% hatchability. Similar results have been reported for domestic fowl (*Gallus gallus*) by Tejning,[12] who found that after 28 days of continuous feeding of methylmercuric dicyandiamide at rates of 18.4 mg/kg and 9.2 mg/kg, hatchability was reduced to 10% and 17%, respectively, as compared to a control value of 61%.

Successful hatching is related to total accumulation of mercury in the bird and in the egg. Eggs which were laid after a small amount of methyl mercury had been consumed (0-4 mg) had much better success in hatching than those laid after consumption of larger amounts (5-12 mg). This suggests that a certain concentration of methyl mercury, and phenyl mercury to a smaller extent, must be accumulated in the hen's body and incorporated into the eggs before hatchability will be reduced. Tejning[12] reported similar results with domestic chickens, showing that hatchability depends on the concentration of methylmercuric dicyandiamide in the food, number of days the food has been consumed, and the concentration of mercury in the egg.

Phenylmercuric acetate, in comparison with methylmercuric dicyandiamide, is much less toxic. There were no effects on survival, egg production, or food consumption attributed to phenylmercuric acetate. Hatchability was affected, declining at a rate of $0.20 \pm 0.06\%$ for each mg of phenylmercuric acetate consumed; but hatchability did not decline below the control value until 20 mg had been consumed. Calculations of $L.D._{100}$ by Grolleau and Giban[13] also show phenylmercuric acetate to be much less toxic than methylmercuric dicyandiamide.

Although no data are available on the amount of mercury consumed by wild pheasants, Tejning[7] has estimated the average spillage of seed grain in Sweden to be 1% of the total amount planted, with an average mercury concentration of 16 mg/kg. Tejning[7] and Ulfvarsson[14] have shown that the high levels of mercury found in Swedish pheasants can be attributed to the amount of grain left on the ground after spring and fall planting.

In the past, recommended dosages for the use of methylmercuric dicyandiamide in the United States have ranged from 10 mg/kg for cereal grains to 82 mg/kg for corn, peas, soybeans, and navy beans. Based on recommended dosages for wheat and corn, and an average daily consumption of 60 grams, it would take a wild pheasant hen 6.5 days and 0.8 days, respectively, to consume 4 mg of methylmercuric dicyandiamide. The 4 mg level is the point at which hatchability declines below the control value. Consumption of more than 4 mg would seriously decrease hatchability and would result in a cessation of egg production if approximately 16 mg were consumed. We believe that methylmercuric dicyandiamide could limit pheasant numbers if treated seed is available.

References

1. Petoskey, M. "Effects of Mercury Treated Grains on Pheasants," Paper presented at Michigan Acad. Sci. Arts and Letters, Ann Arbor, Michigan (1948).
2. Leedy, D. and C. Cole. "The Effects on Pheasants of Corn Treated with Various Fungicides," *J. Wildl. Mgmt.*, *14*(2), 218-255 (1950).
3. Carnaghan, R. B. A. and J. D. Blaxland. "The Toxic Effects of Certain Seed-dressings on Wild and Game Birds," *Vet. Rec.*, *69*(2), 324-325 (1957).
4. Heuser, G. F. "Feeding Chemically Treated Seed Grains to Hens," *Poultry Sci.*, *35*(1), 161-162 (1956).
5. Smart, N. A. and M. K. Lloyd. "Mercury Residues in Eggs, Flesh, Livers of Hens Fed on Wheat Treated with Methyl Mercury Dicyandiamide," *J. Sci. Food Agr.*, *14*, 734-740 (1963).
6. Borg, K., H. Wanntorp, K. Erne, and E. Hanko. "Alkyl Mercury Poisoning in Terrestrial Swedish Wildlife," *Viltrevy*, *6*(4), 301-379 (1969).
7. Tejning, S. "Mercury in Pheasants (*Phasianus colchicus*) Deriving from Seed Grain Dressed with Methyl and Ethyl Mercury Compounds," *Oikos*, *18*(2), 334-344 (1967).
8. Hamburger, V. and H. L. Hamilton. "A Series of Normal Stages in the Development of the Chick Embryo," *J. Morphol.*, *88*, 49-92 (1951).
9. Labisky, R. F. and J. F. Opsahl. "A Guide to Aging of Pheasant Embryos," *Ill. Nat. Hist. Sur.*, *Biol. Notes No. 39*. (1958).
10. Steel, R. G. D. and J. H. Torrie. *Principles and Procedures of Statistics.* (New York: McGraw-Hill Book Co., Inc., 1960).
11. Labisky, R. F. and G. L. Jackson. "Production and Weights of Eggs Laid by Yearling, 2-, and 3-Year-Old Pheasants," *J. Wildl. Mgmt.*, *33*(3), 718-721 (1969).
12. Tejning, S. "Embryonic Mortality and Hatching Frequency in Artificially Incubated Eggs from Hens Fed with Treated Grain," *Oikos Suppl.*, *3*, 56-59 (1967).
13. Grolleau, G. and J. Giban. "Toxicity of Seed Dressings to Game Birds and Theoretical Risks of Poisoning," *J. App. Ecol. Suppl.*, *3*, 199-212 (1966).
14. Ulfvarson, U. "Mercury, Aldrin and Dieldrin in Pheasants," *Srensk Kemisk Tidskrift*, *77*(2), 235-246 (1965).

Dose-Response Relationships After Exposure of Swine
to Organo-Mercurial Compounds

L. Tryphonas

In western Canada, grains contaminated with organo-
mercurial fungicides constitute a major known source of
mercury poisoning in domesticated animals entering the
human food supply. It is known that different species
react quite differently to organo-mercurials; for example,
chickens appear to be relatively insensitive, while cattle
appear to be quite sensitive to poisoning by organo-
mercurials. This could have public health implications,
since some species might achieve relatively high body
burdens of an organo-mercury compound without showing any
detectable signs of mercury poisoning. This fact, and the
need to know more about the pathology of organo-mercurial
poisoning in domestic animals, prompted our studies with
alkyl and aryl mercury compounds which were initiated in
Saskatoon in 1965.

These studies were conducted in swine with two alkyl
compounds: methylmercuric dicyandiamide (MMD) and ethylmercuric chloride (EMC). We also studied on aryl compound,
phenylmercuric chloride (PMC). The dosages ranged from
0.19 to 4.56 mg of Hg/kg administered daily. MMD produced
clinical disease at about 0.76 mg Hg/kg/day, EMC produced
disease at about 0.38 mg Hg/kg/day, and PMC produced disease
only above 2.28 mg Hg/kg/day. PMC caused predominantly
kidney damage. Macroscopically the kidneys appeared yellow
and swollen. Microscopically there were attempts by the
kidney to regenerate, but ultimately the animals died
because of renal failure as a result of necrotic changes.
In addition, PMC causes a necrotic enteritis which also
contributes to the death of the same animals.

By contrast, the alkyl mercury compounds affect the
brain. The cerebrum is decreased in volume, while the
cerebellum maintains approximately normal size. There is
necrosis in the deeper cerebral cortical lamina. "Holes"
appear in the cortical substance, due to the destruction
and cytolysis of neurons. The process appears to be
progressive as the disease advances. There is a proliferation of glial cells. The observed severe polioclastic
changes may in part be produced by occlusive arteriolar
lesions. Some arterioles in affected areas demonstrate
fibrinoid degeneration and necrosis. These changes make
the vessels nonfunctional and produce additional destruction
of brain tissue.

The effect of alkyl mercury compounds on the kidneys
is not as severe. The most severe lesion observed in the
kidney was a hydropic degeneration of the tubular epithelium.
With higher doses, there were also some effects on the
gastrointestinal tract, such as edematous changes in the
mesocolon and necrotic colitis.

In summary, this study confirms the relatively higher
toxicity to swine of alkyl mercury compounds as compared
with aryl mercury compounds. Alkyl mercury compounds primarily affect the brain, while the aryl mercury compounds
primarily affect the kidneys. Other organ systems are also
affected. Mercury compounds stored in these affected tissues can, under certain circumstances, become important
problems to public health.

Detection and Appraisal of Subclinical Intoxications

Leonard J. Goldwater

The occurrence of overt or classical manifestations of
occupational poisoning due to mercury (or to other chemicals)
represents a failure of industrial hygiene and is no longer
acceptable as a means of detecting intoxications. This
obviously dictates that means must be sought to recognize
adverse effects at an early or subclinical stage. Advances
in biochemistry, particularly enzymology, have opened up
promising avenues of investigation. Refined methods of
measuring metals in biological materials have revealed the
presence of mercury where formerly it had been thought to
be absent. The significance of this latter point is
illustrated in Figure 66.

When it was possible to detect mercury only in the
higher ranges, that is, at the right hand end of the curve
in Figure 66, the demonstrated presence of the metal was
always likely to be associated with biological injury.
Hence, if no injury were found, it was assumed that mercury
was absent. At least theoretically, this simple "all or
none" concept is no longer tenable; furthermore, it is not
unreasonable to assume that minute amounts of mercury might
be found to play a beneficial role in biological processes,
just as been found to be the case with several other metals
and elements. This hypothetical range of favorable effect,
however, is almost certainly very narrow.

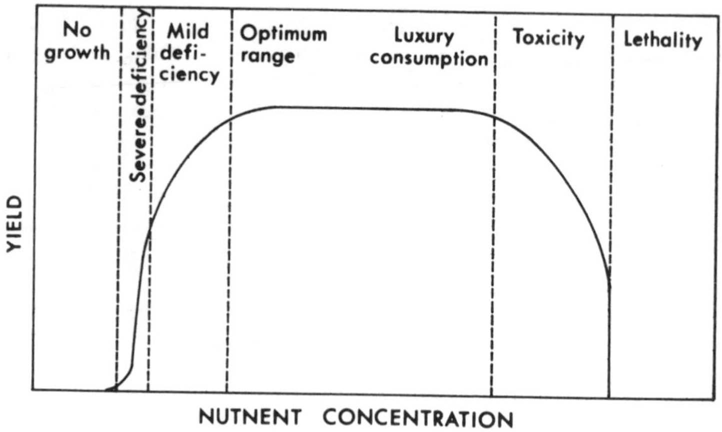

Figure 66: Idealized Diagram of Growth of an Organism as
a Function of the Concentration of an Essential
Nutrient. After P. F. Smith, <u>Ann. Rev. Plant. Physiol.</u>
13, 81 (1962).

Tests with Little or No Value

Before investigating the newer methods of detecting
subclinical intoxications, let us consider some older
methods, of which measurement of mercury in urine is one
of the most widely practiced. There is little or no doubt
that high levels of exposure will, in a general way, be
reflected by high levels of urinary mercury. The same is
true for blood, hair, saliva, and other biological materials. However, high urine levels, which simply reflect
absorption, are by no means regularly associated with
evidence of intoxication. Their value is further vitiated
by the great fluctuations which occur in any individual
from hour to hour and from day to day, as illustrated in
Tables 70 and 71.[1]

Studies of mercury in blood are of no greater value
than those of urine as indicators of subclinical or even
of clinical intoxication. Alkyl and some alkoxyalkyl
mercury compounds have greater affinity for blood cells
than do inorganic and phenyl mercurials, which means that,
for the former, blood levels may be more useful than urine
levels in measuring the extent of absorption.[1]   Mercury
concentrations in saliva tend to parallel those in blood.
As far as urine and blood are concerned, there is overwhelming

Table 70

Fluctuations in Urinary Excretion of Mercury in a
Single Individual Exposed to Mercury Vapor

	Air		Urine		
Day	Estimated average mg Hg/m^3	Range mg Hg/m^3	24-hour volume $(ml)^a$	Range gamma Hg/l	Total $Hg/24$-$hour^b$
Monday (pm)	0.425	0.20–1.00	434	225–345 (4)[c]	229.6
Tuesday	0.343	0.13–0.70	910	180–870 (6)	470.2
Wednesday	0.187	0.10–0.45	968	158–457 (6)	375.2
Thursday	0.189	0.10–0.55	570	360–1020(4)	431.0
Friday	0.166	0.10–0.65	843	165–555 (5)	268.6
Saturday			605	4.5–358 (4)[d]	109.2
Sunday			642	168–615 (3)	223.5
Monday (am)	0.190	0.10–0.45	481	203–398 (3)	

[a]Urine volume per minute = 0.15 ml to 2.60 ml
[b]Hg per minute = 35–882 nanograms
[c]Numbers in parentheses = voidings
[d]Sample voided during an evening of liberal intake of beer.

Table 71

Fluctuations and Variations in Urinary Excretion of
Mercury in Six Individuals Having Identical Conditions of
Exposure to Phenylmercuric Benzoate

Day	G	C	GL	O	R	F
Monday	108–367	84–451	69–388	27–292	22–120	0–25
Tuesday	105–322	160–472	22–282	198–607	2–78	0–21
Wednesday	69–315	195–546	12–483	87–552	21–150	0–60
Thursday	120–451	214–441	15–214	33–472	0–112	0–33
Friday	185–315	189–732	3–234	30–456	0–81	0–37
Saturday	138–309	210–441	22–303	66–337	3–247	0–78
Sunday	229–309	243–528	3–451	12–112	0–49	0–49
Monday	57–288	385	37–45	97–138	15–27	0–2

evidence that there is nothing like a "critical" level of
mercury which is or is not regularly associated with
clinical or subclinical manifestations of adverse effect.
In this connection, host factors, some of which are listed
in Table 72, are probably of importance.

Table 72

Host Factors Which May Affect Response to Toxic Agents

age	genetic make-up
sex	work habits
race	permeability of skin
nutritional status	permeability of lungs
medical care	endocrine status
personal hygiene	intestinal flora

Severe poisoning with mercuric chloride is known to
result in major injury to the kidneys, resulting in
albuminuria and total kidney failure. Low grade absorption of some mercury compounds may cause a slight increase
in the excretion of protein and, rarely, a nephrotic
syndrome. Detection of the subclinical albuminuria requires quantitative analysis, as the ordinary routine
tests are not sufficiently sensitive.[2] This quantitative
analysis is of some value, but, because of its complexity,
it does not lend itself to use when large numbers of
individuals are to be examined on a recurring basis.

Biochemical Tests

Because of the known affinity of mercury for sulfhydryl-
containing enzymes, biochemical changes based on this
affinity have been sought. Among the substances studied
may be mentioned coproporphyrins, delta-aminolevulinic acid,
lactose dehydrogenase, serum phosphoglucose isomerase, and
serum glutathione reductase. Some of the published reports
suggest that further work may result in useful findings.[3,4]

Reports of enhancement rather than inhibition of enzymatic action attributable to mercury are not numerous but
do exist. Perhaps if investigators were more alert to the
possibility of beneficial effects, more such observations
would be made. At certain concentrations of mercury in the

substrate, the detoxification of diisopropyl fluorophosphate[5] and of procaine[6,7] have been assisted. More interesting is the effect of mercury on 2,3-diglycerophosphatase, one of the enzymes concerned with oxygen transport. In consonance with the principle illustrated in Figure 66, there is evidence that low concentrations of mercury may enhance and higher concentrations inhibit the activity of 2,3-DGP.[8,9]

A study of mercury poisoning in the hat industry was made in 1936, although not published until much later.[10] Among the findings was the presence of strikingly high hemoglobin values in the hatters having the heaviest exposure to mercury. This unexpected occurrence at first suggested the possibility of technical error, but this was ruled out by careful checking of reagents and instruments. The values are given in Table 73 and Figure 67, reprinted

Table 73

Percentage Distribution of Hemoglobin Values
in Three Groups of Workers

Hemoglobin *(g per 100 cc)*	*Control* *(81 persons)*	*Mercury* *(281 persons)*	*Benzol* *(180 persons)*
Less than 11.0	0	0	1
11.0 to 11.9	0	0	3
12.0 to 12.9	2	1	9
13.0 to 13.9	27	4	35
14.0 to 14.9	44	15	33
15.0 to 15.9	22	16	13
16.0 or more	5	64	6

from an earlier publication; they include observations on other groups of workers for comparison. Other hematological findings, incidentally, were within normal limits.

The possible connection between the oxygen transport functions of 2,3-DPG, the effects of mercury on this enzyme, and the high hemoglobin values in hatters is obvious. Mercury levels in blood were not measured in these workers, but exposures and urinary mercury were high. Inhibition of the delivery of oxygen to tissues, resulting in anoxia,

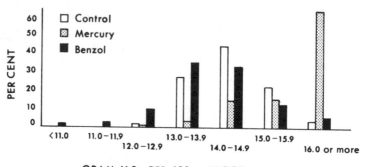

GRAM H.B. PER 100 ml BLOOD

Figure 67: Percentage Distribution of Hemoglobin Values in Workers Shown in Table 73.

could be reflected in a compensatory increase in hemoglobin. This theory seems to be worth testing as a possible indicator of subclinical intoxication.

References

1. Goldwater, L. J. "Occupational Exposure to Mercury: The Harben Lectures, 1964," J. Royal Inst. Pub. Health and Hyg., 27, 279-301 (1964).

2. Joselow, M. M. and L. J. Goldwater. "Absorption and Excretion of Mercury in Man: XII. Relationship Between Urinary Mercury and Proteinuria," Arch. Environ. Health, 15, 115-159, 1967.

3. Goldwater, L. J. and M. M. Joselow. "Absorption and Excretion of Mercury in Man: XIII. Effects of Mercury Exposure in Urinary Excretion of Coproporphyrin and Delta-Aminolevulinic Acid," Arch. Environ. Health, 15, 327-331 (1967).

4. Taylor, W., H. A. Guirgis, and W. K. Stewart. "Investigation of Population Exposed to Organomercurial Seed Dressings," Arch. Environ. Health, 19, 505-509 (1969).

5. Mazur, A. "An Enzyme in Animal Tissues Capable of Hydrolyzing the Phosphorus-Fluorine Bond of Alkyl Fluorophosphates," J. Biol. Chem., 164, 271-289 (1946).

6. Beutner, R., J. Landay, and A. Lieberman. "Evidence for the Local Effect of Mercurial Diuretics," Proc. Soc. Exp. Biol. and Med., 44, 120-122 (1940).

7. Haury, V. G. "Protective Action of Mercury and Lead Salts Against Procaine Convulsions," Proc. Soc. Exp. Biol. and Med., 46, 309-310 (1941).

8. Rapoport, S. and J. Leubering. "Glycerate-2,3-diphos-
    phatase," J. Biol. Chem., *189*, 683-694 (1951).
9. Rapoport, S., J. Leubering, and R. H. Wagner, "Ueber
    die Quecksilber-Aktivierung der Glycerinsaure-2,3-
    diphosphatase," Hoppe-Seyler's Z. Physiol. Chem., *302*,
    105-110 (1955)
10. Goldwater, L. J. "Blood Studies on Workers in the Fur-
    Felt Hat Industry," Monthly Review, N.Y. State Dept.
    of Labor, *29*, 1-3 (1950).

Approaches to the Detection of Subclinical Mercury
Intoxications: Experience in Minamata, Japan

Tadeo Takeuchi

On the basis of pathological findings observed in
autopsy cases, three types of Minamata disease have been
differentiated. The first was a complete type of Hunter-
Russell's syndrome that was characterized by ataxia,
dysarthria, concentric construction of visual fields,
deafness, and sensory disturbance in the extremities. The
second was an incomplete type that showed only one of the
signs of the Hunter-Russell syndrome, or a few other
nervous signs. Finally, the third, a latent type, showed
no clinical symptoms. The relationships of these three
types of Minamata disease are shown in Figure 68.

In the Minamata area, almost all patients who were
clinically diagnosed as having Minamata disease belonged
to the complete or first type. However, many cases also
showed signs of the incomplete type, particularly those
that showed only signs of a polyneuritis-like symptom or
a few other signs, without the constriction of the visual
fields and ataxia. These cases have not been diagnosed
clinically. According to Tokuomi *et al.*,[1] this type could
not be definitely established as Minamata disease because
similar nonspecific symptoms also occur in other nervous
disorders.

Because lawsuits by patients against the industrial
companies involved damage claims, a more definitive diagnosis
was needed. Therefore problems of differential diagnosis
emerged. Patients who showed doubtful nervous signs were
not diagnosed until an autopsy could be performed. Furthermore, especially in the higher age brackets, the nervous

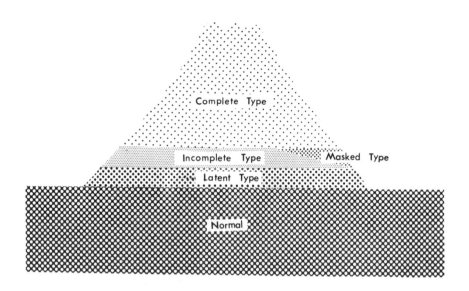

Figure 68: Relationship of Various Types of Minamata
    Disease in Human Beings, Based on Pathological Findings

signs from the incomplete type of Minamata disease could be
masked by the signs of other nervous symptoms, particularly
cerebral vascular disorders. For this reason Takeuchi
named this incomplete type the "masked Minamata disease."
    Latent Minamata disease also was found in a victim who
died after a gastric hemorrhage. A detailed autopsy revealed that this individual had eaten fish and shellfish
caught both inside and outside of Minamata Bay. Moreover,
a cat that lived at this individual's home also suffered
from Minamata disease. The autopsy revealed a decrease of
nerve cells in both calcarine regions. A distinct decrease
of granular cells in the cerebellum was apparent. Analyses
of the tissues showed mercury in the brain (2.12 ppm),
liver (7.99 ppm), and kidneys (28.12 ppm), similar to
findings in other chronic cases of this disease.
    The number of patients afflicted with Minatama disease
has been documented with increasing frequency since the
disease was first recognized in 1953. Fifty-three cases
had been reported by 1956. By 1960, the number of cases
had risen to 88, and then to 111 in 1962. Recently ten
new patients were added, to give a total of 121 documented
cases. Moreover, on the basis of pathological diagnoses,

the number of cases will probably increase as previously doubtful patients who reported nervous signs and numbness of the limbs and fingers may eventually be found to have structural evidence of the disease.

As the symptoms are more widely recognized, the greater susceptibility of the human fetus to Minamata disease will result in a reappraisal of infant cases. To date, 23 cases of fetal Minamata disease have been described, but only one of the mothers was diagnosed as having Minamata disease. New patients will quite likely also be diagnosed from the latent Minamata disease group on the basis of pathological investigations.

Pathological Changes Due to Minamata Disease

From a pathological standpoint, Minamata disease produces relatively characteristic changes. Typically, the granular cells in the cerebellum begin to disappear under the Purkinje cell layer, and nerve cells decrease in both calcarine regions. It is important to note that these changes were found in individuals who had no clinical signs of Minamata disease except for numbness in the early stage. According to Takeuchi,[2,3] methyl mercury may involve nerve cells in the preferential areas of the brain cortex. In these areas, the nerve cells have a tendency to disappear gradually from the small areas. This appears to be a function of the mercury concentration in the tissues. In some cases the loss of nerve cells has been proven to have occurred in a certain region, but clinical signs failed to appear in the patient. Therefore, it is probable that the number of disturbed and lost nerve cells has to drop below a certain level before neurological signs are clinically apparent. A gradually increasing degree of neurological disturbance seems to depend on an accumulation of organic mercury over time. Presumably, this is important in the pathogenesis of Minamata disease.

Detection of Subclinical Organic Mercury Intoxication

An important practical problem is how to detect subclinical organic mercury intoxication. In our laboratories it was considered that the sural nerve biopsy is most useful for diagnosis with mercury determination, because it tends to be most easily disturbed in sensory peripheral nerves.

Visual microscopic examination reveals a relative increase of smaller fibers below 3μ and a decrease of normal

size fibers (2 peaks of 5µ and 11µ) with collagen proliferation. The most conspicuous findings were observed on
electron micrographs, which demonstrated an incomplete
regeneration of nerves with abnormal, smaller fibers and
with incomplete formation of myelin. This was very characteristic, except for various degenerative and reparative
processes.

These characteristic findings were also clearly shown
in cases of the incomplete type of Minamata disease which
had not been clinically diagnosed. It is quite apparent
that many subclinical cases of the Minamata disease are
difficult to detect, but the electron-microscopic observations of sural nerve tissue may be useful in the detection
of subclinical cases.

Besides using biopsy specimens of the sural nerve in
cases with numbness of the limbs, subclinical diagnosis
should also be attempted by determining the levels of
mercury in human hair. The correlation of Minamata disease
with increasing mercury in hair was noted in Niigata where
new patients appeared among persons whose hair contained
more than 50 ppm mercury.

References

1. Tokuomi, H. *et al.* "Clinical Investigation on Minamata
   Disease," in Minamata Disease (Shuhan Co., 1968), pp.
   37-72.
2. Takeuchi, T. *et al.* "Minamata Disease and Its Pathological Changes Following More Than Ten Years," Nippon
   Iji Shinpo, *2402*, 22-27 (1970) *Japanese*.
3. Takeuchi, T. "Pathology of Minamata Disease," in
   Minamata Disease (Shuhan Co., 1968), pp. 141-252.

Mercury Concentrations in Human Tissues Among
Heavy Fish Eaters

R. F. Korns

The New York State Department of Health has undertaken
a variety of large-scale explorations of mercury levels in
fish, municipal water supplies, sewage effluent, etc., and
to a lesser extent in human tissues. This brief paper
deals with the studies of limited material from selected
human populations. The cold vapor atomic absorption technique was used throughout.

In view of the initial focus of concern on fish from
the Great Lakes, it was deemed most pertinent to examine
specimens of hair from a group of individuals known to be
fishing these waters intensively, and for whom such fish
represented a substantial and frequent item in the diet.
Locating such persons along the shores of Lake Erie in New
York State and obtaining the samples presented some problems. Most of the subjects were Negroes or Puerto Ricans.

Table 74

Mercury in Hair from Consumers of Fish from Lake Erie
August 1970

Area Fished	Fish Eaters*			Non-fish Eaters		
	No.	Mercury ppm Range	Average	No.	Mercury ppm Range	Average
Dunkirk	8	0.7-4.9	2.7	4	0.8-1.9	1.1
Upper Niagara	4	0.7-6.7	4.8	1	-	0.04
Lower Niagara	10	0.7-11.6	4.3	2	0.7-0.8	0.7
Total	22	0.7-11.6	3.7	7	0.7-1.9	0.9

*Fish eaten at least 3-5 times per week

The findings are presented in Table 74. A total of 22
heavy fish eaters and 7 comparable control subjects from
the same populations, who ate no fish, were studied. Mercury levels as high as 2.0 ppm had been found in fish
recovered from the Dunkirk area and from the upper and lower

Niagara River (above and below the falls). Some effort was
made to identify the species and size of fish customarily
eaten, but in general, the fishermen were not very selective.
One person, found to have 11.6 ppm of mercury in her hair,
ate these fish seven days a week and occasionally more than
once per day. Although it may be argued that all of these
findings are probably within normal limits, the levels of
mercury in the hair of fish eaters (average 3.7 ppm, with
a range from 0.7 to 11.6 ppm) seem to be clearly higher
than among the controls (average 0.9 ppm, with a range
from 0.7 to 1.9 ppm).

Table 75 presents the mercury findings in a collection
of miscellaneous human tissues obtained from the Buffalo
region in August, 1970, as an initial step toward exploring
the occurrence of this element in relevant population groups.

Table 75

Mercury Levels in Assorted Human Tissues
Buffalo Region--August, 1970

Source of Specimen	Type of Tissue	No.	Mercury Level Range ppm	Average ppm
Stillbirth	Liver	10	0.02–0.10	0.06
Fetus (11–19 weeks)	Liver	43	<0.01–0.39	0.06
	Brain	6	<0.05	0.05
Mother	Whole blood	16	<1.0–2.5*	1.0*
Patients with senile dementia	Hair	10	<0.04–1.8	0.33

*Mercury level expressed as μgm/100 ml.

The rationale for selecting these particular subjects is
not especially cogent. The known excess of mercury in the
fetus as compared to the exposed mother suggested the collection of most of these samples. The coincidental
implementation of a new abortion law in New York State
made such studies readily feasible. It had been hoped to
limit these examinations to tissues from mothers who were
heavy consumers of fish from Lake Erie. Actually, this

proved impracticable, so that the tissues collected are from mothers and abortuses, none of whom were exposed to lake fish. The levels of mercury in mothers' blood, fetal liver and brain, and stillbirth liver are, in general, remarkably low.

One other group was sampled, namely a few patients diagnosed as having senile dementia of fairly recent clinical onset. Admittedly, such a study design could hardly shed light on the difficult question as to whether lifetime ingestion of low levels of mercury might produce such senile changes. On the other hand, this first step was deemed to be useful. The uniformly low levels found in the hair from these subjects are at least worth mentioning.

Epidemiological Approaches to the Study of Subclinical Effects of Mercury Intoxication

I. T. T. Higgins

Introduction

This paper will review ways and means which an epidemiologist might use to study the problem of subclinical mercury intoxication. I was asked to direct my attention more specifically to the question: What does of mercury is safe? A "safe" dose is assumed to be one which produces neither clinical effects nor any subclinical alterations which may presage serious implications. Clinical effects, which would be fairly easy to discuss, are excluded by these terms of reference. I shall try as far as possible, therefore, to concentrate on subclinical changes and their potential or actual implications

The Epidemiological Approach to Subclinical Mercury Intoxication

There is nothing unique about the epidemiologist's approach to the problem of mercury intoxication. He may be more conscious than others of the importance of defining the population he is studying, but that is all. For the rest he follows steps that any scientist would take (Table 76). He defines and measures subclinical effects; he relates these to dosage in order to establish the dose/response

Table 76

Summary of Epidemiological Approach

---

1. Select populations for study.
2. Define subclinical effect.
3. Measure subclinical effect.
4. Measure dose.
5. Establish dose/response relationships.
6. Determine characteristics other than dose which differentiate affected from unaffected.
7. Determine long-term implications of exposure, subclinical and clinical disease.
8. Measure the effects of intervention and control on subclinical symptoms and signs and on blood, urine, or hair concentration.

---

curve; he looks for ways in which affected persons differ from unaffected persons other than in relation to dosage; he determines the long-term implications of exposure, subclinical and clinical disease; and finally, he assesses the effects of any intervention. He speculates about mechanisms of action, though for the most part he leaves the study of mechanisms to laboratory or other workers.

Definition of Subclinical Effects

A subclinical effect is one which does not take a person to a clinician, but which can be detected if it is carefully looked for using appropriate means. Symptoms, signs, and special tests which might indicate mercury intoxication are indicated in Table 77. Those listed under inorganic mercury intoxication were derived from the paper by Smith and his colleagues;[1] those under organic mercury intoxication resulted from discussions with Dr. Bertram Dinman of the University of Michigan.

However, most of the symptoms described are nonspecific. It would be surprising if they proved to be satisfactory and usable indices of mercury intoxication. Whether they are usable or not for this purpose depends on the following criteria: discrimination, reproducibility, validity, simplicity, and acceptability. Let us consider each of these criteria.

Table 77

Subclinical Effects of Mercury Intoxication

Inorganic:
    Loss of appetite
    Loss of weight
    Objective tremor
    Insomnia
    Shyness
    Nervousness
    Dizziness
    Frequent colds
    Diarrhea
    Sore gums
    Albuminuria

Organic:
    Fatigue
    Headache
    Impaired power of concentration
    Impaired memory
    Tingling or numbness of fingers or mouth
    Clumsiness. Ataxia. Dysdiadochokinesis
    Inability to speak clearly. Dysarthria
    Concentric defect of visual fields
    Audiometric defects

Organic and Inorganic:
    Concentrations in blood, urine, hair

(a) Discrimination

The first consideration is the degree to which the test differentiates persons who are exposed to mercury from persons who are not. An important extension of this is the degree to which the test differentiates persons who are exposed to different dosages of mercury. In their study of chlorine workers exposed to inorganic mercury, Smith and his colleagues[1] showed that loss of appetite and a subjective history of weight loss discriminated well between persons who were exposed to mercury and others who were not. Furthermore, within the exposed groups, the proportions who responded positively increased steadily with increasing dose level (Table 78). Other symptoms discriminated less

Table 78

Number and Percentage of Workers Affected
According to Level of Mercury Exposure

	Mercury-exposed Workers					Controls
	Time-weighted Average (mg/m^3)					
	<.05	.06-	.11-	.24-.27	Total	
Number	334	145	61	27	567	382
Per cent with:						
Loss of appetite	3.6	4.1	11.5	85.2	8.5	1.3
Loss of weight	7.8	10.3	16.4	92.6	13.4	2.6
Objective tremor	6.6	7.6	9.8	51.9	9.4	6.8
Insomnia	7.2	7.6	11.5	44.4	9.5	5.5
Shyness	6.3	8.3	19.7	18.5	8.8	3.9
Nervousness	16.8	14.5	21.3	29.6	17.3	8.6
Diarrhea	1.2	3.4	6.6	0.0	2.3	1.1
Frequent colds	9.0	11.0	18.0	0.0	10.1	2.4

Smith, *et al.*[1]

certainly between the various groups, or, as in the case of
fatigue and headache, failed to discriminate. How well
these symptoms would differentiate between similar exposure
groups in the community, as opposed to the occupational
setting, is debatable. Clearly, in Smith's study, those
who were exposed to mercury knew of their exposure. Moreover, they were probably also aware of the approximate
degree of exposure. This knowledge could have influenced
their responses to questions. Provisionally, however, it
would appear reasonable to record the symptoms listed under
inorganic mercury intoxication as subclinical effects.

We are on even less sure ground when considering the
symptoms listed under organic mercury intoxication. Those
which appear to be most usable, such as tingling or numbness of the fingers or mouth, ataxia, difficulty in speech,
constriction of the visual field, and so on, are clinical
manifestations. Is there any evidence that they may be
present yet sufficiently mild not to take a person to a
physician? Symptoms such as fatigue, headache, impaired
power of concentration, and impaired memory are symptoms
which I would not like to have to rely on. These thoughts
prompt the question: Are there any subclinical symptoms

or signs of organic mercury intoxication other than the
detection of mercury in body tissues and fluids? Are there
any changes in the electroencephalogram, for example? What
about changes which have been shown to occur in the electro-
myogram of persons exposed to mercury? Are there any tests
of enzyme inhibition which might be used? I believe the
epidemiologist's role should usually be one of using tests
suggested by others rather than devising new ones. At the
moment, epidemiologists are very much in need of sound suggestions from clinicians or laboratory workers about
potentially usable tests.

(b) Reproducibility

The second criterion of a usable test is that it should
have good reproducibility. This means that, if a subject
is tested on two occasions, the results should be in rea-
sonably close agreement. This consistency should apply
equally well if the test is applied by the same observer
on the two occasions or by different observers.

Reproducibility to questions depends largely on the
precision of the wording of the questions. Sound question-
naire design, adequate instructions, training and testing
of interviewers are all important in obtaining optimum
reproducibility.

(c) Validity

The test should be valid. This means that, in addition
to discriminating between exposure groups, a positive test
carries implications on the subsequent incidence, course,
progression, and mortality of the disease. I realize that
a subclinical effect differs in one respect from a preclinical effect: There is no implication that it will
progress to clinical disease. If exposure to mercury is
reduced or eliminated, the subclinical effect will cease
to be present. Validation of subclinical effects by subsequent disease history is less satisfactory than, say,
validation of preclinical effects in relation to the
development of cancer. However, the progression of a
subclinical effect to a clinical state is presumably the
main reason for anxiety. Consequently, prospective observation of the group to determine long-term implications
seems to be essential.

(d) Simplicity and Acceptability

These are desirable attributes of any test. They are
obvious and mentioned only for completeness.

Estimation of Dose of Mercury

A person's dosage of any substance is usually measured
by measuring the concentration of the substance in the
environment at different times and in different places and
then relating this to the duration of that person's exposure
at these different times and places. In the case of mercury
exposure, a community study requires that the concentrations
of mercury in the air, water, food, and working environment
are integrated with residential, occupational, and dietary
histories to provide an estimate of dosage over some specified period of time. Such a procedure may provide a
reasonably accurate estimate of a person's dose in certain
limited circumstances--when exposure is mainly due to the
consumption of one type of food, for example, or in the
occupational setting. But even in this latter situation,
problems often arise through contamination of clothes or
of cigarettes, or through ingestion of unmeasurable amounts
of mercury due to faulty hygiene. The inaccuracy inherent
in assessing dosage from multiple sources in the community,
and the labor involved in taking adequate dietary, occupational and residential histories are such that most
epidemiologists would cry out for something better. In
the case of mercury, it would seem infinitely preferable
to use one's own personal monitor--one's hair. This provides a good estimate of the dosage of mercury during the
past six months or so, provided such technical difficulties
as contamination by mercury in hair dressings can be over-
come. Variations in concentration along the length of the
hair provide some indication of variations in dosage at
different times. It also appears to be possible to differentiate between exposures to inorganic mercury and to
methyl mercury from hair samples. Thus, we are much better
off in asessing a person's dosage to mercury than we are,
say, in assessing his dosage of air pollution.

Dose/Response Relationship

Whether dosage is assessed by integrating measured
concentrations of mercury with lifetime exposures or by
measuring the mercury concentration in hair, dose/response
relationships are studied by plotting one's estimate of
dosage against the proportions of subjects showing the
subclinical effect or effects. One has not a single dose/
response curve; rather, one has a family of dose/response
curves for each effect. Graphs A to D in Figure 69 indicate

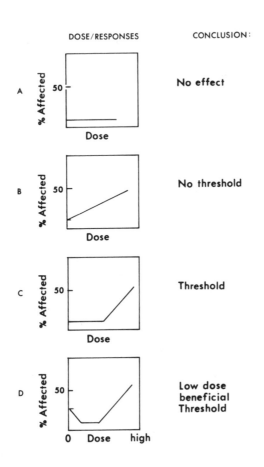

DOSE/RESPONSES   CONCLUSION:

A — No effect

B — No threshold

C — Threshold

D — Low dose beneficial Threshold

Figure 69: Dose/Response Relationships from Exposure to Mercury

the main relationships which might be detected. The conclusions to be drawn from each naturally differ.

In graph A, there is no relationship between dosage and the proportion of persons affected. If this curve were to be confidently established, mercury could be ignored. In graph B, there is a progressive increase in

proportions affected with increasing dosage. There is no
indication of a threshold and no evidence of an acceptable
minimum dosage. All mercury is undesirable. In graph C,
there is a progressive deterioration after some threshold
level is exceeded. An acceptable dosage would be below
this threshold, the precise level being determined by any
safety factors which may be included. Finally, in graph
D the curve suggests again that, once some threshold is
exceeded, there is deterioration; but there are beneficial
effects of lower dosage.

Populations for Study

Two types of population are suitable for studies of
mercury intoxication:
1. occupationally exposed groups
2. general communities living in areas where
    environmental levels are high.
The advantages of studying an occupationally exposed
group are that the group is usually readily accessible,
can be studied quickly and relatively cheaply, provides a
good range of exposures (some of which may be sufficiently
high to produce symptoms or other subclinical effects), and
is often amenable to control measures and measurement of
their efficacy. Environmental sampling can be readily
carried out at appropriate sites within the plant. The
main disadvantages are the lack of really satisfactory
controls and the possibility that those who have become
affected even subclinically may leave the occupation and
seek work elsewhere. Suitable occupations include laboratory workers, makers and repairers of scientific instruments,
dentists and dental hygienists, and persons engaged in the
manufacture and use of mercury-containing pesticides and
fungicides.

The major concern about mercury intoxication at the
present time is, however, less with potential occupational
exposures than with the risks of general communities exposed
to high mercury levels as a result of pollution. The definition of such populations is harder, more expensive, and more
time-consuming than the definition of occupationally exposed
groups. Before it is attempted, it is essential to have
some clear indication that a sufficient number of the inhabitants of any area which might be suggested for study
have been exposed to significant levels of mercury. Two
potentially useful screening tests are available to help
in the selection of suitable communities: concentrations
of mercury in either the blood or in hair. Samples of hair

could be obtained from barber shops. Blood specimens from
hospital admissions or out-patients, or more representative
samples from premarital or pregnancy blood tests, might be
examined.

The procedure leading to the choice of community might
be somewhat as follows: A number of villages or other
communities in the vicinity of the Great Lakes might be
considered. Samples of hair would be obtained from those
attending barbers in the neighborhood. Premarital, pregnancy, and hospital blood samples would be obtained for
mercury estimations. If hair and/or blood samples revealed
values above some predetermined level, the community would
be selected, defined by census, and a survey carried out.

Characteristics Other than Dosage Which Differentiate Affected from Unaffected

Among those persons experiencing a similar dosage there
is a variety of response. Some are affected, others are
not. The explanation for this variation must lie either
in inborn characteristics (genetic or constitutional) or
in acquired characteristics (personal habits or other
environmental exposures). An important area of epidemiological research is determining ways in which affected and
unaffected persons experiencing similar doses differ in
these respects.

Long-Term Implications of Exposure, Clinical and Subclinical Disease

What are the long-term implications of exposure,
clinical disease, and subclinical effects of mercury intoxication on subsequent morbidity, disability, and
mortality? Rather little interest has been directed at
assessment of the implications of clinical mercurial
poisoning, let alone the implications of subclinical
effects. A high case fatality rate and very high long-
term disability rate is known to have occurred in the
Minamata epidemic.[2] Much less is known about the outcome
of other episodes of mercury poisoning. For example, has
anyone ever followed up the population of the felt hat
industry?[3] Is anything known about the subsequent course
of the detectives in the Lancashire constabulary?[4] What
happened to children with pink disease (acrodynia) once
regular doses of calomel for teething were stopped? Can
the decline in nephritis mortality during the past half
century be related to a reduction in calomel ingestion

over the same period?   It is equally important to try to determine whether persons with any subclinical manifestations of mercury intoxication or with high levels of mercury in body tissues or fluids have any excess morbidity or mortality. Is their life expectation reduced? Do they become unduly disabled? Do they have any increase in chromosome abnormalities? Is there any evidence that their children are more prone to genetic defects? Do they have any excess of congenital malformations? These questions require that adequate follow-up of populations which are studied for mercury intoxication should be carried out.

Effect of Control Measures

What are the effects of instituting measures for prevention and control? Wherever possible, I should like to see rigorously designed studies in which control measures are randomly assigned in some areas but not in others, and the effects compared. Such a study might be feasible in the chlorine-producing plants studied by Smith and his colleagues.[1] The effects of reduction in mercury exposures in randomly selected plants would be assessed by changes in the prevalence of symptoms, and in blood and urinary mercury levels in treated and untreated plants. The subsequent mortality and morbidity of the workers would be ascertained.

Studies of this kind, of course, raise serious ethical questions as well as practical considerations. More often, one has to be content with the less scientifically satisfactory comparisons of groups before and after the institution of control measures.

In conclusion, I believe that whatever subclinical effects can be demonstrated in man are a relatively small, though certainly very important, part of the wider ecological problem of mercury intoxication. We need to keep this wider view in deciding what community emissions of mercury into the environment are tolerable.

References

1. Smith, R. G., A. J. Vorwald, L. S. Patil, and T. F. Mooney, Jr. "A Study of the Effects of Exposure to Mercury in the Manufacture of Chlorine," Am. Indust. Hyg. Assoc. J., 31, 687-700 (1970).
2. Nomura, S. "Epidemiology of Minamata Disease," in Minamata Disease (Shuhan Co., 1968), pp. 5-35.

3. Bloomfield, J. J. and J. M. Dallavalle. "Application of Engineering Surveys to Hatter and Fur Cutting Industry," J. Indust. Hyg. and Tox., *19*, 115-116 (1937).
4. Agate, J. N. and M. Buckell. "Mercury Poisoning from Fingerprint Photography, an Occupational Hazard of Policemen," Arch. Ind. Hyg. and Occup. Med., *1*, 364 (1950).

Biological Effects of Mercury Compounds
Discussion Paper

Contributions by: T. W. Clarkson, B. D. Dinman, J. C. Gage, L. J. Goldwater, H. Guirgis, D. I. Hammer, R. Hartung, R. Henderson, S. Herman, I. T. T. Higgins, A. Hinman, A. Jernelöv, E. Kahn, R. Klein, C. Kramer, L. T. Kurland, D. J. Lisk, H. B. Lovejoy, J. A. McGroarty, N. Nelson, L. J. Nicholson, J. F. Shea, R. G. Smith, T. Takeuchi, D. J. Tessari, L. Tryphonas, J. F. Uthe.

Industrial hygiene studies into the human toxicity of inorganic mercury and mercury vapor took place at an early date, and presently provide much important reference material. Present studies into the effects of mercury vapor on man near or at the threshhold limit value (TLV) point out some of the problems in measuring very subtle effects.

In the study of the effects of low concentrations of mercury vapor on man, weight losses reported in questionnaires were significantly correlated with dose. But subsequent examinations of actual weight records in some of the chlorine plants did not substantiate these reported weight losses, so that in some instances they must be regarded as subjective weight losses only. The incidence of the subjective weight loss was, however, substantial, in that 25-50% of the exposed people claimed that they had experienced weight losses.

There are some important differences in the absorption and distribution of ionic mercury and metallic mercury vapor. Both materials produce significant accumulations of mercury in the kidney, but the mercury concentration in the brain, though fairly low, is about 10 times higher in

brain after exposure to vapor.[1] While much of the vapor
is oxidized to the divalent ion in the red cells, enough
mercury vapor can be transported with the blood during the
15 seconds that the blood moves from the lungs to the
brain because the metallic mercury vapor is quite lipid
soluble.

It is exceedingly important to be aware of the compound
of mercury that is producing the exposure, since the various organic and inorganic compounds can have drastically
different rates of absorption, distribution, and toxicity.
Experiments with CBA-strain mice demonstrated that Hg^{++}
may be absorbed only to the extent of 1% from the gastrointestinal tract, while CH_3Hg^+ may be 98% absorbed by the
same route.

It is not fully known whether the mammalian intestinal
flora or the normal biochemical processes can convert inorganic mercury to methyl mercury in man. However,
presently available evidence mitigates against this. In
mice fed ratioactive mercuric chloride, 98% could be
accounted for as inorganic mercury at the end of the test.
To date, no methyl mercury has been detected in mammals
after the ingestion of inorganic mercury.

Different organo-mercury compounds have different
stabilities *in vivo*. Methyl mercury appears to be the
most stable. Methoxyethyl mercury is readily degraded,
and so is phenyl mercury, which is normally classed as a
stable compound. However, *in vivo* the phenyl group is
hydroxylated in the para position in the liver, and subsequently this less stable compound falls apart. The
symptoms of renal failure and gastric enteritis produced
by phenyl mercury compounds bear some resemblance to the
action of mercuric chloride.

Methoxyethyl mercury is also less toxic than methyl
mercury, and does not normally produce paralysis in rats
and mice. However, at this time it would not be wise to
generalize those findings to all the other alkoxyalkyl
mercurials. Much of the organic and inorganic mercury in
the intestines seems to be associated with proteins.

It has long been recognized that Hg^{++} and $R-Hg^+$ ions
react readily with proteins, especially with sulfhydryl
groups. Divalent mercuric ions can form cyclic mercaptides
with two adjacent sulfhydryl groups, while $R-Hg^+$ ions can
be used to obtain quantitative titrations of sulfhydryl
groups. In light of this, it is not surprising that the
sulfhydryl-containing enzymes phosphohexose, phosphoglucose
isomerase, and glutathione reductase in blood are inhibited.
Inhibitions such as these have been reviewed by Webb.[2]

However, some enzymes which do not contain any sulfhydryl groups can also be affected by mercury, presumably by reactions with amino or carboxyl groups.

The inhibition of 2,3 diphosphoglyceryl dehydrogenase (2,3DPG-ase) by mercury has interesting implications for the oxygen transport by hemoglobin. When 2,3DPG-ase is inhibited, there should be an accumulation of 2,3DPG in the red cell. When this occurs, there exists a potential for blockage by 2,3DPG at the γ-protein of hemoglobin, which in turn tends to reduce the oxygen-carrying capacity of hemoglobin. With such impairment of the oxygen-carrying capacity, a feedback mechanism responding to hypoxia appears to stimulate hemoglobin synthesis. Such a hypothesis could explain the increase in hemoglobin reported above by Goldwater.

Methyl mercury cannot be readily removed from fish tissue. Westöö[3] reported that there were no demonstrable losses of methyl mercury during cooking. The preparation of fish meal from pike produces losses amounting to only 15-20% of the mercury, even when the final drying temperatures are as high as 177°C (350°F). When fish is repeatedly extracted with isopropanol, the resulting powder still contains all the mercury.

The findings of chronic methyl mercury poisoning in man in Minamata and Niigata present an important source of data for evaluation. The diagnoses in Minamata did not detect milder cases, and were at first conducted in the face of considerable antagonism and opposition. Studies of the Niigata cases were much more refined and milder cases were detected. But, for those reasons, the findings from Minamata and Niigata are not fully comparable as to the frequency of occurrence of mortality and various symptoms.

The transmission of methyl mercury in mothers' milk may contribute to the onset or progress of Minamata disease but it should still be possible to differentiate pathologically between the fetal and infantile forms of the Minamata disease. The fetal *in utero* form of the disease demonstrates hypoplastic and dysplastic changes in the brain which occur while the brain is being formed in the fetus. A different change occurs when the exposure takes place after birth.

Data presented in this section by Takeuchi indicate that the ingestion of 20 mg of mercury as methyl mercury daily for about one month would ultimately produce Minamata disease. By comparison, crude estimates of the amounts of methyl mercury ingested by the people in Alamogordo indicate that approximately 40 mg mercury were ingested over

a three month period. Not all members of the family
became ill.

The fishermen in Minamata who were affected by Minamata
disease derived most of their protein from seafood. They
also ate the livers of fish, which contained 2-3 times
higher concentrations of mercury. However, the significance
of this dietary habit is doubtful because liver accounts
for only 5-10% of the entire weight of the fish.

The most important difference between inorganic and
methyl mercury poisoning is the irreversibility of the
neurological symptoms in the case of poisoning by methyl
mercury. Complete recovery has been noted for inorganic
mercury poisoning characterized by very severe ataxia. On
the other hand, since methyl mercury poisoning produces
brain lesions and damage to neural structures which cannot
regenerate, symptoms are irreversible unless compensatory
pathways can come into play to counteract mild symptoma-
tology. For this reason, antidotal therapy with BAL and
penicillamine can only prevent deterioration, but not cure
neurological symptoms. Even this requires additional
study, because it is not known how BAL and penicillamine
affect the transport of methyl mercury to the brain in
man, while they improve urinary excretion. Antidotal
therapy may be useful before symptoms fully develop, but
the effects on organ distribution must be investigated
before this can be recommended without reservation. This
is especially true since animal studies have shown that
BAL can increase the concentrations of mercury in the
brain.[4]

The concentrations of mercury in cerebrospinal fluid
(CSF) were very low in Japanese studies, but they experienced some technical difficulties in the collection of
these specimens. The CSF in the Alamogordo cases contained
about 3.3 ppm mercury. The study of CSF mercury levels in
comparison to concentrations in liver and other organs may
be important in assessing the function of the blood-brain
barrier in the generation of Minamata disease, and the
degree of protection which may be afforded by detoxication
mechanisms in the liver.

The analysis of hair for mercury appears to provide a
good system to monitor mercury levels in the human population. However, a number of important details must be
tested to improve the utility of this analysis. Optimal
methods for the removal of surface contamination from hair
must be devised. Hair-blood ratios appear to vary with
the concentrations found, and must therefore be better
defined. One of the hair specimens analyzed for the

Alamogordo cases contained 2400 ppm of mercury with an average of 877 ppm for all cases. These are very high levels which cannot readily be compared to whole blood levels because only serum mercury levels were measured for these cases. The value of many monitoring studies could be greatly increased by including measurements of methyl mercury in blood.

The detection of subclinical intoxications by methyl mercury is difficult. It is essential to find new sensitive and specific early signs which can be used to provide warnings before the occurrence of gross irreversible neurological deficits. Many suggested signs, such as weight changes, may turn out to be sensitive, but definitely lack specificity.

There is a great need for long term studies and follow-ups to elucidate such questions as genetic defects as described by chromosome breakage, and the detection of subtle motor and psychic dysfunctions in relation to mercury exposures, especially for methyl mercury.

References

1. Magos, I. "Mercury-Blood Interaction and Mercury Uptake by the Brain After Vapour Exposure," Env. Res., *1*, 323-337 (1967).
2. Webb, J. L. Enzyme and Metabolic Inhibitors. Vol. II (New York: Academic Press, 1966), pp. 729-983.
3. Westöö, G. "Methylmercury Compounds in Animal Foods," Chemical Fallout (C. C. Thomas Publ., 1969), pp. 75-96.
4. Berlin, M., L. G. Jerksell, and G. Nordberg. "Accelerated Uptake of Mercury by Brain Caused by 2,3 dimercaptopropanol (BAL) after Injection into the Mouse of a Methylmercuric Compound," Acta Pharmacol. Toxicol., *23*(4), 312-320 (1966).

INDEX